GW00646600

Remodelling Medicine

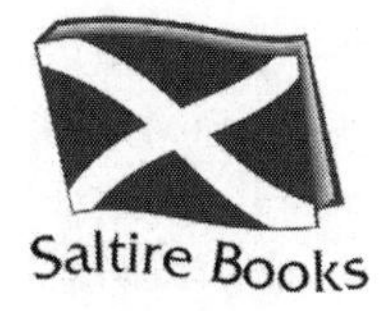

Saltire Books Limited, Glasgow, Scotland

Remodelling Medicine

Jeremy Swayne
BA(Oxon), BM, BCh, D(Obst)RCOG, MRCGP, FFHom.

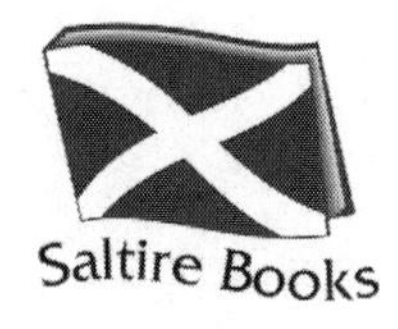

Saltire Books Limited, Glasgow, Scotland

Published by Saltire Books Ltd

18–20 Main Street, Busby, Glasgow G76 8DU, Scotland
books@saltirebooks.com www.saltirebooks.com

First published in 2012

Typeset by Type Study, Scarborough, UK in 9¼ on 13½ Stone Serif
Printed by Information Press Ltd, Eynsham, Oxford, UK

ISBN 978-1-908127-00-6

A catalogue record for this book is available from the British library

For Saltire
Project Development: Lee Kayne
Editorial: Steven Kayne
Designer: Phil Barker
Graphics: Rebecca Bloom, Barnaby Swayne
Cartoons by Mike Flanagan (flantoons@btinternet.com)
Indexing: Lawrence Errington

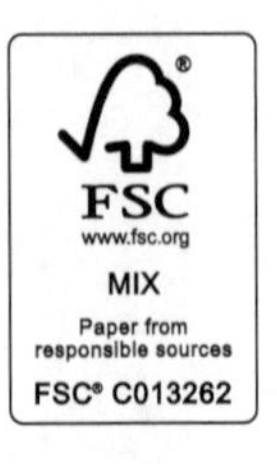

FSC MIX

The timber or fibre in the product is a mixture of some/all of the following:

Timber from an FSC®-certified forest
Post-consumer reclaimed material
Controlled Sources, which exclude unacceptable forestry

CONTENTS

FOREWORD
by Professor David Haslam

Sometimes medicine is very straightforward. Whether you fracture your femur, rupture your aorta, or block your coronary arteries, the response of the medical profession is fantastically skilled, technically complex, and theoretically relatively simple. There is a problem. It needs fixing. And medicine can fix it. It is a real tribute to the advancement of science and many of us will be truly grateful for such skill.

But not all medicine is like that. Of the million consultations in UK General Practice every single day, a relatively small proportion will deal with clear cut pathology. Both in primary and secondary care, our patients present with an extraordinary mixture of fears and concerns, symptoms and alarms. We screen the healthy, protecting some but worrying others. Over the past decades, life expectancy has progressively improved, therapies have become more effective, and our patients have become more worried and concerned about their health than ever. What is going on? What are we trying to do?

Logic might have predicted that as healthcare evolved, as more diseases were prevented, and as everyday access to health information became ever more available, then doctors and nurses would have seen their workload diminish. In fact, the very opposite has happened. In my work as a doctor, as every year went past I seemed to become busier and busier. In any other walk of life, this would cause us to stop and think. Are we doing the right things? What exactly are we trying to achieve? What is going wrong? And as costs go up year on year, such questions become ever more critical.

Jeremy Swayne's remarkable book could not be more timely. Authoritative and challenging, the author poses questions that have to be answered. As a profession we need to stop, and we need to think. After all, if we go on doing what we've always done, we will just achieve more of the same. Unusually – and that in itself is puzzling – the author stresses that healing needs to be our raison d'etre. Healing isn't soft and fluffy; it's what the medical profession is for. As Dr Swayne says "the fact that the concept of healing is in large part philosophical and abstract is no excuse for not grappling with it as a fundamental theme of health care and all medical education."

What is healthcare trying to do? Are we succeeding? And are we doing it in the most effective way? These aren't small questions. But they are certainly worth asking.

Professor David Haslam, CBE, FRCGP, FRCP, FFPH
President, British Medical Association, 2011–12
Past President, Royal College of General Practitioners

FOREWORD
by Professor Gene Feder

By convention, a manifesto is short and a textbook is long. So it is unsettling to hold a 490 page tome that is essentially the former wrapped in the latter. That feeling is wholly appropriate, because unsettling the reader is an implicit aim of this book. More accurately, it articulates why so many clinicians and patients are unsettled by the current shape of medical practice and health care policy. And it then lays out characteristics of a remodelled medicine, partly answering the question: what would different look like? Jeremy Swayne's diagnosis of medicine's malaise focuses on the corrosive effect of the biomedical model on the healing vocation of doctors. Running through the book is an extended argument with a model that has dominated medical practice and education for over a century. Swayne consciously (sometimes self-consciously) places himself in a tradition of dissidence, critiquing the limitations of the biomedical model from *within* the medical profession, and drawing on the work of other medical dissidents, such as Eric Cassells, George Engel, Howard Brody and Iona Heath. Like his predecessors (and contemporaries, as he has been writing about healing and medicine for 30 years), he both celebrates the achievements of scientific medicine and demonstrates why its hegemony makes it difficult for doctors to engage with the person of the patient on their path through illness and death. Swayne synthesises philosophical premises, ethical insights, and empirical evidence with his own experience as a doctor and patient. Although the reader senses the urgency behind the text, the tone of the book is balanced and modest, like Swayne's ideal doctor, even when he is proposing radical changes to practice. And it is these changes that are the engine of the book or, more in keeping with Swayne's predilection for organic metaphors, its heart. His proposals for re-modelling the medical model encompass methods that enhance the contextual effects of treatment, help patient's find meaning in their pre-dicament, and limit diagnostic and treatment interventions to appropriate settings. His catholic choice of exemplars for the remodelling includes occupational therapy, rehabilitation medicine and some complementary therapies. This part of the book is bursting with ideas and surprising juxtapositions, such as the necessary precariousness of medical practice and the need for "humble hubris" in our engagement with patients. As a researcher, I missed a discussion of how we could evaluate which components of re-modelled medicine are effective. Swayne shows that there are different types of evidence without being clear about how we decide that a treatment works or not beyond contextual effects. Most doctors and many patients want to know that. Swayne generally underestimates science's self-critical/correcting processes and the potential of evidence-based medicine to tackle over use of diagnostic methods and treatments. I hope that guidelines will still have a place in re-modelled medicine, but no longer as performance targets.

Gene Feder
Professor of Primary Health Care
University of Bristol, UK

PREFACE

Ambition

A colleague who read a first draft outline for this book remarked that it was ambitious, by which I took him to mean that it was over ambitious. He was referring chiefly to the scope of its subject matter, and he was right. It is now considerably more modest. But it is still ambitious in other respects.

First, because it is intended to make people think; to persuade people to rethink our approach to healthcare; to provoke debate; to make a difference. Over the years others have written books, articles and academic papers with the same intention. But the biomedical bias in health care that has been the focus of criticism has not shifted. If anything it has intensified. So in its intention to be more effective in promoting the 'remodelling' process it is certainly ambitious. If it is to be successful, it must amongst other things help to remedy, or at least mitigate the problems described in Chapter 9, 'Medicine in crisis?', including the increasingly prohibitive cost of modern Western medicine.

Secondly its ambition is to be readable and read by a wide range of people involved in or concerned about medicine and healthcare: academics and educators, practitioners of all kinds, commentators, and above all patients (who are all of us) – general readers to whom health care matters personally rather than theoretically.

Its third ambition is to rekindle medicine's healing vocation. This is ambitious because it invites an understanding of human nature in health and illness that is at odds with the materialist and secular culture of our time and the reductionist tendency in science. It insists that the goals, values and ideals of medicine can only be fully realised in terms of what one of the doctors I have quoted calls 'the aspirations of the human spirit', as well as 'the biological imperatives' of life.[1]

Those are its three ambitions. Ambitions that I approach, I hope, with the 'humble hubris' that will be described later.

Politics

The question, 'What are the goals of medicine?', is at the heart of this book. The answer it presents, in a very small nutshell, is that they are chiefly concerned with healing and the relief of suffering. The heart of health care is the care of patients, but its ability to achieve its goals depends to a great extent on the various factors that constitute the context of care. One of these is the health care policy of the government of the day.

When two thirds of the book was already written the U.K. general election produced a government whose policies are very different to those of its predecessor. The implications of its most radical policy for this 'remodelling' project are touched upon in the first part of the introduction. But some of the less dramatic changes, such as its attitude to targets and guidelines, affect a number of the issues raised throughout the book. Some of the criticisms of the distortion of health care resulting from political approaches to health promotion for example, or to the embedding of biomedical targets in health care policy, may be mitigated by the change of emphasis introduced by this government. But they remain relevant examples of the kind of interaction between medicine and society that can subvert the goals of medicine. If a particular criticism becomes less pertinent under the evolving policy of the present government, it should be read in that sense.

Sources

Later I explain how my personal view of the need for medicine to be remodelled was increasingly informed and supported by the reading I undertook as the book developed. The numerous and various sources that I quote are evidence of this. My original literature search yielded only one reference arguing on behalf of *greater* emphasis on the biomedical approach. The lack of any body of argument supporting the biomedical model is not surprising, however, because it is not necessary. The model is taken for granted. "We use the medical model because the medical model is what we use."[2]

But the literature supporting what I have called the remodelling of medicine is extensive, far more so than even my references suggest, and constantly emerging week by week in medical journals and the press. So much so that there is a considerable amount of material that I have not included, chiefly because I would never have got the book finished if I continued to weave it into the text. I have not gone out of my way to be selective of this material. It represents a real and strong current in medical thought. There is no substantial argument in favour of the status quo. I have just been playing what is in front of me, as the saying is.

The omission of precise page numbers for the books I have cited is not laziness. If the quotations prompt you to follow them up, then the book as a whole deserves to be read, or at least browsed, to appreciate the full weight of the argument and gain full value from it. The exploration of this book's themes in the writing of others has been stimulating, often exciting, and sometimes inspiring. I hope I have done justice to them, and that bringing their voices together in this way will accelerate the momentum for change that they represent.

Humanity

The most highly rated aspect of care reported in the *British Medical Journal* study of what makes a good doctor, and quoted in Chapter 8, was "humaneness". This quality is obviously fundamental to medicine's vocation and goal, and it is why 'learning to do medicine' (Chapter 18) must be rooted in the humanities as well as in good science. To give you a flavour of what this means, and why it is a theme that underpins the whole argument in this book, I recommend a play and a film. The play is *State of Nature*, by Simon Turley,[i] also available as a book.[3] Its essence is captured in this abbreviated excerpt from a review by Anne Taylor in the *British Medical Journal*:[4]

State of Nature was commissioned by the company Theatrescience, which describes itself as a "rolling laboratory" of new plays and workshops aimed at breaking down barriers between arts and sciences and exploring the implications of biomedical science for society. At the core of its productions lies the idea of transforming scientific debate into a human story, opening up biomedical topics to greater public engagement and redefining them as matters of the heart as well as of the head. It is difficult to imagine a finer example of the realisation of this ambition than this play, which has Patrick (the patient's) story pulsing through it. (Professor) Anthony Pinching worked closely with Turley as scientific adviser. He made sure that the science was right but also enabled a "deeper authenticity," underpinned by patient narratives and stories of his own and others' clinical experience.

The film is *Patch Adams* (Universal Studios, 1998; DVD 820 415 2.11), starring Robin Williams. It is based on the true story of a contemporary

i http://tinyurl.com/39chorp

doctor whose insistence on humaneness and humour in the relationship with patients, and his capacity to make them laugh, in defiance of the narrow scientific ethos of his medical school, nearly sabotaged his medical education. It does indeed "combine side-splitting humour", and not a few tears, "with an inspiring story that transcends the traditional comedy". Even if you have seen the film, please watch it again. And if you haven't got the DVD please get it; it is not expensive. It does half my work for me.

An apology

You will find that this book is very doctor centred. Its concern is the well-being of patients, but its focus is chiefly the responsibility of doctors for achieving this. This doctor dominance is probably an accurate reflection of the balance of power within the biomedical model. But it is something of a distortion of the true picture; and certainly not a reflection of what a better model of medicine should look like. To overstate the case, but not a lot, it is as though doctors are at the centre of the medical solar system, with the allied professions and services held in orbit around by their magnetic pull. The implication being that without the medical profession they would fall away and lose their place in the firmament. In fact the medical firmament is not a solar system. The reverse is true. Without the energy and influence of those other planetary professions and services, it is the medical profession that would be lost.

So if you are a nurse, or an occupational therapist, or speech therapist, or a provider of any of the skills or services on which doctors depend, be reassured. This book is not neglectful of you. In fact it should become apparent that you have a vital contribution to make to the remodelling process. For example, in *The Healing Tradition*, David Greaves suggests, "The traditional disposition and role of nurses may also provide them with the potential to act as archetypal healers in the community, which would seem of vital importance now that they are beginning to be employed as first-line practitioners in primary care".[5] But reflecting the undercurrent of dis-ease throughout this book, he also warns, "The fact that their education and training are becoming increasingly driven by technical procedures could, however, be fatally damaging to this possibility".

During my hospital training and early years in general practice I soon learned how essential are nurses, health visitors, pharmacists and others to a doctor's effectiveness, and even survival. Later, while working on the development of a shared terminology for health care, my doctor-centric horizon was further enlarged by acquaintances with the work of those others, including occupational and speech therapists.[6] Their approach to patient care, their medical models, taught me a lot, and already represents many of the principles that I will suggest are to be given greater prominence in a new more general model of medicine. Examples of these models are given in Chapter 13.

But the doctor-centred biomedical model is the problem. And hence, what doctors do is inevitably the primary focus of attention.

References

1 Fitzpatrick, M. *The tyranny of health.* Abingdon: Routledge; 2001.
2 Haslam, D. Who cares? *British J Gen Pract.* 2007: 987–993.
3 Turley, S. *State of Nature.* Cardigan: Parthian; 2010.
4 Taylor, A. The illness is the side story. *Br Med J.* 2011; 341 c6970:54.
5 Greaves, D. *The Healing Tradition.* Oxford: Radcliffe Publishing; 2004.
6 Swayne, J. A common language of care? *J Interprof Care* 1993; 7:29–35.

ACKNOWLEDGEMENTS

Any 'reflective practitioner' must acknowledge their debt to the many patients whose willingness to entrust us with your 'stories of sickness' has been the source of so much that we have learned that has been of real value in the practice of our craft. You have helped us to learn compassion, to apply our knowledge and skills effectively and appropriately, and to acquire the wisdom without which knowledge and skill may be wasted, or even dangerous. Because this book is the product of 40 years reflection, this debt to my own patients is huge.

The degree of trust that patients show is often humbling. A recurring refrain has been the admission, "This is the first time I have ever told anybody that in my life". 'That' is invariably some particularly intimate, painful or precious piece of the story that has been essential to my understanding of their predicament; to the proper diagnosis of their illness, certainly, and their disease often. And, more importantly perhaps, essential to their understanding of themselves. For this trust I am deeply grateful. It has helped me to develop whatever resources I have of the humble hubris I recommend later in the book.

Over the years, a parallel source of knowledge, skill and wisdom has been, of course, the colleagues who have shared their experience and have personified good practice and genuine care. And also the doctors, nurses and other practitioners whose patient I have been, and who have shown me the combination of compassion and expertise that exemplify the right balance of *scientia* and *caritas*. There have been contrasting instances in my experience as a patient, and of colleagues, when these qualities have not been shown. But even these are instructive, and have been greatly outnumbered by instances of conspicuous skill and care, often in busy and stressful situations. The good experiences are the foundation for my confidence that the remodelling that is the theme of the book is an evolution that most healthcare practitioners desire and would like to achieve because it is an inherent part of their vocation.

The importance of these acknowledgements is to emphasise the personal aspect of the argument that I am making. Not just in terms of my personal experience, but because medicine is all about persons. It is about you and me, the patient and the practitioner who are the people at the heart of the therapeutic process, the healing relationship.

The book has had a long gestation and many people have contributed to its conception and ante-natal care. First amongst these was Gene Feder, whose enthusiasm for one of my original papers on this theme in 1976 did much to encourage me in my continuing exploration; as did a characteristic hand-written letter from the late George Godber at that time, and the approval of Denis Pereira Gray, then editor of the Journal of the Royal College of General Practitioners, who published one of those papers.

But those who have assisted its safe delivery deserve particular thanks. These must include the many authors whose work I have cited and who have inspired and informed my own thinking. Every reference serves as an implicit acknowledgement of my debt to them. Amongst these, David Haslam and Iona Heath, successive Presidents of the Royal College of General Practitioners have been particularly influential. James Willis, another senior member of the College was especially encouraging and constructively critical in commenting on early drafts of some chapters. David Greaves read every chapter as it was completed, and his feedback not only helped me to achieve greater clarity in some important passages, and to keep me honest to my purpose, but made me braver in expounding some of its essential principles than I might otherwise have been. So too did Paul Dieppe, whose combination of scientific rigour and holistic vision has been immensely encouraging, and whose detailed criticism prompted many improvements in the manuscript.

Fellow members of the group mentioned in the Prologue to Part 5, who together have been exploring what a more integrative and holistic approach to medicine really means, and how to promote it, have contributed more than they may realise to the book's progress. My thanks to Liz and Trevor Thompson, Michael Connors, Lesley Wye, Michael Evans, Catherine Zollman, Gene Feder, Charlotte Paterson and Paul Dieppe; and particularly David Owen and David Peters, who helped to set up the group, and with whom I have wrestled with these questions on many other occasions. George Lewith, too, has been generous in his help whenever called upon.

Other friends and colleagues whose encouragement and comments have been much appreciated include Jill Paxton and Tim Harlow.

I am grateful to Jan Alcoe and the Editor of *Holistic Healthcare* for permission to use the Wellbeing diagram (Figure 12.4) and to Elsevier Global Permissions for use of Figure 15.1 and Appendix 15.1; to the Editor of the *British Medical Journal* for the many citations to its authors; and to

Colin Tudge for the original concept of the 'Biomedical Filter' cartoon in Chapter 2. I cannot overstate my appreciation of the help of the Library staff at the Royal College of General Practitioners. I would have been lost without it.

Much of the discussion of healing that occurs in various sections of the book is brought together in an article on The Concept of Healing In *The Fairacres Chronicle*, Summer 2011 (Oxford: SLG Press).

It has been a pleasure to work with Steven Kayne and the team at Saltire Books on the editing and design of the book. Without my lovely wife Clare's tolerance of my lark-like predilection for starting the working day at 5.00a.m., and her remarkable ability to translate my handwriting into typescript, the book would never have reached a publisher in the first place.

ABOUT THE AUTHOR

Jeremy Swayne gained a degree in physiology and studied pre-clinical medicine at Oxford, continuing his studies at St George's Hospital (where he produced the hospital revue) qualifying in 1966. After the Wessex General Practice Vocational Training Scheme he entered general practice in Somerset in 1969, and started his own practice in the Forest of Dean in 1976, the year in which his first papers exploring the relationship between medicine and healing were published. His interest in psychological illness was complemented by increasing awareness of the spiritual dimension of health and illness.

He was introduced to homeopathy in 1978 and began to apply its methods within routine GP consultations. In 1983 he left full time general practice, combining in various permutations over the next 10 years or so – work in a mental handicap service in Bristol, NHS clinic sessions at Bristol Homeopathic Hospital, organising courses in homeopathy for GPs in the South West, promoting research in homeopathy, private practice, GP locum work, and developing medical terminology for the Read Codes. He was Dean of the Faculty of Homeopathy from 1997 to 2003, responsible for all aspects of its academic programme for doctors, and helping to develop education and training for other healthcare professionals.

Jeremy was ordained in the Church of England in 2000, and has worked as a part time parish priest. He has a role in the Christian Healing Ministry, and an active interest in the relationship between Science and Theology.

He is author of *Homeopathic Method: Implications for Clinical Practice and Medical Science*, and Editor of *Churchill Livingstone's International Dictionary of Homeopathy*.

Happily married since 1965 he takes great delight in his family. His favourite recreation is walking through the English countryside; he and Clare celebrated their 30th wedding anniversary by walking from Wells Cathedral to Norwich Cathedral. His chief eccentricity – a spell as a member of the Forest of Dean Morris Men. His 'famous five minutes' – the performance of a comic song to celebrate the 900th anniversary of the Battle of Hastings, on the Today programme on BBC Radio 4.

DEDICATION

This book is dedicated to those who have been mentors to me, or who have influenced my vocation in ways of which they may be completely unaware; some of them no longer living to be embarrassed by being implicated in this way. They include Sister Edmé, Ian Hazlewood, John Horder, Martin Israel, Alistair Jack, Mother Jane, Marshal Marinker, Mother Mary Clare, Robin Pinsent, John Polkinghorne, Jim Thompson, Andrew Winser.

INTRODUCTION

The Problem

The way we do medicine

> The established medical model must change if it is to have a healing influence in society. It must be more provisional and exploratory than dogmatic and absolute, it must have as its central driving force the eliciting of positive experiences of well-being, it must be conducive to human flourishing, and it must safeguard personal 'wholeness'.[i] (Adapted from Keith Ward[1])

There is something wrong with the way we do medicine in the developed Western world; or at least, in that part of it represented by medicine in the UK.

But that is not a particularly original remark. There have been recurrent suggestions within and without medicine for many years that medicine is in crisis; and 'dissident voices', particularly among doctors, challenging the direction that modern medicine has been taking as later chapters will confirm. Indeed the mission statement of the College of Medicine launched in October 2010, whose aims embrace many of the goals of medicine discussed in this book, includes a section – 'The Crisis in Medicine' – which begins with the words 'Something has gone wrong with healthcare'.[2]

This is not simply a matter of health service organisation or funding. Those thorny issues may compound the problem, but are a reflection of it rather than a cause. The problem is more fundamental. It has to do with the goals of medicine.[3] It has to do with our understanding of the nature of suffering and of healing. And it has to do with safeguarding personal wholeness.

I joined the dissident voices in 1976, ten years after I qualified; publishing a number of articles whose general theme was expressed in a nutshell

---

i The actual quotation, from *The Case for God,* reads ". . . the established religions must change in the modern world if they are to be forces for good. They must be more provisional and exploratory than dogmatic and absolute, they must have as their central driving force the eliciting of positive experiences of transcendence, they must be conducive to human flourishing, and they must safeguard freedom of belief."

by the title of one of them – 'Medicine and Healing: A broken marriage?'[4,5,6] The intervening years have been spent exploring that theme; leading to the conclusion that there *is* something wrong with the way we do medicine, and that it has something to do with that separation.

The rest of the book examines the justification for reaching this conclusion; asks why it is that medicine continues on this misdirected path despite the warnings of those within the profession who share the dissident view; and seeks a solution in the form of a better model of medicine – not one that abandons the gains of the past, but one better tuned to medicine's vocational goal.

In fact, there has been lively, if sporadic criticism of the medical model, the principles that govern western medicine, since modern scientific method began to influence medical practice at the beginning of the last century. This criticism, though perhaps not widespread, is as prevalent now as it ever was; in mainstream medical journals and in the media, as well as in conversation between healthcare practitioners and between patients. Put simply and crudely it represents a tension between the undoubted power and achievements of biomedicine – medicine based on controlling disorder in the human biological machine, and the need and the desire to understand illness and disease as a more diffuse and subtle aspect of the human condition – a complex threat to the human *person*, and to respond accordingly. This perspective, usually described as a more holistic approach, is a part of all good medicine, but it is difficult to reconcile with the dominant biomedical perspective. It has been reflected in some developments in medical education, but it has made very little difference in practice.

In short, continuing criticism of the medical model has not made a significant difference, despite the level of unease that it represents. As the past President of the Royal College of General Practitioners suggests, "We use the medical model because the medical model is what we use, even though it may not always be appropriate".[7] This book proposes that change, perhaps amounting to a minor revolution, really is needed if medicine is to evolve rather than merely advance on the same narrow front. By this I mean the sort of *metanoia* or change of mind-set that the American philosopher Thomas Kuhn (1922–1996) describes when he discusses the process of change and the obstacles to progress in his book *The Structure of Scientific Revolutions*.[8]

The boundaries of knowledge

My GCE Advanced Level zoology teacher exhorted us repeatedly – irritatingly, but of course quite rightly, to "Know what you know. Know what you *don't* know. Then *know* what you don't know." This is excellent advice for pursuing a syllabus and passing exams. Reference to the syllabus tells us what is to be known so that we can determine those bits of it that we do or do not know. But it is not a good precept for science, where the limits of what is knowable cannot be known. We can continuously extend the boundaries of what we already know, but the real excitement, challenge and purpose of science is to explore what lies beyond the horizon of the known. For the same reason, it is not a good precept for medicine. Or, rather it is an even worse precept for medicine, because medicine not only deals with questions that science can legitimately ask and hope to answer, even though they may lie beyond the immediate horizon. It also deals with questions of human experience, value and meaning that occupy a different landscape altogether from that bounded by the legitimate horizon of science.

Medicine cannot afford to pursue a syllabus based on what is already securely known, the set curriculum of medical science, however magnificent its achievements. It must not do so because it excludes not only subject matter that could be accessible to science but that has not yet been explored, but also everything that belongs to that other landscape not accessible to science, which is nevertheless the whole context within which science operates.

In his book *A Guide for the Perplexed*,[9] EF Schumacher puts it like this:

> (Our) maps of . . . knowledge . . . show (only) things that allegedly (can) be proved to exist. The . . . principle (seems) to be 'if in doubt, leave it out'. . . . It occurred to me, however, that the question of what constitutes proof was a very subtle and difficult one. Would it not be wiser to turn the principle into its opposite and say. 'If in doubt, show it prominently?' After all, matters that are beyond doubt are, in a sense, dead; they do not constitute a challenge to the living. To accept anything as true means to incur the risk of error. If I limit myself to knowledge that I consider true beyond doubt, I minimise the risk of error but I maximise, at the same time, the risk of missing out on what may be the subtlest, most important and most rewarding thing in life.

The question of what constitutes proof will be a theme of Chapter 10.

Medical dis-ease

To all intents and purposes, the history of modern medicine can justly be described as triumphant. Its investigation of disease processes, and its increasing control over them has had remarkable and welcome consequences. Medical practice and medical science appear in many respects to be in robust good health. But the dis-ease felt by many actively engaged in medicine, and some prominently so, reflects the undercurrent of dis-ease within it . The diagnosis of this dis-ease will be discussed fully in due course, but in brief symptoms of two related syndromes can be discerned. These are paradigm paralysis and scientific tunnel vision. They have to do with the inability or reluctance to see beyond the immediate horizon of medical and scientific endeavour and achievement.

The limitations of medicine

As later chapters will confirm, I am not at all disillusioned about modern western 'scientific' medicine, the biomedical model – subject to its limitations. On the contrary, I have used it, benefited from it, and admire it – subject to its limitations. My reservations are implied in the phrase 'subject to its limitations', and in the use of the word 'scientific' above in inverted commas. It is those 'limitations' that need, I suggest, to be more honestly acknowledged and more fully explored, as does the narrowness of the concept 'scientific', in our appraisal of modern medicine. Those are two of the key issues to be explored in later chapters.

The whole experience

In your experience as a patient (and I address this question to medical colleagues as well, in their own experience as patients) what has been the balance between medicine's ability to comprehend and respond to the *whole* of that experience? How adequate and appropriate has medical science been to answer all the questions about your illness that have concerned you?

Of course, the answer to those questions will depend on the context. If you have been seriously injured in an accident, the answers may be 100% favourable to the biomedical approach and the medical science that is brought to your immediate aid. If you have a heart attack the biomedical approach and the science that underpins it may still deserve a high approval rating, indeed it may be life-saving. But there may be some questions to which the answer is vague or incomplete. Why me, exactly? Why then? What is the whole story of this event? How will/may/should the future story unfold? If you have a chronic illness – hormonal, rheumatological, neurological, psychological perhaps, the answers are likely to be a great deal more vague

Self-regulation and healing

Modern western scientific medicine has been so successful, and has come to dominate our thinking about healthcare to such an extent that we might be forgiven for wondering how the human race ever survived and evolved to this extent, without it. In fact, of course, no organism would have survived and established itself without the capacity to recover from and repair the damage caused by its environment or its competitors, or from disorder within itself. The capacity to do so by preventive and prophylactic means, or by processes of self-regulation and self-healing has been an evolutionary imperative.

Even today, the amazing achievements of modern surgery would be impossible without the inherent resources of body tissues for self-healing and repair. And in terms of the recovery of the *person* from trauma or disease, the same is true of our psychological and spiritual resources.

Remodelling

The achievements of modern medicine are wonderful, but they are leading us astray in our search for a more comprehensive understanding of illness and disease, and for a more complete and appropriate response to it. The exploration of what a new model might look like begins in Chapter 3, and is completed at the end of the book. But we can briefly anticipate its essential features here.

A new model of medicine will not be composed of any new parts. All the necessary elements are already there, even if some are marginalised. But it will comprise familiar elements in a new structure, a new order. And its key components will be well recognised but too little valued elements of healthcare. These are that a fully effective response to illness and disease must take account of the person as a whole, and not be focused exclusively on the affected parts; must take account of the whole narrative of the illness, which may have social and environmental themes, and not just the immediate event. Secondly, an effective response will mobilise and maximise the self-regulating self-healing potential of the patient. This is in any case a component of all medical care, and can be encouraged by a variety of subtle stimulus, including the all-important placebo or 'contextual healing' effect.[10,11]

These two core elements of healthcare are not at all controversial. But to promote them as primary goals of medical culture, education and practice, and healthcare policy, will require a very considerable effort of will and imagination. It will require a redeployment of resources and some restructuring of the process of care. It will also require some humility on the part of all who have a vested interest in maintaining the status quo; the intellectual, clinical, political or commercial power that the structure of the existing model confers. Modern medicine is successful and powerful, and does confer power on those who plan, manage and practice it. The reordering of power, even quite slight, that remodelling will involve, might be difficult for some to accept.

The requirements for remodelling may be summarised as follows:

- Will and imagination.
- Redeployment of resources.
- Restructuring of the process.
- Reordering of power.
- Humility.

Political change: the playing field and the goal posts

While I was writing the concluding chapters of this book in 2010, the coalition government in the UK published the most radical plan for the reorganisation of the National Health Service since its inception. Critics see this as yet another 'redisorganisation', destabilising the service and likely to cause chaos. Supporters see it as admittedly risky but potentially transformative of a service that has become bogged down in bureaucracy and hamstrung by central control that has deprived clinicians of the freedom to practise in the best interests of the individual patient. The proposed change will turn the National Health Service upside down, fundamentally altering the political and economic context of care, and placing the decisions about the process of care in the hands of primary care physicians (general practitioners) and their teams, and local stakeholders. The intention is to make the process of care as responsive to the needs of the individual patient as possible.

Theoretically, these changes in context and process are conducive to the remodelling recommended in this book, and depending how events unfold, could provide a different frame of reference for some of the criticisms it presents. The proposals afford general practitioners the opportunity to remedy the dis-ease within medicine which many among them have been diagnosing for many years, and whose symptoms and causes are described in these pages. It provides the opportunity to redress the balance between medicine's dominant biomedical methodology and its neglected holistic and humanistic goals. It provides the opportunity for a narrowly rigorous use of evidence to be modified by the informed empiricism and more subtle 'mindlines' of primary care practice (Chapter 10). It allows the therapeutic relationship whose core principles and essential importance are described in Chapter 16, and which has potentially its most formative influence in primary care, to become the springboard for change in the whole dynamics of healthcare. The instinct that exists within primary care towards holistic practice and integrative practice (Chapter 16), and the promotion of self-care and 'enablement' (Chapters 12 and 17), can be fully mobilised. The sense of being part of a community of care that used to prevail in general practice can be revived and extended; not only to refresh and consolidate the relationship with specialist medicine and other mainstream health care professions, but to develop the relationship with complementary practitioners who are part of the reality of contemporary health care, and part of the landscape of most local healthcare communities.

These are just some of the possibilities that could facilitate the remodelling that this book is all about. That many general practitioners are willing and able to take quite radical initiatives, despite the misgivings that many have expressed about the new policy, is evident in the use that has been made of the opportunities for practice based commissioning of services made possible by the previous government.[12] This encourages the belief that such a major revolution in the NHS as the new policy proposes could make room for the minor revolution, or metamorphosis, that I am arguing for. It already promises to remedy some of the problems identified in this book that were more plainly evident when I embarked upon it. But new policies will not promote any creative remodelling of medicine unless structural change in the Health Service is accompanied by the change in the ethos and culture of medicine that this book recommends; unless medicine rediscovers its proper goals and virtues, its healing vocation. A change of playing field will make little difference if the goal posts remain the same.

Models and Paradigms

The model

Why is it appropriate and helpful, in fact necessary, to discuss what is wrong with the way we do medicine in terms of a model? Why is this book a critique of the medical 'model'?

The ideas, knowledge and beliefs that shape our lives are represented by models (patterns for what we construct and do), paradigms (patterns for what we think and believe), and plausibility constructs (patterns that determine our view of the world). These are three different but closely related ways in which we construe the world and our experiences, and manage our lives. They have changed and evolved throughout human history, and they affect and are affected by every aspect of life, from religion through science to business and commerce. They certainly influence the practice of medicine and the provision of healthcare in the United Kingdom and the western world in general. Human history is a story of constant change in these patterns of life. The pace of change has not been constant. There have been bottlenecks in the flow of knowledge, ideas and insights and their cultural and social effects. Established patterns of thought have sometimes been reluctant to give way to new insights until the dam bursts and a new momentum is established. The evolution of Western medicine, as briefly outlined in Chapter 2, has been a part of this continuous process. Medicine has been repeatedly remodelled, chiefly in relation to developments in philosophy or science, but undoubtedly also in relation to social and cultural influences.

Models

A model is a representation. It may represent something that has existed in the past, or that that already exists; or something we are in the process of creating, an experimental design, or a flight of imagination. It may be used to preserve or maintain a tradition or traditional form, to promote a particular style or form, or to suggest or introduce innovation. There are conceptual models – most purely in mathematics; experimental models – to test new ideas; design models – from which new products can be built; and working models – which may represent the way things already are, or demonstrate what a new product will look like.

Models influence us – our thinking and/or our behaviour. Their influence may be positive or negative; role models are a case in point. A model may be fashionable or unfashionable, old fashioned or modern. Models on a catwalk promote new fashions, or revive old fashions that have once again become fashionable. They are also a representation of one kind of feminine beauty, some might say a distorted kind, which has considerable influence on female behaviour.

A model has power and influence. It may be progressive or reactionary, healthy or unhealthy, susceptible to change or resistant to change.

Generally speaking, a model is a representation with a concrete form or a practical application.

Paradigms

A paradigm is more theoretical. The meaning of the term is somewhat vague. Originally it described a set of grammatical examples, but its meaning has become broader and looser. In its very broadest sense it can be applied to a theoretical world-view. But it is most commonly understood to mean a conceptual framework or mind-set that determines how we approach the questions and challenges that life presents to us. That is the sense in which it is used here, and more particularly the sense in which

Thomas Kuhn used it to explore the nature of progress in science.[8] To be useful a paradigm must represent a clearly defined set of concepts or ideas that provide a framework for the investigation or practical application (modelling) of those ideas. The term paradigm should not be used to embrace a nebulous collection of ideas, or to excuse sloppy thinking.

Plausibility constructs

If 'model' is primarily a practical concept and 'paradigm' theoretical, 'plausibility construct' is primarily a cultural concept or world view. It embraces the influence of culture, including philosophy, religion and science, on statements about, and explanations of belief and experience. It determines the way we make sense of things, which may differ greatly between different societies, and even different individuals. It is akin to what is called 'constructivism', a belief about knowledge that asserts that the reality we perceive is constructed by our social, historical, and individual contexts, so that there can be no absolute shared truth.[13]

There is a circular and synergistic relationship between these three dynamics of human progress (Fig I.1). For example Galileo pursued his studies of the solar system within the social and cultural milieu of the Christian Church and its ruling institutions and the dominant philosophical influence of Aristotle. That milieu constituted the plausibility construct for people's view of the natural world and the place of humans in the cosmos. This gave birth to a paradigm, a set of principles that dictated the relationship of the earth to the other heavenly bodies, an astronomical paradigm, from which a working model of the earth, the sun and the planets could be created. Galileo realised empirically that the workings of the solar system did not fit that model. His model required a new paradigm,

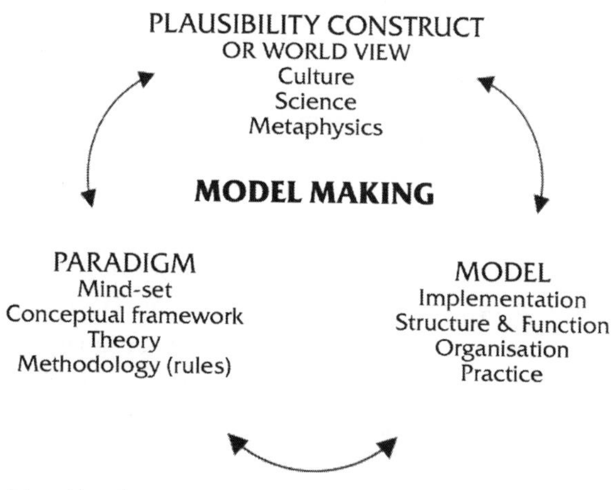

Figure I.1 Model making 1.

new astrological principles that set the world in a different relationship to the other heavenly bodies – no longer the centre of the universe. This challenged the plausibility construct of the day, to Galileo's considerable discomfort. But the new model prevailed, the paradigm shifted, and the cultural acceptance of what was plausible changed.

By contrast the 'swinging' '60s, in Europe and America, represented an upheaval in the social and cultural milieu that made 'plausible' certain beliefs, intellectual and political attitudes – paradigms, that gave rise to new models of behaviour, student politics and clothes, amongst other things.

At the beginning of his book, *Medicine and Society*, published in 1973, the British physician Henry Miller quotes the statement by Rudolf Virchow (1821–1902) that "Medicine is a social science and politics nothing else but medicine on a grand scale."[14] This observation is worth pondering, but here it is representative of a number of commentators who have seen medicine as always, to some extent at least and possibly to a large extent, influenced by the plausibility construct of the time; its paradigm inextricably entangled with other social and cultural trends and forces. In his analysis of the past 200 years history of medicine in America, for example, sociologist Stephen Lyng, relates the rise of modern scientific medicine explicitly to the influence of big corporations, including the petrochemical industry and its pharmaceutical offshoots.[15]

Quite apart from the obvious investment opportunities arising from an expanding pharmacological approach to medicine, Lyng claims that the corporations saw in scientific medicine an opportunity to shift the responsibility for well-being related problems in the work force from themselves onto the medical profession, because what had previously been construed as social problems were now susceptible to a medical interpretation. Be that as it may, the investment by big corporations in scientific medical education greatly enhanced and accelerated its development, and hence the growing dominance of the biomedical model. The biomedical paradigm suited the plausibility construct of the burgeoning industrial society, which in turn helped to foster a particular model of medical practice.

In another example it is suggested that the popularity of complementary and alternative models of medicine is primarily a consequence of a reaction against modernism.[16] The argument seems far-fetched to me, and I think there are better ways of construing that phenomenon. But it nicely exemplifies in principle the inter-relation of plausibility constructs, paradigms and models of health care.

The power of paradigms and models

> Our minds operate in such a way that models grab ideas and take them over, giving them a shape and solidity which is false – useful, for sure, but false. Obviously useful but less obviously false. (James Willis[17])

Paradigms and models are powerful things that can have positive and negative effects, in medicine and medical research as in other spheres of life. "Models are ways of constructing reality, ways of imposing meaning on the chaos of the phenomenal world. The models physicians use have decisive effects on medical behaviour. The models determine what kind of data will be gathered; phenomena become 'data' precisely because of their relevance to a particular set of questions (out of the possible sets of questions) which is being asked. Once in place, models act to generate their own verification by excluding phenomena outside the frame of reference the user employs. Models are indispensable but hazardous because they can be mistaken for reality itself rather than as but one way of organising reality."[18]

We could replace the word 'model' with 'paradigm' in this quotation, because many of the virtues and dangers of models and paradigms apply equally to both. Paradigms, though, are more powerful because they command the mind and are the foundations on which models are built. They are of great value because they give coherent expression to ideas. They allow us to work constructively with those ideas, to build models upon them, and to set standards of performance for those models. Thomas Kuhn applied the concept to science in exploring the way that scientific attitudes and beliefs, and the research and development programmes that follow them, become established. The scientific paradigm determines the parameters of what he called "normal science", the precepts and methods gaining consensus within the scientific community of the day. It determines not only the current view of reality, but also the sorts of questions that can be asked, the methods that can justifiably be used to resolve those questions, and the form that potential answers will take.

A helpful description of the process is provided by Peter Lipton in his book *Inference to the Best Explanation*: Scientists acquire through their education a stock of exemplars – concrete problem solutions in their speciality – and use them to guide their research. They pick new problems that look similar to an exemplar problem, they try techniques that are similar to those that worked in that exemplar, and they assess their success by reference to the standards of solution that the exemplars illustrate. Thus the exemplars set up a web of 'perceived similarity relations' that guide future research, and the shared judgements are explained by the shared exemplars.[19] (See Figure I.2.)

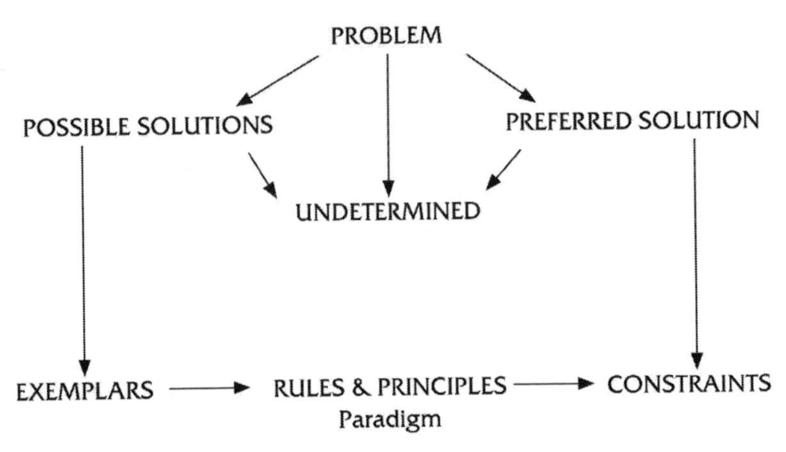

Figure I.2 Undetermination.

The limits and dangers of paradigms

A paradigm is a conceptual framework, adequate for its time but not eternally true, and essentially metaphysical because it is a framework of ideas and values. It is contingent upon other circumstances, including the social and cultural influences that have been mentioned, and cannot claim to represent permanently an objective reality. Lipton's description of Kuhn's theory of paradigms is in the context of a discussion of 'undetermination' – a state of affairs in which the rules or principles that govern a particular problem-solving process constrain the solution in such a way as to leave it actually undetermined; or in simpler language, according to the *Concise Oxford Dictionary*, undecided. But a paradigm can be difficult to shift. Which is why the book in which Kuhn developed his paradigm thesis is called *The Structure of Scientific Revolutions*. Once a paradigm is established, it tends to consider itself self-evidently true and perceives no need to justify itself from first principles.

There is an obvious relationship between paradigms and knowledge. Because no paradigm is eternally true, it will eventually give way to new knowledge. But the paradigm, while it holds sway, will dictate the terms on which new knowledge may be acquired. As John Heron explains: Any method of enquiry presupposes an enquiry paradigm. This implies and depends on a set of basic beliefs about the nature of reality and how this reality can be known. These are *the philosophical presuppositions of the method* that are not derived from the method itself and inevitably the continued use of the method will show up the limitations of its underlying paradigm.[20] (My italics.)

And paradigms and the search for knowledge must be tempered with wisdom. T.S. Eliot's words, "Where is the wisdom we have lost in knowledge? Where is the knowledge we have lost in information?" are pertinent.[21] It is easy to mistake information for knowledge. Knowledge is not just information, and it does not itself confer wisdom. It embraces information and its proper function is to develop wisdom, but it must also sometimes be subordinate to wisdom. Wisdom is more than knowledge; it is knowledge become truly fruitful in enriching life. Thomas Merton, the Christian monk, wrote a prayer for peace that was read in the U.S. House of Representatives in 1962, the year of the Cuban missile crisis at the height of the cold war. It included an intriguing and though-provoking line that prays for "Wisdom in proportion to our Science". A scientific paradigm must be tested by knowledge, even while it sets the tests for new knowledge. But it must also be tested by wisdom. The key question is, 'Is this paradigm truly life enhancing?'

But paradigms operate in more mundane settings too, if the business community will forgive that aspersion. Here is a definition taken from training material that was being used by the Whitbread Group some ten years ago: 'All organisations operate by an accepted set of rules and traditions. Some are formally spelled out in writing; others are accepted for use over time. These rules and traditions are known as a paradigm. A paradigm establishes the pattern for how we work and live, how we interact with customers and how we react to changes occurring around us. Our paradigm or pattern tells us what is accepted and what is unusual. It helps us make sense of the world. Some rules and traditions are positive; others get in the way of us being able to recognise and act on opportunities. A positive paradigm helps us to act and react in a future-focussed way. Paradigm paralysis blinds us to opportunities and change. To know if your paradigm is positive or negative, you must first be aware of what it is.'

'Paradigm paralysis': a nasty condition – resistant to new knowledge, and whose most serious symptom is tunnel vision, or even blindness; as in Step 3 of the McNamara fallacy, which we will encounter again in Chapter 10: 'The third step is to presume that what can't be measured easily really isn't important. This is blindness.'[22]

Paradigm paralysis is a diagnostic term coined by Joel Barker, an American whose vocation is to treat it where he finds it within business organisations, and prevent it if he can.[23] Barker uses the term paradigm in much the same sense as in this book, to describe a mind-set or conceptual framework. He proposes that paradigms are essential. They establish rules and principles that allow us to work, and live effectively. They impose order on systems that might otherwise be unruly or inefficient. They provide an environment for creativity – *while they remain valid.* But, as already stated, they do not remain eternally valid. They are a staging post on a continuing journey towards new horizons. The problem is, as Barker explains, that if we are not careful we become conditioned by our paradigm. It conditions our expectations, so that we cannot see beyond the immediate horizon. He goes on to demonstrate how paradigms that have worked well in business can inhibit innovation if they become too rigid. He describes how Swiss watchmakers could not 'see' the advantages of the quartz mechanism because it did not fit their paradigm. The Japanese, of course, did. And he characterises the Japanese as good innovators because of their freedom from the restrictive effects that paradigms can come to have.

Barker says what are needed in any organisation, or any system that works to a particular paradigm, are 'paradigm pioneers'; people who are restless within the prevailing paradigm, and have a tendency to peep over the perimeter fence and see what lies beyond, what might be coming next.

The dissident voices within present day medicine are its present day paradigm pioneers. Hippocrates, Galen, Paracelsus, Pasteur and Harvey were amongst medicine's earlier paradigm pioneers. But there is a difference. The dissident voices of today are not pioneers of a new frontier. They are not exactly pioneers at all, they want to reclaim territory which has always been there. They are not struggling to establish a new paradigm, but for the re-emergence of an old one.

If a paradigm holds the middle ground between the cultural and social milieu that makes it plausible, and the model that is built upon it and by which it is put into practice, what are the plausibility structure, the paradigm, and the model of modern Western medicine?

The Plausibility Structure

> Current societal values do not, on the whole, support or nurture relationships. Our Western society, on the contrary, values individual accomplishment above community, science over art, analysis over synthesis, technological solutions over wisdom. In such a context, all of us suffer diminished capacity for spirituality and love. (Moira Stewart[24])

It is beyond dispute that we live in an age of technology and consumerism, a secular age and a materialist age. Of course, the spirit of the age does not define all who live in it, nor all its social and cultural institutions. But the attitudes and expectations of very many people, perhaps of all of us to some extent, are certainly affected by those trends, and conditioned by them. We live in an age of continuing rapid development in science and technology that seems to make all things possible; developments that offer the promise that we will increasingly be able to manage all the predicaments of life with their help. At one end of the scale we look forward to engineering an explanation for the origin of the universe, at the other to making repairs in faulty tissues and DNA sequences. Understanding the machinery of the universe, and controlling the machinery of life, seem to be at our fingertips.

This is the ruling spirit of the age. It determines our plausibility structure, our attitudes to what is acceptable and what makes sense. And this is the plausibility structure within which the scientific biomedical model operates. But it is not, of course, the whole story. There is a cultural undercurrent flowing against this tide, which is not only reflected in the dis-ease within medicine that I have described, but in the artistic, ecological, interpersonal and spiritual awareness of people. This undercurrent is strong, and imparts momentum to the remodelling process. And because the bond between medicine and society is so strong, reciprocal evolution in medicine will in turn be to the benefit of our whole culture. A theme we will return to in Chapter 17.

The Paradigm

The modern western medical paradigm is the analytic scientific method. This is based on the study of natural phenomena to discover their component parts in the finest detail, and the functional relationships between those parts; whether they are elementary particles in the nucleus of an atom or genetic particles in the nucleus of a cell. It can, perhaps, be traced back to the conception of French mathematician Pierre Laplace (1749–1827) of – "science pursuing the ideal of absolute detachment by representing the world in terms of its exactly determined particulars". It also involves the study of factors that influence the condition or behaviour of the component parts, and of factors that can be used to control or manipulate their condition or behaviour. The description, explanation and application of this knowledge, all theories and procedures based upon it, must be rigorously tested, subjected to what has been called destructive analysis, to prove their validity. There are two primary rules for this testing. One is that the proposition should be framed in such a way as can be falsified, proved wrong, the rule attributed to Karl Popper.[25] The other is that a satisfactory test of the proposition (it is not falsified) must be reproduced in other independent tests. A corollary of the first rule is that factors that might confuse the outcome of the test, the confounding variables, must be controlled and eliminated as far as possible.

This paradigm has made possible staggering advances in science in general and medicine in particular. We are able to control and manipulate body structure and function, and the disease processes that affect them in remarkable ways. And most of us will have benefited from this at some time. The limits of the paradigm are that it reduces the phenomenon that is the object of study from its state as a complex integrated entity responsive in various ways to its circumstances and environment, to an assemblage of parts isolated from the multiplicity of other factors that impinge upon it. But these limitations are a prerequisite to the precision with which the investigation can be carried out.

Another characteristic that is claimed for the scientific paradigm, and which can be perceived as a strength or a limitation, is that it is value-free, detached, objective. This claim is made sometimes vehemently, but as will be discussed later, is false.

Cosmology

David Greaves suggests that 'cosmology' is a more helpful concept than 'paradigm' for exploring the evolution of medicine, and particularly its future evolution.[26] His reasons are that cosmology embraces moral and cultural as well as scientific and technical matters, theory and practice, while paradigm refers only to theory; and that Kuhn's concept of paradigm involves relatively rapid shifts, whereas changes in cosmologies occur over longer periods of time, as in the transition between the two main eras of Western medicine mentioned later, in Chapter 2.

The bigger picture

Figure I.3 sketches out the relationship between the two contrasting patterns of thought and practice that influence the way we do medicine in the UK that will be explored in this book. The fact that they are contrasting, and sometimes competing, does not mean that they are mutually

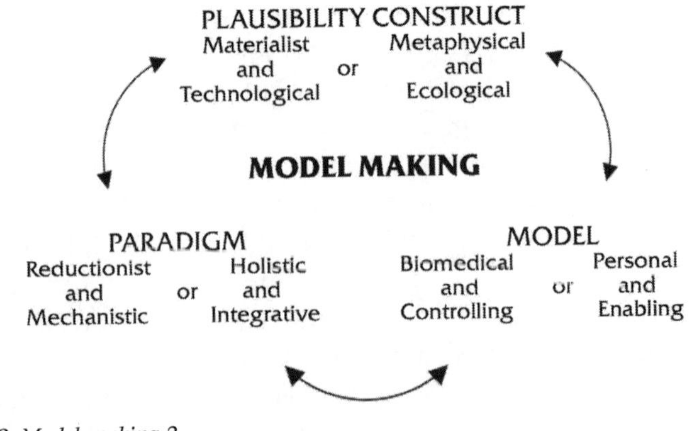

Figure I.3 Model making 2.

exclusive. On the contrary, the point is made in the discussion of the holistic perspective in Chapter 12 that they are essentially complementary. At issue is the imbalance in our culture, and particularly our medical culture, between the two pairs of concepts in each part of the cyclical relationship shown in the figure, and the dominance of those in the left hand pair.

The Model

For the reasons given in the above account of its underlying paradigm, the modern medical model is commonly known as the biomedical model, sometimes the biomechanical model. It is the practical application of the paradigm to the study, understanding, diagnosis and treatment of human disease, and to understanding the factors that predispose to disease (epidemiology) and their prevention (public health, health promotion). It usually works by trying to identify a specific bodily disorder, attributable to a specific cause, which is susceptible to a specific intervention. In the process, what is often a poorly defined subjective illness is reduced to a recognisable and treatable disease.[ii] "Illness is what the patient has on their way to see the doctor and a disease is what they have on the way home."[27]

We may feel uncomfortable to be identified with the plausibility construct of medicine as I describe it, but who would want to abandon the paradigm or the model? That would be nonsense. But they do have limitations; in some cases severe limitations.

The biomedical model is dominant, but has not had it all its own way. The ambivalent or frankly critical comments quoted already and elsewhere in the book reflect the continuing discomfort at its dominance, within and without medicine. They may be reflected to some extent in what is now included in medical school curricula, but they have not significantly affected what actually happens on the ground. Reasons for resistance to change are discussed in Chapter 11, and underpinning these, and examined in Chapter 10, are our attitudes to truth, proof and evidence; above all because evidence has become the big enforcer of the medical paradigm.

---

ii To simplify a semantic problem that often causes confusion: by contrast with illness and disease, sickness is illness or disease referred to in terms of its social impact. Consider terms like 'Sick room', 'Sick leave', 'Sick note', 'He's sick!', or even 'Sick joke.' These distinctions are teased out more fully in the discussion of the story in 'Being a patient', Chapter 8.

References

1 Ward K. *The Case for Religion*. Oxford: One World; 2004.
2 College of Medicine Policy Document. Available from the College of Medicine 19, Buckingham Street, London WC2N 6EF and online at www.collegeofmedicine.org.uk
3 Cassell E. *The Nature of Suffering and the Goals of Medicine*. New York: Oxford University Press; 2004.
4 Swayne J. An uncertain healing. *World Medicine* 1976 November 17th; 74–85.
5 Swayne J. Medicine and healing: A broken marriage? *New Society* 1976 September 2nd; 491–492.
6 Swayne J. On our best behaviour. *J R Coll Gen Pract.* 1976; 26:560–564.
7 Haslam D. Who cares? *Br J Gen Pract.* 2007; 57(545):987–993.
8 Kuhn T. *The structure of scientific revolutions*. Chicago: University of Chicago Press; 1996.
9 Schumacher E. *A Guide for the Perplexed*. London: Sphere; 1998.
10 Miller F K. The owner of context: reconceptualising the placebo. *J R Soc Med.* 2008; 101:222–225.
11 Moerman D. *Meaning, medicine and the 'placebo effect'*. Cambridge: Cambridge University Press; 2002.
12 Cassidy J. Commissioners doing it for themselves. *Br Med J.* 2010; 341:c4488.
13 Kuper A, Reeves S, Levinson W. An introduction to reading and appraising qualitative research. *Br Med J.* 2008; 337:404–407.
14 Miller H. *Medicine and Society*. Oxford: Oxford University Press; 1973.
15 Lyng S. *Holistic Health and Biomedical Medicine*. New York: State University of New York Press; 1990.
16 Lejeune S. In: Ernst E, editor. *Healing, Hype or Harm? A critical analysis of complementary or alternative medicine*. Exeter: Societas; 2008.
17 Willis J. *Friends in low places*. Abingdon: Radclife; 2001.
18 Eisenberg L. Disease and illness: Distinctions between professional and popular ideas of sickness. *Cult Med Psychiat.* 1977; 1:9–23.
19 Lipton P. *Inference to the Best Explanation*. Abingdon: Routledge; 1991.
20 Heron J. The placebo effect and a participatory world view. In: Peters D. *Understanding the placebo effect in complementary medicine: theory, practice and research*. London: Churchill Livingstone; 2001.
21 Eliot T. *Collected Poems 1909–1962*. London: Faber and Faber; 1963.
22 Handy C. *The Empty Raincoat*. London: Random House; 1995.
23 Barker J. *Paradigms: The business of discovering the future*. New York: Harper Collins; 1992.
24 Stewart M. Reflections on the doctor–patient relationship. *Br J Gen Pract.* 2005; 55(519):793–801.
25 Popper K. *The Logic of Scientific Discovery*. Abingdon: Routledge; 1992.

26 Greaves D. Reflections on a new medical cosmology. *J Med Ethics* 2002; 28;81–85; 2002.

27 Heath I. *The Mystery of General Practice*. London: Nuffield Provincial Hospitals Trust; 1995.

part 1

A CHRONIC DIS-EASE

1

THE CHALLENGE

Summary

- The challenge confronting contemporary Western medicine is to reconcile its huge achievements with the limitations that its methods impose on our understanding of illness and our response to it.
- Clinical experience, in general practice in particular, emphasises the diversity of illness in the community, and as part of people's everyday lives; its multifaceted and multi-factorial nature, and the diagnostic and management problems and uncertainty that this creates.
- At the heart of the challenge is a separation between medicine and healing; between medicine as a means of controlling disease processes and manipulating body functions, and healing as a process of enabling self-regulation, reintegration, insight and new growth.
- Time and opportunity to tell the whole story is often 'whole-making' and therapeutic in itself; allowing patients to see themselves, and be seen, as a unique person with an individual problem.
- The challenge is to achieve the right balance between the power and sophistication of medical science and the power of the human organism and personality to restore and repair itself, because in our commitment to the first we have lost sight of or devalued the second:

> Some of medicine works extremely well because it treats people as being all the same; and some of medicine works very well because it treats people as all being different. Physicians must constantly juggle these two ways of seeing their patients. (Howard Brody[10])

A point of view

The original motive for writing this book was a point of view. It was a personal view based on the 40 years in clinical practice that have shaped my understanding of healthcare. For me, that challenge has been to reconcile the huge achievements of modern western medicine with the limitations that its methods impose on our understanding of illness and our response to it. The sense of challenge, and the perspective that informs it, are certainly personal, although I knew them to be shared by other doctors and healthcare practitioners, and by patients and commentators. What I did not appreciate until I began to explore the literature relating to the medical model (crudely, the way we do medicine), was the extent to which both the sense of challenge and the perspective are so widely shared. Nor did I appreciate how persistent they have been throughout the 100 years during which orthodox scientific medicine has risen to its present pre-eminence. This will be apparent from the many quotations and references I have used that illustrate how others perceive or experience it. It has been a fascinating study, revealing on the one hand admiration and gratitude for the power and achievements of medical science and technology, and on the other grave misgivings about the narrowness of the vision of human healing and health care that they represent, and the limitations of their ability to explain and manage illness and disease in all its complexity.

The references to contemporary commentaries in medical journals and the media often reflect the misgivings of people engaged in routine front-line healthcare at the present design of the medical model. The *British Medical Journal* in particular, one of the most widely read mainstream medical journals, reflects this trait. So as it has developed the book has become less of a personal view; rather an attempt to draw together and articulate strands of thought and experience from many sources; to offer a more comprehensive and compelling critique of the prevailing medical model than has been attempted hitherto, and perhaps a braver exploration of how the model might evolve.

The doubts that have shaped my point of view arose quite early in my GP career, but on reflection were probably triggered by an experience soon after I qualified:

> Mick was a retired Merchant Seaman in his 60s from Liverpool. He was in hospital for repair of an aortic aneurysm, a dilatation of the main artery from the heart, which could rupture at any time with fatal results. It had been a chance finding on a chest X-Ray for a cough. He was a smoker. He had travelled the world as a seaman and lived a colourful life. Venereal disease had been an occupational hazard to which he had succumbed at some time, possibly contributing to the development of the aneurysm.

As a very junior House Surgeon it was my job to 'clerk' him when he arrived; to record his medical history and give him a general physical examination. Although he had given informed consent, it turned out that he had little understanding of what was wrong with him and why he was there; nor of the risks of surgery. He was amusing, cheerful and full of life. Knowing the seriousness of his situation and realising how little he understood the implications, it was difficult to know quite how to pitch the conversation.

An operation of this complexity was an uncommon event, and the prospect excited considerable interest within the hospital. It would be a severe challenge for the surgeons, and there was a mood of eager anticipation. The observation gallery of the operating theatre was well attended.

But Mick died during the operation.

It was a great shock to me; partly because I had liked him so much and enjoyed his company during our very brief acquaintance, but also because of my dismay that as I saw it, naively perhaps, personal care had been subordinated to medical heroics.

After hospital jobs I went on to join the Wessex General Practice Vocational Training Scheme. This was a pioneering scheme lead by one of the founder members of the Royal College of General Practitioners, which was still quite a young institution at that time. The course introduced us to the reality of medical life outside hospital – the diversity of illness in the community, its multifaceted and multi-factorial nature, and the diagnostic and management problems and uncertainty that this created. It made us aware of patients as people, and their illness as part of their everyday lives – rather than as the 'cases' we had encountered in hospital medicine, isolated from the context of their lives. We began to understand the psychological dynamics of illness, and the pastoral nature of much medical care in the community. This was in the 1960s, and medical education is more broadly based now, but at the time this was eye-opening stuff. As well as gaining a new perspective of health care we were encouraged to reflect on the experience. I became more aware of the meaning of my sense of vocation as a doctor, and as my early years in general practice progressed I found I was facing the challenge I have described.

The broken marriage

I experienced this as a separation between medicine and healing; between medicine as a means of controlling disease processes and manipulating body functions, and healing as a process of enabling self-regulation, re-integration, insight and new growth. The welcome, often life-saving, and increasingly indispensable power of medicine to control seemed to be at the expense of some equally important, sometimes perhaps more important, more subtle, more creative, more whole-making function of health-care.[1,2,3]

Experience over the years strengthened my appreciation of the validity of both these aspects of medicine – the power to control and the need to enable. But it also increased my sense of the divergence between them. I experienced satisfaction and gratitude for what modern medicine could achieve for my patients (and indeed for my family and myself). But I was also increasingly aware of what it could not achieve; and of what more might be achieved by other means; approaches to health care other than the repertoire of interventions that medicine provided and that my medical education had equipped me to use. I began to explore this challenge by setting up a new practice with fewer patients that allowed me to provide more consultation time but still within the context of routine general practice; time for a more thorough clinical appraisal, but more importantly time to hear more of the patient's story – the story of the illness and of the life experience from which the illness arose (see Figure 1.1).

It was evident that the opportunity to tell the story was often 'whole-making' and therapeutic in itself; an opportunity for patients to see themselves, and be seen, as a unique person with an individual problem. And the fuller narrative that often emerged revealed dynamics in the illness, and in the history and circumstances, that made a more complete and relevant therapeutic response possible. It also helped the patient to make more sense of the problem, to find some meaning in it, and feel more in control of it.

Later the introduction of the homeopathic method to my repertoire alongside conventional care provided additional evidence of the remarkable degree of self-regulation and self-healing that is possible. The therapeutic effects of this approach, particularly any specific effect of the homeopathic medicines, are not yet fully explained and are often attributed, usually dismissively but sometimes correctly, to placebo or contextual effects.[4] But apart from anything else it provides an excellent means of eliciting the story, with all the therapeutic benefits to which I have alluded. What really matters, and what impresses me regardless of how it is achieved, is the difference it makes to the patient.

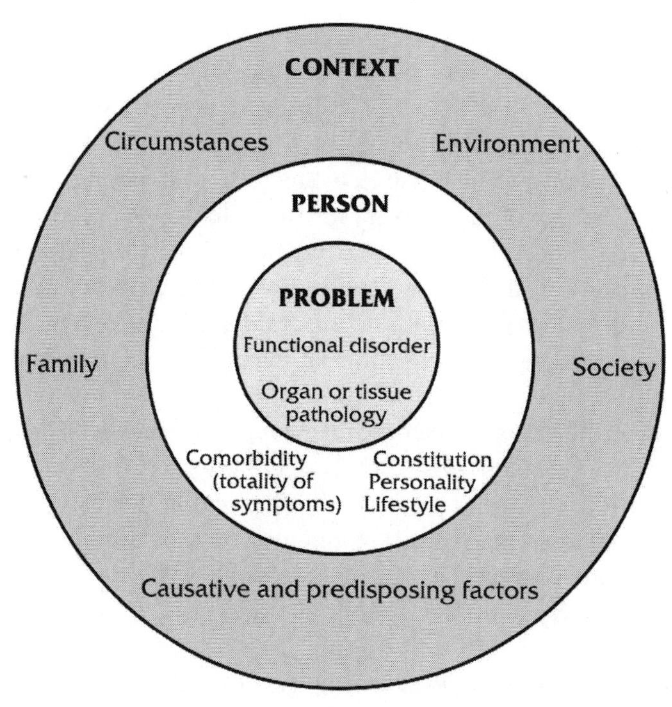

Figure 1.1 *The whole story.*

I am deeply appreciative of the power of medical science to alleviate disability and manage disease, and often awestruck at its sophistication. I am also deeply appreciative and awestruck at the often astonishing power of the human organism and personality to restore and repair itself. This book is about achieving the proper balance between those two powers. It argues that we have got the balance wrong because in our commitment to the first we have lost sight of or devalued the second; that to get the balance right we need to revise the medical model and shift the scientific paradigm that underpins it. The momentum for change has been present for a long time. The book articulates the rationale for change and seeks to increase that momentum.

Keeping the balance

But to what extent is it *practically* possible to develop and implement a medical model that reconciles and integrates the personal and biological dimensions of healthcare, not to mention the public health dimension? To develop a model that reconciles and integrates the control of disease processes with the enabling of healing processes? In an early document setting out its vision for general practitioner vocational training, 'The Future General Practitioner', the Royal College of General Practitioners (RCGP) urged that all diagnosis should be composed "*simultaneously* in physical, psychological and social terms" (my italics).[5] That is a tall order in itself. But having, where possible, achieved it, to respond accordingly to the mixed dynamics of the problem identified in this way is an even taller order. The RCGP ideal "encouraged a truly holistic practice to develop, such that the disease and the person could not easily be dissected in the name of a spurious biological objectivity".[6] But this frame of reference did not readily accommodate the disease, the pathological entity that would be the focus of the medical intervention.

Discussing the limits of scientific medicine to comprehend the nature of suffering, the American physician and Professor of Public Health Eric Cassell writes, ". . . if medicine is to achieve its enduring goals . . . we must clarify what kind of knowledge is represented by knowing who a person is, and mediate any conflict that exists in medicine between the two kinds of knowledge, which we call the *scientific* and the personal". (emphasis in the original).[7]

London GP Iona Heath, President of the Royal College of General Practitioners 2009–2012, describes the problem in this way:

> The general practitioner, while actively using the generalisations of biomedical science has a constant duty to refocus on the individual, the detail of their experience and the meaning they attach to that experience. . . . We cannot see the particular patient and the generalisation simultaneously. At any given instant, we have to choose one way of seeing or the other. If we are to maximise our understanding, if we are not to become stranded and impotent at one pole of the dualism, we must learn to oscillate our gaze.[8]

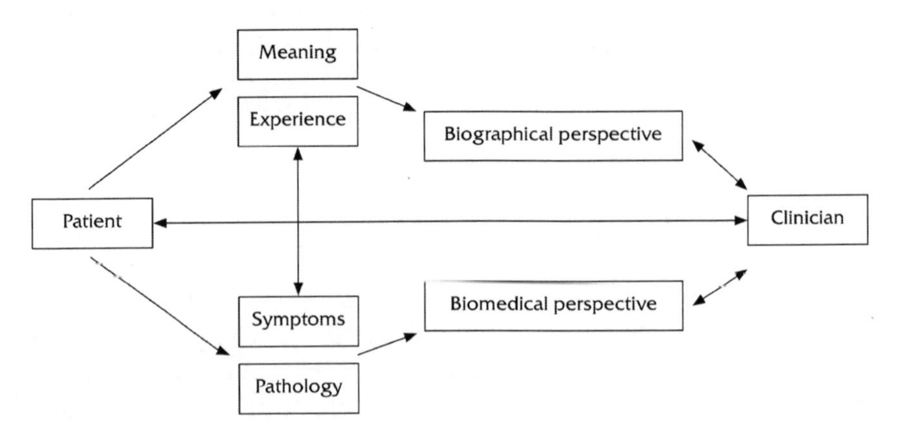

Figure 1.2 *The dichotomy in clinical practice.*

Many healthcare practitioners face the same challenge, not only general practitioners (see Figure 1.2).

Dr Heath writes eloquently here and elsewhere about the tension between the personal qualities in healthcare that do so much to enable the healing resources in the patient and the demands of the biomedical method.[9] Here she represents these as two poles of a dualism that seem to have contradictory and mutually exclusive properties. Each requires our attention and respect, but we cannot focus our gaze *simultaneously* on both. We have to oscillate between them with as much agility as we can. The American Physician Howard Brody, makes the same point: "Some of medicine works extremely well because it treats people as being all the same; and some of medicine works very well because it treats people as all being different. Physicians must constantly juggle these two ways of seeing their patients."[10]

David Warriner, commenting on John Macleod's book, *Clinical Examination* says, "The most inspiring doctors have breathtaking vision, one moment passively surveying the patient's entire human condition, the next seamlessly zooming in to the minutiae of their pathology".[11,12]

This theme – the problem of reconciling and integrating these two apparently conflicting perspectives of illness, these apparently competing approaches to patient care – recurs throughout this book. It is nicely encapsulated in the title of an essay, *Narrative based medicine in an evidence based world*,[13] that directly addresses this problem and that will be referred to again in the discussion of evidence in Chapter 11. As the book proceeds we will explore how a remodelling process might constructively shift the balance between these poles – the biomedical, analytical and controlling aspect of medicine and its personal, descriptive and enabling aspect – and achieve a better harmonisation of the two.

References

1 Swayne J. An uncertain healing. *World Medicine* 1976 November 17th; 74–85.

2 Swayne J. Medicine and healing: A broken marriage? *New Society* 1976 September 2nd; 91–492.

3 Swayne J. On our best behaviour. *J R Col Gen Pract.* 1976; 26:560–564.

4 Miller F G, Kaptchuk T J. The power of context: reconceptualising the placebo. *J R Soc Med.* 2008; 101:222–5.

5 RCGP. *The future general practitioner.* London: Royal College of General Practitioners; 1973.

6 Marinker M. Sense and sensibility. (In: Marinker M, *Sense and sensibility in medicine.* London: BMJ Publishing Group; 1996.

7 Cassell E. *The Nature of Suffering and the Goals of Medicine*. New York: Oxford University Press; 2004.
8 Heath I. Uncertain clarity: contradiction, meaning and hope. *Br J Gen Pract*. 1999; 49:651–657.
9 Heath I. *The Mystery of General Practice*. London: Nuffield Provincial Hospitals Trust; 1995.
10 Brody H. Diagnosis is treatment. *J Fam Pract*. 1980; 10(3):445–449.
11 Warriner D. Medical Classics: Clinical Examination, by John Macleod. *Br Med J*. 2009; 338:b1786.
12 Douglas G, Nicol F, Robertson C. *Macleod's Clinical Examination*. 12th edition. Edinburgh: Churchill Livingstone; 2009.
13 Greenhalgh T. Narrative based medicine in an evidence based world. In Greenhalgh T H. *Narrative Based Medicine*. London: BMJ Books; 1998.

2

EVOLUTION AND STRUGGLE

Summary

- The early history of medicine reveals the slow pace of its evolution over the course of at least 4,500 years up to the 16th century when it increased rapidly. The rise of orthodox scientific medicine to its present pre-eminence has been most rapid and most conspicuous during the past 100 years.
- As the pace accelerated, most examples of change and resistance to change were small perturbations in the flow of medical history. But there have been episodes of more pronounced struggle, as between vitalism and mechanism, miasmatic theory and germ theory.
- A watershed was the emergence of a professional and scientific orthodoxy. But a dissident tendency has been present throughout.
- A common denominator of this tendency is an approach to patient care that is responsive to the whole nature of individual patients and the mixed dynamics of their lives and illnesses.
- This dis-ease became increasingly pronounced in the 1970's. Criticism has focused on the pressure to accommodate the human narrative of illness in a biomedical framework, narrowing the way that doctors think about patients, and creating tension between *scientia* and *caritas*.
- This 'evolutionary struggle' has been at least latent in the hearts and minds of many doctors and other healthcare professionals and patients for a long time.
- The dominant model of Western medical science and practice has served us well, often dramatically well. But if the undercurrents of dis-ease are to be taken seriously a new vision for medicine is needed, and a changed model.

The rise of scientific medicine

The rise of orthodox scientific medicine to its present pre-eminence has been most rapid and most conspicuous during the past 100 years. I have described the difficulty that I and others have found in reconciling the remarkable and welcome achievements of this biomedical model with other more subtle and personal aspects of health care, but it is helpful to put this in a brief historical perspective.

The early history of medicine reveals the immensely slow pace of its evolution over the course of at least 4,500 years up to the 16th century when the pace increased rapidly. This is why David Greaves prefers to talk about slow moving 'cosmologies' rather than 'paradigms' in relation to the evolution of medicine.[1] He quotes another author's suggestion that there have been two main eras of Western medicine since ancient times which can be associated with dominant medical cosmologies – humoral medicine, dominant from 200CE (Galen's time) to 1600 CE, and biomedicine dominant from 1800 CE to the present, with some two centuries of transition from 1600–1800 CE.

Examples of key events over the course of the transitional years and leading into the biomedical era include: The detailed anatomical work of Vesalius; the turbulent and pioneering influence of Paracelsus (1493–1541) shown in Figure 2.1, which stimulated the progression from pharmacy, the giving of plant medicines, to pharmacology, the study of their active constituents; the eventual isolation of bioactive chemical compounds and

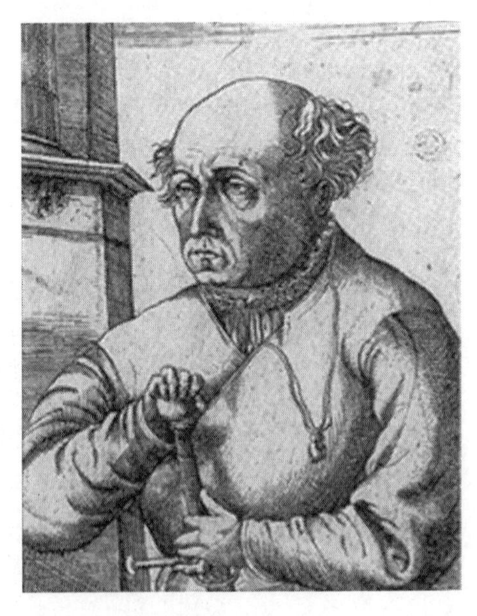

Figure 2.1 *Paracelsus: paradigm pioneer.*

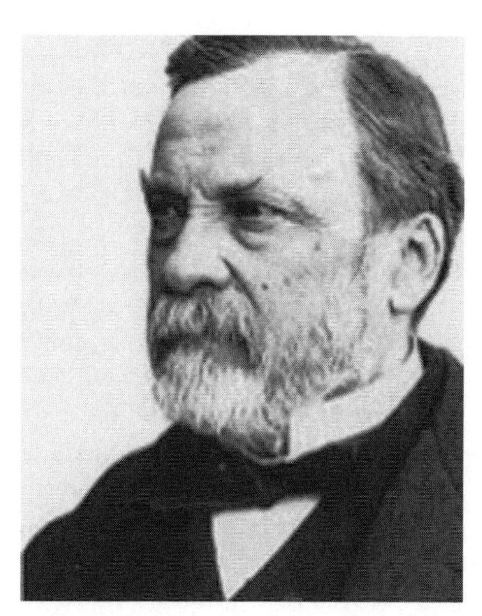

Figure 2.2 *Louis Pasteur (1822–1896).*

the understanding of their specific action; the birth of the germ theory of disease, microbiology, and the concept of specific causation of disease.

This period also embraced the pioneering work of William Harvey on the circulation of the blood (1628) and his insistence on experiment as a source of reliable knowledge, echoing the earlier precepts of Francis Bacon (1561–1626). It included the invention of the microscope, which made it possible to examine the tissues of the body in detail (for example, Malpighi's treatise on the lungs, published in 1661). And, beginning with the work of van Leeuvenhoek around 1671, made visible the 'animalcules', including bacteria, whose role as infectious organisms and agents of disease was later demonstrated by the experiments of Louis Pasteur (1822–1896) shown in Figure 2.2 and Robert Koch (1843–1910).[2]

Although the pace of change accelerated, and there was certainly controversy, there was still continuity. Paracelsus upset the medical apple-cart, and despite his influence became persona non grata to the profession. Even Harvey's description of the circulation of the blood had been regarded as heretical at first. But these and other examples of change and resistance to change (discussed in Chapter 13), were small perturbations in the flow of medical history. A more significant and systemic change, however, beginning much earlier in the 11th Century, had been the adoption of medicine into the universities and the creation of medical schools, leading to the creation of a medical elite that excluded practitioners without the approved academic qualifications.

The period of the 16th to the 19th centuries saw scientific medicine becoming established, but it was also a period of increasingly 'heroic' medicine. Knowledge of anatomy and pharmacology, but limited knowledge of physiology, encouraged the use of interventions which were surgically crude, dangerous and painful, and pharmacologically toxic. They were also not very effective.

In the course of this continuing cumulative process of medical evolution there have been episodes of more pronounced struggle. The challenge presented by the progress of scientific medicine in the last century, that I describe in Chapter 1 is the most recent, but there have been others. One occurred during the first half of the eighteenth century and still has resonance today. It took the form of the debate between vitalism and mechanism, in which the mechanistic argument eventually prevailed much assisted by the demonstration of the electrical properties of living organisms, when "many (came to regard) the superior properties of living entities as deriving not from some super-added transcendental principle but from innate organisation".[2] David Greaves points out an irony here, however, in that the vitalist principle (that the nature of living things cannot be explained only in physical and material terms) is integral to a proper understanding of the work of both Harvey and Sydenham, another 17th century pioneer of modern medicine later dubbed 'the English Hippocrates', a fact that is missing from familiar accounts of their achievements.[3]

The second was the struggle between the germ theory of disease (specific diseases caused by specific organisms), demonstrated finally in the years 1878–88 by Pasteur and Koch, and the miasmatic theory (diseases caused by poisoned air). Florence Nightingale eventually adopted the germ theory of disease, but her pioneering work during the Crimean War (1854–56) involved the heroic pursuit of hygiene in the military hospitals to mitigate the ill effects of miasm, not the spread of germs. At the same time, in London John Snow (1813–58) was demonstrating the water-born nature of Cholera infection in the face of a general consensus that it was a miasmatic disease, and before its cause by microbes was proved by Pasteur in 1879.[2]

In the 19th century we begin to see a trend in the evolution of medicine that provides the background to the struggle that I suggest is going on today (Box 2.1). This trend had two main elements:

- As medicine moved into the 20th Century and medical science became more sophisticated and effective, its focus became progressively narrower. Its success was achieved by analytical and investigative methods that interpreted disease processes in terms of demonstrable abnormalities of body structure and function resulting from single identifiable causes, and by the development of techniques to manage those biological processes. This narrowing of the focus of medical endeavour onto the *biological* components of illness that made effective intervention possible, directed attention away from the *biographical* context within which illness often needs to be understood.

- The establishment of a medical elite that had originated with the representation of medicine within the universities, the creation of medical schools and the birth of a medical orthodoxy, was consolidated. From a state of lively, if not chaotic competition between members of the medical elite themselves, as well as between the elite and the unqualified practitioners, emerged a unified and regulated profession, promoting a medical orthodoxy rooted in the natural sciences, and capable of exercising increasingly powerful and effective control not only over bodily disorder, but also over the ethos and practice of medicine. This was much to the general good, but also encouraged a certain narrowness of mind towards nonconformist ideas that might fruitfully challenge that control.

BOX 2.1 *Trends in the evolution of medicine*

- Biographical perspective (illness).
- Analysis and investigation.
- Abnormality of structure or function (disease).
- Single identifiable cause.
- Technological remedy.
- Medical orthodoxy.
- Medical elite.
- Biomedical perspective.

A distinctive conceptual framework and methodology of medical science underpinning distinctive and dominant modes of medical practice was established that has achieved staggering advances in the treatment of disease.

The contemporary struggle

The complete ascendancy of scientific medicine, that is medicine based on the insights and methods of the natural sciences as well as its own particular researches in anatomy, physiology, bio-chemistry and microbiology, was achieved some 100 years ago. A defining moment was the publication of the Flexner report in America in 1910, which formally established there a state of affairs that had finally become a fait accompli in Britain with the passing of the Medical Act of 1858, and the setting up of the General Medical Council; namely an education and qualification in the medical sciences as the prerequisite of orthodox medical practice.

But the element of struggle becomes apparent from the outset because the development of modern scientific medicine was accompanied by the emergence of the 'dissident' tendency (Box 2.2), to which I have already referred. This reflected, in various ways, something of the dislike of the old heroic medicine, and something of the liking for traditional, 'folk' or 'domestic' methods of treatment that we might call 'low tech' medicine. It reflected, too, something of a dislike of the growing exclusiveness of orthodox scientific medicine. And it reflected a preference for an approach to illness that was not narrowly focused on physical biological disorder but emphasised more strongly a whole person approach to medical care. In addition to these general tendencies, not only amongst patients, but also amongst some providers of health care, a number of methods of treatment began to provide alternative or complementary, and increasingly competitive, forms of medicine that seemed to satisfy these inclinations. Some were developed within the Western health care culture, for example homeopathy and osteopathy. Others were adopted from other cultures, for example Traditional Chinese Medicine.

BOX 2.2 *The emerging 'dissident tendency'*

Human story	–	Disease process
Biography	–	Biology
Caritas	–	Scientia
Low-tech medicine	–	Heroic medicine
Diversity of method	–	Exclusivity of method
Uncertainty	–	Certainty
Alternative	–	Orthodox

Dissident voices have been plainly heard throughout the forty years of my own lifetime in medicine, within the medical profession itself as well as from outsiders concerned at the turn of events. They represent a sort of underground movement, struggling to promote what has been called a 'counter system' in the face of the success and power of the dominant medical model.[4] It is an intriguing struggle with implications for science and clinical medicine, but with political, economic, cultural and philosophical ramifications as well. Until recently it has been a low-key struggle for hearts and minds, and often only within the hearts and minds of individuals directly concerned with it.

The dis-ease in medicine

The struggle has to do with what one might call the science of the human organism, and unease at the way that medicine applies that science. I have described how my own experience of hospital medicine and general practice had bred concerns of this kind in me, and my recruitment to the ranks of the 'dissident voices.' But I already knew I was not a lone voice. A number of other voices encouraged me to try to make mine heard. The first of these was the psychiatrist Michael Balint, whose book, *The Doctor, his Patient and the Illness*, and whose early GP co-workers, greatly influenced my generation of general practitioners and developments in medical education as well.[5] Balint taught GPs to recognise the psychological and pastoral elements of the doctor-patient relationship, and to use these therapeutically – an insight and skill not altogether unfamiliar, but marginalised by the priorities of medical science. In those early years in general practice I also came across three critiques of contemporary medicine from very different sources: a paper questioning the state of medical 'engineering', by John Powles,[6] a booklet published by the Office of Health Economics (OHE), called *The Health Care Dilemma*[7] and the briefly notorious *Medical Nemesis* by theologian, philosopher, historian and scourge of the 'Industrial Society' Ivan Illich. For all its faults, Illich's book struck a few chords with me with its analysis of 'the limitations of medicine'.[8] The OHE booklet, rather like Illich but quite independently and with no cross-reference, challenged the medical profession's assumptions about its role in healthcare. Another 'voice' that resonated with me was that of a number of general practitioners in the 1970's, deeply uneasy at the high level of psychotropic drug prescribing in general practice, which still prevails today of course, and the medicalisation of social ills that this represents.

Common to these critiques and the continuing unease that they reflect, has been the belief that *in general* western medicine is based on too limited an understanding of human nature, of the disease processes and healing processes that affect human well-being, and of the ways in which these may be managed – the biomedical model. I emphasise *in general* because individual doctors have always been aware, and often humbly aware of the limitations of their science to comprehend the complexity of human nature, and of the importance of their art in making good those limitations. It is an irony that the great majority of doctors do have a real care for the whole person of their patient, and know perfectly well that tinkering with the mechanism, whether surgically or pharmacologically, which is often all that their circumstances or their training permit, is only a very partial response to the disorder that is presented to them. (See also 'The paradox' in the Prologue to Part 2.)

If this causes any loss of job satisfaction there are of course many other compensating factors in medical practice. And surveys suggest that some 80% of NHS patients express satisfaction with the care they receive, which probably compares pretty well with consumer satisfaction in any organisation. Nevertheless, in reflective moments many doctors will acknowledge a degree of vocational dis-ease due to the constraints that the nature of medical practice imposes upon them. There is for example inevitable frustration, even if subliminal, in having to prescribe a battery of different medicines for a patient's various complaints; particularly when some are required to counteract the adverse effects of others. And despite their level of general satisfaction, patients frequently express unhappiness at these constraints.

The illness, the disease and the story

> The physician must understand that the patient's story is not an intrusion but a legitimate requirement for the clinician's effectiveness. (Eric Cassell.[9])

A particular source of dis-ease results from the need to fit a human story into a biomedical framework, and particularly within the constraints of a service that is designed around the biomedical model. This is described by American physician Howard Brody in his book *Stories of Sickness*.[10] The book examines the place of illness and the role of medicine within the broader narrative of a person's life, and discusses the errors and limitations that affect the practice of medicine if this context is neglected. He writes, "The ritual need to devalue story telling in medicine may take several forms; and as is often the case, the patient may be blamed for the results. Overworked and harried physicians display little tolerance for any information from patients that is not already formulated as, or at least partly translatable into, the standard medical history".

Associate Editor Christopher Martyn commented in the *British Medical Journal* in 2009, "(I) wonder how often communication between doctors and patients fails . . . because doctors fit what patients say to them into an inappropriately exact medical framework".[11] Conrad Harris, Emeritus Professor of General Practice at Leeds, develops this theme, pointing out how much may be missed as a result from the scientific point of view.[12] Writing for general practitioners he says, "What we expect to find is powerfully conditioned by what we have learned. This sets the limits of what we ask our patients about and the extent to which we are prepared to ignore anything they tell us that is not required by, or does not fit, a pattern with which we are familiar". He goes on to say: "It is easy to forget that every patient presents us, in a sense, with a research project". Hearing the story and observing the natural history, careful attention to what the esteemed physician Sydenham (1624–1689) described as being "the march of events in the development of the disease", are the essential prerequisites for effective patient care, for discovering what more is to be known about illness and disease, and for the doctor's job satisfaction. (Although Sydenham himself regarded diseases as distinctive biological states or entities, rather than individual phenomena.)

The theme recurs in various forms in the work of other doctors. Iona Heath, writing about *The Mystery of General Practice*, says, "All aspects of human existence are the legitimate concerns of the general practitioner provided they are presented as a problem by the patient. This means that the GP is obliged to deal with the complexity of each individual. . . . Each person and each context is unique and this is the joy and the challenge of general practitioner care". But, "Scientific medicine's emphasis on disease has tended to invalidate the individual's experience of illness. . . . Distress and unease that do not fit the pattern are belittled and ignored".[13] How the doctor responds to the story of that experience will have a significant impact on the patient, "Whenever we listen, we choose what we will hear, and in that choice *we communicate the relative value* we attach to what we choose to hear and what we choose to ignore"[14] (my italics). Elsewhere, reflecting Conrad Harris's remark, she writes, "(GPs) work at the point where the territory of human suffering meets the map of medical science, and there is always a gap between the map and the territory. . . . The possibility for new knowledge and creative thinking about old knowledge exists in the gap and only through exploring the gap can we hope to improve the map".[15]

A fascinating insight into the working of this biomedical filter is provided by a study of patients' 'unvoiced agendas' in general practice consultations by Christine Barry and colleagues.[16] Their research involved interviews with patients before seeing the doctor to elicit their agendas – the issues they hoped to raise with the doctor or that the consultation would address – comparing these with what audio-tapes of the consultation and follow-up interviews with the doctor and the patient revealed. The pre-consultation interviews were designed to encourage the patients to 'present their full selves', and were obviously much more leisurely than a GP consultation. But the interesting point is the way that patients are 'present' in two different ways in the interview situation and the medical situation. Referring to work from other sources they describe the two presences as two voices: the voice of medicine, in which the consultation is conducted, and the voice of the 'lifeworlds', which is largely left outside the consultation.

The 'lifeworlds' are described as being a contextually grounded experience of events and problems expressed in everyday language, the everyday 'presence' of the patient. The presence that the authors have described earlier as socially and contextually situated, thinking, feeling people, with their own ideas on their medical condition and opinions and possible criticisms of medical treatments. They say this translation suggests that in the consultation the patient is most commonly construed as a 'biomedical' entity – that is, a person with disconnected bodily symptoms, wanting a label for what is wrong and a prescription to put it right. Of the 35 patients whose consultations were studied in this detail no one had only one agenda item, and most had five or more. But within the consultation it was predominately the biomedical issues that were voiced and heard. Only four of the patients voiced their whole agenda. And 14 of them subsequently

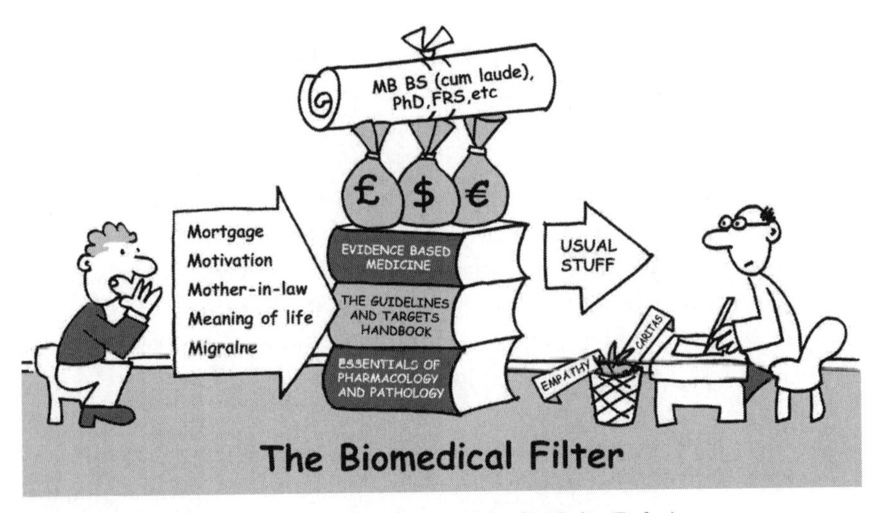

Figure 2.3 'The Biomedical Filter' (based on an idea by Colin Tudge).

experienced at least one problem arising from their unvoiced agenda. The various constraints of GP consultations, particularly time, obviously affect the extent to which the agenda is voiced, but the biomedical focus of the encounter is certainly one of them.

A step in the direction of greater awareness of patients' agendas and greater appreciation of patients' stories is the recent creation of *Cases Journal*. Writing in the *British Journal of General Practice*, its editor asserts that, "We believe that every interaction with a patient is unique and that every case offers an opportunity to learn."[17] He suggests that doctors might ask the patient to write up their own case at the same time, betting that a comparison of the two would yield surprises, from which something new and unexpected may emerge. Equally important and influential could be the patient experience website www.healthtalkonline.org.

How doctors think

An analysis of this tendency to disregard the story, and of its roots in medical education, is summarised in a review in the *British Medical Journal* of the book *How doctors think* by Jerome Gloopman, an American oncologist and haematologist.[18,19] He attributes most errors of diagnosis and treatment to errors of thinking, which include: 'attribution errors' – in which thinking is guided by stereotype and shuts out possibilities that might contradict that preoccupation; 'availability thinking' – the tendency to judge the likelihood of an event by the ease with which relevant examples come to mind; and 'anchoring' – where a doctor doesn't consider multiple possibilities but quickly and firmly latches on to a single one. He believes that a defence against the discomfort of uncertainty is built from a culture of conformity and orthodoxy that begins in medical school, and something he calls 'diagnosis momentum' – when an authoritative senior doctor has fixed a label to a problem it usually stays firmly attached. And he identifies additional obstacles to creative thinking as 'commission bias' – the tendency towards action rather than inaction, 'search satisfaction' – the tendency to stop searching for a diagnosis once you find something, and 'vertical line thinking' – the hackneyed 'inside the box' variety.

Petr Skrabanek and James McCormick accepted the charge of scepticaemia laid against their book *Follies and Fallacies in Medicine*, and hoped to infect others with this 'sceptic' condition as a remedy for the 'errors of doctrine' in medicine that they were addressing. They were concerned with a slightly different set of 'obstacles in the path of rational thought and enquiry' than Gloopman's, but in their definition of scepticaemia as, "An uncommon generalised disorder of low infectivity. Medical school education is likely to confer life-long immunity", they make a similar attribution of cause.[20]

Another example of the constraints that make it so difficult for doctors to think for themselves, to think outside the box (almost, one might think, a caricature of the problem), is described in an anguished letter to the *British Medical Journal* from a Health Service manager turned doctor who has seen both sides of the dilemma. After describing the effect of clinical guidelines and performance indicators that expose patients to unnecessary admissions and investigations, and that prevent junior medical staff from seeing, learning and practising good clinical medicine, he goes on to say, "I now have to write up my assessment of a patient on a standard proforma, although the same sized box obviously does not fit every patient. Through standardisation the nuances of the consultation, the backbone of individual care, are lost. But so are my opportunities to use my ability to think, a skill crafted at university – in my case on behalf of my patient".[21]

Scientia and *caritas*

Engaging with the story of sickness is also a pre-requisite of the *caritas* that the motto of the Royal College of General Practitioners essentially allies to the *scientia*. It could be that the increasingly rigorous academic criteria for entry to medical school, and the education required to equip students for it, are not conducive to the development of *caritas*. At the same time, however, changes in medical school curricula are exposing students to a more patient-centred rather than disease-centred experience. There is more emphasis on the psychosocial factors in the story of sickness, and insights from the humanities as well as the sciences are encouraged. Despite, or even because of these changes, if students mature into the ideally 'reflective practitioner', they may find themselves having to suppress an uneasy sense that their repertoire of knowledge and skills does not properly equip them for the challenge that illness presents to them in the real world. And the scope for *caritas* is limited by the demands of *scientia*, particularly when those demands are politically generated.

The irony is compounded by the fact that most progress in medicine, and its increasingly accelerating progress, is technological. There is real excitement and satisfaction in medicine's increasing power to control and manipulate body function, and to engineer solutions to hitherto intractable problems. And there are obviously many reasons to be thankful for it. But for all that, the uneasy feeling remains in the minds of many patients and many doctors, that there should be more to it than this.

The remodelling movement

The explicit and public proposition that a new perspective in medicine is needed was already around at the time that my own dissident tendency developed, though I was not aware of it. It came in a paper explicitly titled 'The Need for a New Medical Model: A challenge for Biomedicine', published in *Science* in 1977.[22] George Engel, who was at the time Professor of Psychiatry and Medicine at the University of Rochester, New York, points out that the first effort to introduce a more holistic approach into the undergraduate medical curriculum in the USA had been initiated 55 years before. He offers perhaps the first persuasive blueprint for a new model of medicine, the biopsychosocial model. Some years later, Brody remarked how relatively modest had been the interest shown either in affirming or criticising that model in the intervening years.[23] There has been increasing interest in the mixed dynamics of health and illness in the last 30 years. And there is greater pluralism within health care as a whole as a result of the integration within some mainstream practice and the availability outside it of so called complementary and alternative methods. But there is little sign that the dominant biomedical model is yielding to change. In fact recent advances in biological and medical science, and in medical technology are tending to reinforce that dominance.

But the model has never won wholehearted acceptance. Abraham Flexner's report for the American Medical Association in 1910 effectively enshrined the sciences in the curriculum of American medical schools.[24] It confirmed the ascendance of the biomedical model, and lead to the dissolution of medical colleges that did not satisfy those standards or otherwise conform; including, incidentally, many colleges that provided a pathway for women into medicine.[25] But he emphatically resisted the misapprehension that the methods of scientific medicine, which his report established were "in conflict with the humanity which should characterise the physician in the presence of suffering",[26] and he lamented that scientific medicine in America – young, vigorous and positivistic – is today sadly deficient in cultural and philosophic background.[27] It is reported that he later felt that the uniformity of medical education stifled creative work. In the years after his report was published, he became increasingly disenchanted with the rigidity of the educational standards that had become identified with his name.[28]

Engel's paper contrasts biomedicine with a more holistic approach. The nature and validity of holism as a model for medicine, or as an aspect of such a model, will be discussed later. But the introduction of the concept at this point, implying an approach to patient care that is responsive to the whole nature of the patient and the mixed dynamics of her or his illness, characterises the key common denominator of the tendency that I have described as 'dissident'. And it reflects the ambivalence towards narrowly scientific medicine that has been a constant tendency amongst a significant proportion of the medical profession itself; predominately family doctors, because the medical model does not fit easily with the traditions of family medicine.

In *Holistic Health and Biomedical Medicine* Stephen Lyng analyses the perceived shortcomings of the biomedical model and contrasts it with the perceived virtues of what he calls a 'counter system', which with some reservations largely corresponds to a holistic model.[4] And writing of American doctors, post-Flexner, he says, "For the large group of physicians who served the vast majority of the population . . . there was little to be gained by placing medicine on a scientific footing. . . . Generally speaking, what patients wanted was a therapeutic approach that dealt with illness by attending to the many different dimensions of their life – biological, psychological, social and spiritual. . . . (These physicians) resisted (attempts) to bring science into medicine because they perceived that the scientific model would move medical practice away from the very things that had traditionally helped them to keep their patients".

This ambivalence, even frank disenchantment, with the constraints and expectations of the modern medical model, is reflected in the earlier quotes from Brody, Harris and Heath. It is at the heart of the dis-ease within medicine, its present dilemma. The practice of medicine, if it is to serve a healing purpose, requires a high degree of artistry that can only be developed, practised and effective within a holistic and narrative perspective. But it is dominated by a biomedical model that is subservient to the prevailing scientific paradigm whose 'truth' is very much more circumscribed.

Another cause of the disenchantment with the medical model in the United Kingdom has been the progressive reorganisation of general practice, and the imposition of performance targets in all areas of medicine. This exemplifies the extent to which, inevitably in a politically accountable national health service, biomedicine has become entangled with politics; another issue we will return to later. But disenchantment arises when, as Iona Heath writes, politicians and health service planners try to place general practitioners at the centre of the system without properly understanding the essential transactions of the discipline: the intimate interaction between the individual patient and the generalised doctor.[13]

One way and another, the contemporary 'evolutionary struggle' has been at least latent in the hearts and minds of many doctors and other healthcare professionals and patients for a long time, and seems likely to persist. The voices urging a change in the model, at least of emphasis if not altogether of direction, have also been persistent and sometimes urgent. After reflecting on the issues for 40 years, I am persuaded that a more determined attempt at remodelling medicine is appropriate and timely. Western medicine is ruled by a particular model of medical science and medical practice. It has served us well, often dramatically well. But if the undercurrents of dis-ease and dissatisfaction are to be taken seriously a new vision for medicine is needed, and a changed model. This is not an 'out with the old – in with the new' argument. The remodelling will confirm and preserve all that is good and indispensable of what already exists. As implied in the introduction, it is likely to involve a reordering, a shift in priorities, a change of emphasis. But it will only actually displace what it is shown can be done better. Or that can be done as well by other means that carry fewer disadvantages. Or, in some cases, that is preferred for various reasons even if its proven efficacy is less.

Remodelling or metamorphosis?

I have described the present state of western medicine as an evolutionary struggle. But I have already indicated that the dis-ease that is the most prominent symptom of the struggle, is found, and always has been found amongst members of the medical professions themselves. This may be true even of some of those who most vehemently defend the status quo in the face of challenge from proponents of other models; their vehemence perhaps a defence against insecurity bred of an unacknowledged unease at the way things are. So the struggle to which I allude, may in fact be more in the nature of a metamorphosis than an evolutionary process; the struggle of a healing vocation to escape from a biomedical straightjacket.

The implication of the book is that a new and *unifying* model of medicine is possible, an aim comparable perhaps to the physicists' search for a unifying theory of everything, and perhaps as elusive. Quite a few models have been proposed, and in some disciplines and clinical settings developed to represent either the whole or parts of the complex endeavour that is healthcare. Examples are discussed in Chapters 13 and 14. But a model that is comprehensive, satisfying, and above all useful may be very hard to achieve. It will have to take account of the complex human beings (you and I) that medicine exists to serve, the various needs it has to meet, the services it has to provide to meet them, and the social and political structures within which that provision has to be made. Of course, the words 'has to' imply both certainty about these things and an imperative in fulfilling them. But a remodelling process requires that we challenge existing certainties and imperatives, and may require that we abandon some of them, such as assumptions about the role of medicine as a repository of all ills, as some of the critics of thirty years ago implied that we should. As David Greaves suggests at the beginning of his book *Mystery in Western Medicine*, what is required is "a deep-seated reflection which recognises and faces up to the false assumptions of the past, and is prepared to rethink questions about the nature of medicine and the goals of health care".[29]

References

1 Greaves D. Reflections on a new medical cosmolgy. *J Med Ethics* 2002; 28;81–85.
2 Porter R. *The Greatest Benefit to Mankind*. London: Fontana; 1997.
3 Greaves D. *The Healing Tradition*. Oxford: Radcliffe Publishing; 2004.
4 Lyng S. *Holistic Health and Biomedical Medicine*. New York: State University of New York Press; 1990.
5 Balint M. *The Doctor His Patient and the Illness*. London: Pitman Medical; 1968.
6 Powles J. On the limitations of modern medicine. *Science Medicien Man*. 1973; 1:1–30.
7 OHE. *The Health Care Dilemma*. London: Office of Health Economics; 1975.
8 Illich I. *Limits to medicine: medical nemesis the expropriation of health*. London: Boyars; 1976.
9 Cassell E. *The Nature of Suffering and the Goals of Medicine*. New York: Oxford University Press; 2004.
10 Brody H. *Stories of Sickness*. New Haven: Yale University Press; 1987.
11 Martyn C. Of mondegreens and misunderstandings. *Br Med J*. 2009; 338:b244.
12 Harris C. Seeing sunflowers. *J R Col Gen Pract*. 1989; 39:313–319.
13 Heath I. *The Mystery of General Practice*. London: Nuffield Provincial Hospitals Trust; 1995.
14 Heath I. Uncertain clarity: contradiction meaning and hope. *Br J Gen Pract*. 1999; 49:651–657.
15 Heath I. That by which it is what it is. *Br J Gen Pract*. 2009; 59(562):316–317.
16 Barry C A, Bradley C P, Britten N *et al*. Patients' unvoiced agendas in general practice consultations: qualitative study. *Br Med J*. 2000; 320:1246–1250.
17 Smith R. Why GPs should write case reports. *Br J Gen Pract*. 2009; 59(562):383.
18 Woods D. Living in a box. *Br Med J*. 2007; 334:856.
19 Gloopman J. *How Doctors Think* www.houghtonmifflinbooks.com; 2007.

20 Skrabanek P, McCormick J. *Follies and Fallacies in Medicine.* 3rd edition. Eastbourne: Tarragon Press; 1988.
21 Thomson-Moore A. Doctors' infantilisation. *Br Med J.* 2008; 337:a791.
22 Engel G. The need for a new medical model. *Science* 1977; 196:129–136.
23 Brody H. Diagnosis is treatment. *J Fam Pract.* 1980; 10:445–449.
24 Flexner A N. *Medical Education.* New York: Macmillan; 1925.
25 Spiro H. *The Power of Hope.* New Haven & London: Yale University Press; 1998.
26 Fitzpatrick M. Reclaiming Compassion. In: Ernst E. *Healing Hype or Harm? A Critical Analysis of Complementary or Alternative Medicine.* Exeter: Societas; 2008.
27 Sokol D. Of interviews and examination machines. *Br Med J.* 2010; 341:c6899.
28 di Stefano V. *Holism and complementary medicine: Origins and Principles.* Sydney: Allen and Unwin; 2006.
29 Greaves D. *Mystery in Western Medicine.* Aldershot: Avebury; 1996.

3

MOMENTUM FOR CHANGE

Summary

- For all its achievments the biomedical model is not the complete answer to our ills. There are aspects of human nature and its afflictions that it does not comprehend.
- 'Remodelling' will not be anti-science, but will require that we recognise and acknowledge the limits to the questions which science should expect and be expected to answer.
- It will require 'deep-seated reflection which recognises and faces up to the false assumptions of the past, and is prepared to rethink questions about the nature of medicine and the goals of health care'.
- Amongst the signs and symptoms of change, the growing emergence of complementary and alternative medicine provides a manifestation of a new approach to health care, and of a new understanding of the dynamics of health, illness, disease and healing.
- A more 'orthodox' indication of the momentum for change is the launch of The College of Medicine, committed to a more inclusive, integrated and patient-centred vision of health care.
- All three principle domains of health care – clinical practice, the process of care, and the context of care – are implicated in the remodelling process.
- The key questions: Is medicine a healing vocation? If so, is the model divorced from the vocation, and what can be done about it?

Fitness for purpose

The title of this book implies, and is intended to imply that medicine, modern Western medicine, needs to be remodelled; that it is in some sense or in some degree unfit for purpose. Its aim is to explore to what extent this is true, and how the present medical model could and should change, and the preceding chapters have begun to set out the justification for it.

A key question is that fitness for purpose. A model may be perfectly well suited to one particular purpose, but unfit for others. The present model is focused on the biological machinery of life, and its particular purpose is to analyse, identify and remedy the things that go wrong with it; a purpose that it fulfils extremely well. Not all medical practice is conceived in that way. But the medical practice that most of us will encounter most of the time will be biomedical. In *The Nature of Suffering and the Goals of Medicine* the physician Eric Cassell writes, "The important thing in medical science for the last fifty years is mechanism – how things work or how their abnormalities distort the normal mechanism. . . . Medicine is still talking about how every patient is different (as it has for millennia) but searching for sameness, invariance, and basing its clinical practice on that idea. Witness evidence-based medicine and practice guidelines, both of which have achieved contemporary popularity by treating all patients as though each person with the same disorder is the same".[1]

This model has made possible wonderful advances in medical practice that we would never wish to be without. But it is not the complete answer to our ills. There are aspects of human nature and its disorders and afflictions that are not comprehended by the model, and to which it does not have answers. And from these, because of its power and success, it distracts attention; to our detriment when it is in those aspects of human nature that the illness resides, or from which the disease arises. And because the tools that the model makes available are powerful and successful, they dominate and tend to make redundant more subtle means by which we might enable or assist the better function or recovery or general well-being of the ill person; the placebo effect, for example (Chapter 12).

Unease towards the biomedical model varies from ambivalence to frank criticism, as these quotations make clear:

> More commonly, the term medical model refers to medicine's ideas and assumptions about the nature of illness, notably its natural scientific framework and its focus on physical causes and physical treatments. As such the term is frequently invoked in the context of ideological and political debates and inter-professional rivalries in which the relevance of this particular set of ideas is called into question . . . some prefer the term 'bio-medical model', since it clearly indicates the focus on the biological, and allows that there are other medical models. An alternative model is a 'bio-psycho-social model' encompassing the biological, psychological, and social aspects. (From *A Dictionary of Sociology*.[2])

> The reductionist model of the patient's body has led in part, to a crisis in quality of care in modern medicine, even though it has produced many of today's modern medical miracles.[3]

> What is wrong with the concept of disease is not that there is no malfunctioning part. There may be. Rather, it is that medicine has come to concentrate on it to the exclusion of all else . . . a sort of medical tunnel vision. What is not seen . . . is the sick person in all his wholeness and variability.[4]

> The biomechanical theory is the core of Western medicine, and is often referred to as *the* medical model. The main assumption of this theory is that human beings are machines and doctors are human engineers. . . . The values of the model are utilitarian. The prime purpose . . . is the extension of life, the secondary purpose avoidance of pain and anything which may inhibit pleasure. . . . A useful simplification, of enormous practical value.[5]

> The model's core structure is an analysis by which symptoms and physical signs – the complex, mostly subjective phenomena known as illness – are reduced to a more specific disordered part, the disease, to which science can then be applied. . . . The process is exquisitely designed for its purpose. It works with great precision whenever the disordered part diagnosed fully accounts for the whole illness, and its treatment restores the whole system to health. . . . The achievements of scientific medicine result from its remarkable capacity to analyse and alter disordered parts right down to the molecular level. (But) it is difficult for those of us trained in medical-model thinking to recognise the extent to which the human situation is invariably bypassed by the reductive process of diagnosis and treatment.[6]

There are other models within the broad spectrum of medical practice, particularly within some of the non-doctor professions such as occupational therapy (Chapter 13). But despite the resistance and criticism it has attracted the biomedical model remains dominant. The 'dissident voices' have not achieved any significant change in, so to speak, the balance of power. The remodelling I am exploring is about changing that balance. It is not, I repeat, about abandoning the good that the biomedical model has achieved. The remodelling process is not a competition between alternative models, it is a balancing act and a process of reconciliation and transformation.

Medical science has made discoveries that have enriched human knowledge and increased our awe at the intricacy of human and animal life. It has done wonders for us. A remodelling process will certainly not be anti-science. But it will require that we recognise and acknowledge the boundaries of science, the limits to the set of questions that science should expect and be expected to answer. At the same time, it will require a willingness to acknowledge that in some respects those limits are too narrow; a willingness to apply science to questions that require scientists to 'think outside the box', and to entertain questions to which the apparent answers seem implausible within the existing framework of knowledge. To use a quotation from philosopher Mary Midgeley, to which I will return later, "We do not need to esteem science less. What we need is to esteem it in the right way. Especially we need to stop isolating it artificially from the rest of life".[7]

Medicine has to be responsive to 'the rest of life' that the biomedical model does not comprehend. At present it does so inadequately. That is why we need to remodel.

Scientific medicine

The relationship between medicine and science is explored more fully in Chapter 6, and the reorientation of medical science that remodelling implies in Chapter 18. But before we go any further, we need to deal with a problem and an ambiguity in the use of the phrase 'scientific medicine' that recurs throughout these pages and in much of the literature concerning the medical model. The phrase seems to imply, and is sometimes used to imply some value judgement. I have just argued that there are limits to the questions that science should expect and be expected to answer, but that nevertheless in some respects the present application of science in medicine is too narrow. When the phrase 'scientific medicine' is used approvingly, it is usually applied to aspects of medicine that conform to the prevailing criteria of scientific legitimacy, implying that there are others that do not and are not scientific and therefore not acceptable. When used critically of the medical model it usually refers to the narrowness of its scientific methodology and its unwarranted exclusion of aspects of healthcare and components of medical knowledge that do not readily conform to this conception of science.

Science does have limitations in its search for truth and its exploration of reality. These can be crudely defined as its ability to answer the questions 'What?' (what is going on) and 'How?' (how does it work, how can we control it), but not the question 'Why?' (why is it this way, what does it mean). An example of the exclusive tendency of the more narrowly focused scientific medicine has been to regard the placebo or contextual healing effect, responsible for so much of the spontaneous recovery from illness, as incidental to the specific effects of treatment; as a distraction, to be controlled when studying those effects and not 'proper medicine'. I say 'has been', because the placebo effect is beginning to attract interest and even respect in the medical literature,[8,9] and becoming a legitimate subject for a wider vision of the application of science in medicine. (See 'Natural medicine and natural healing', in Chapter 12.)

By contrast, an example of the dismissive attitude to scientific medicine is the claim of some complementary therapists that their discipline is not amenable to study by the scientific method.

Both these attitudes are wrong. On the one hand, science is capable of embracing broader questions than are commonly regarded as the legitimate focus of its analytical reductionist gaze. Qualitative research is one such method, a branch of science that uses descriptive methods in contrast to the quantitative method that relies on what can be counted and measured. On the other hand, accepting its limitations, there is no human activity that cannot gain some insight from properly designed scientific study. It is the narrow scope, either of the commonly accepted methodology, or of the type of questions that it is acceptable to ask, or of the type of answers that it may seem plausible to pursue, that is the problem. The proper question may be, "What does an examination of the nature of medical knowledge contribute to a deeper and more adequate conception of scientific knowledge and of human knowledge more generally?"[10] We should bear in mind Cassell's statement of the limited ability of medical science to comprehend the nature of suffering, and the implications of this: "If the question of whether someone is suffering is not open to scientific knowledge, then the relief of suffering – medicine's fundamental purpose – cannot be achieved by purely scientific medicine . . . the objective facts, which are the basis of medical science, as essential as they are, are in themselves insufficient to the clinician's task".[1]

This ambiguity of the term 'scientific medicine' may best be resolved by talking about 'orthodox scientific medicine' rather than 'scientific medicine'. The *Concise Oxford Dictionary* defines 'orthodox' as 'holding correct or currently accepted opinions, not heretical or independent minded or original; generally accepted as right or true, in harmony with what is authoritatively established, approved, conventional.' These definitions convey the sense of orthodox medicine's commitment to the accepted, approved, conventional biomechanical scientific model, and the authoritative, and often authoritarian influence of that model on medical thought. But they also imply ('currently', 'generally') the contingent and provisional nature of that authority, which is always subject to revision, as has historically been the case with all orthodoxies. And that is appropriate, because it is surely true that, as David Greaves maintains in his book *Mystery in Western Medicine*, "The search for definitive criteria by which to provide a fixed standard for an absolute division between medicine which should be considered acceptable and unacceptable is misguided".[11]

What will 'different' look like?

So medicine has to be responsive to 'the rest of life' that the biomedical model is inadequate to comprehend, and that the scientific method on which it is based cannot expect or be expected to comprehend. And that is why we need to remodel. But how could a different model make a difference, and what difference could it make?

As Hamlet said, "Ay, there's the rub". Is there any one model of medicine, or indeed many, which will answer to "the heartache and the thousand natural shocks that flesh is heir to"[12] – which seems to be the expectation laid upon modern medicine? It is an expectation that may need to change as part of the remodelling process, as a result of that deep-seated reflection which recognises and faces up to the false assumptions of the past, and is prepared to rethink questions about the nature of medicine and the goals of health.[11]

Remodelling Medicine joins a succession of books, academic papers, commentaries, and medical and lay journalism, particularly over the past forty years, criticising the limitations of the biomedical model and proposing, sometimes pleading for change. But they have made very little difference. There has been some change, but biomedical thinking still dominates healthcare. In 1977, the pioneer 'remodeller', George Engel, reached a pessimistic conclusion as to the success of his challenge to the biomedical model, doubting that "contributing another critical essay (would be) – likely to bring about any major changes in attitude".[13] There has still been no major change within Western medicine as a whole, despite all that has been written on the subject. Why should this book, and any remodelling it proposes, be any more effective? It will only do so by offering arguments that cannot be ignored, and that will provoke lively debate. That is its intention, and my optimism is based on belief in its timeliness.

Signs and symptoms of change (See Figure 3.1)

Although I suggest there is little sign that the dominant biomedical model is yielding to change, rather that advances in medical science and technology continue to reinforce that dominance, I believe there is evidence from the literature and from common experience that momentum for change can be discerned within the healthcare system. There are the dissident voices, critics of the medical model seeking change. There is a greater number, not so vocal, but similarly desiring change; and an even greater number, not seeking change but uncomfortable with the status quo. The

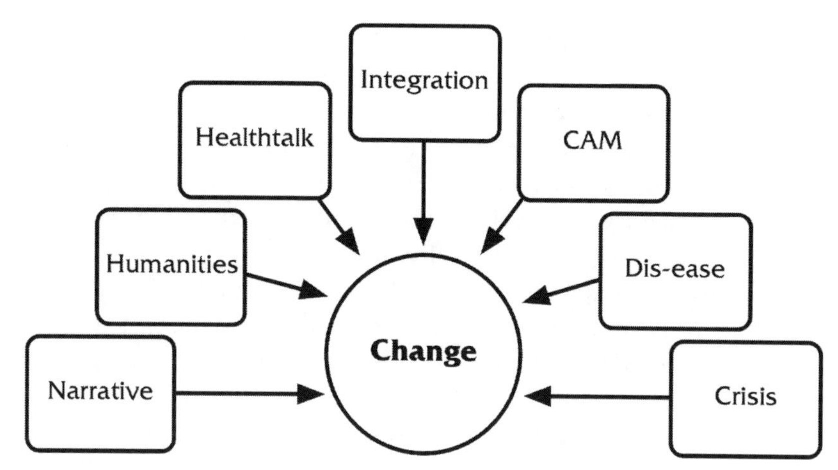

Figure 3.1 *Signs and symptoms of change.*

analysis and the recipe for change presented here are meant to reinforce that momentum. The prevalence (widespread occurrence) of critical voices, amongst doctors in particular, may be low, but the incidence (frequency with which they crop up) is relatively high. This is evident, for example, in the number of articles of a dissident tendency in the pages of the *British Medical Journal* each week. It is by studying and reflecting on the ideas, arguments, insights, and aspirations – the dis-ease of these thoughtful and persuasive critics, that I have sought to configure the model, the stimulus to change, offered in this book. If this is well done it will evoke a response. I would like this response to resemble the 'cascade' by which the physiological response to a stimulus spreads throughout the body, though it will inevitably be a great deal slower. Those who are not receptive, and there are many who will resist, will I hope, nevertheless be provoked to react and to reflect.

Apart from the dissident voices lamenting the status quo, other trends reflect the momentum for change – a growing emphasis on the humanities in medical education, the emergence of narrative medicine with its emphasis on the whole story of the illness, the use of the patient experience website www.healthtalkonline.org that I mention above as a resource in some medical schools, are examples.

One trend that has certainly intensified the evolutionary struggle during the past ten to twenty years has been the growing emergence and popularity of complementary and alternative medicine (CAM). That this phenomenon is being taken seriously in political circles in the UK is demonstrated by the recent creation of the Complementary and Natural Health Care Council (www.chre.org.uk). That it is being taken seriously in medical education is demonstrated by the requirement of the General Medical Council that students be made familiar with at least the basic principles of the leading CAM therapies that their future patients may consult. Summarising its prevalence Edzard Ernst, Emeritus Professor of Complementary Medicine at Exeter University, notes that CAM has become an important topic for public health. Its use is on the increase; in the US and Germany, for instance, about two thirds of the general population now use CAM. Health authorities across the globe now feel the need to deal with the implications of such widespread use. More than half of all WHO member states now have a national office for CAM and 43% support an expert committee on the subject.[14] But this apparent acceptance of a legitimate role for such therapies in mainstream healthcare is by no means universal, and the resistance to it amongst some doctors and medical scientists is fierce. Ernst adds that, "*vis-à-vis* CAM's extraordinary popularity, (the) high level of attention seems justified – but it must be guided by clear thinking. Worryingly this is often not the case".

CAM is a somewhat nebulous concept, poorly differentiated as a coherent group of therapeutic disciplines, and like many aspects of medicine and health care as a whole, arguably more of a social construct than a clinical entity. Nevertheless, it represents for many – patients, doctors and other practitioners, and scientists – an identifiable manifestation, admirable or objectionable according to their point of view, of a new approach to health care; and of a new understanding of the dynamics of health, illness and disease. It has taken the form of a different 'species' of medicine, and there has arisen an element of intense competition between the different species of medical ideology and practice. This is perhaps appropriate and inevitable in an evolutionary process, even if some aspects of it are hardly salutary. The most vociferous proponents of the established conventional model are beset, and seem almost to feel besieged by their CAM neighbours, while some of the latter are struggling for survival. This is a pity, because while the struggle continues in this manner, an opportunity is being wasted and patients are being disadvantaged. The emergence of CAM and the phenomena that it claims to reveal, offer fresh, if not exactly new, but often poorly articulated models of health, illness and healthcare; models that offer a fresh, but again not exactly new, perspective of the human organism and the way it works and relates to its environment, and of the unique person who is that vulnerable organism. For many critics the model and especially the evidence that underpins it, are not persuasive. But it begs intriguing questions, presents serious challenges and offers attractive possibilities that might be expected to excite eager scientific enquiry.

Perhaps the most impressive and immediate evidence of the growing momentum for change in the UK was the launch in October 2010 of the College of Medicine that I mentioned in the Introduction. In the policy document produced to accompany the launch, its president Sir Graham Catto writes: "Over time, the science will change; society's expectations will change. But people and our need for humanity and care when we are ill and vulnerable are unchanging. Healers down the ages, from all caring disciplines, have recognised the importance of treating the patient and not just the specific ailment. The complexity of modern medicine, and the different skills of the members of the multidisciplinary team delivering the care, sometimes obscure that crucial distinction".[15]

Finally, the crisis in medicine that many perceive and the College of Medicine addresses in its policy document, and which is discussed in Chapter 9, lends its own impetus to the momentum for change.

So, one way or another there is good reason to believe that the healthcare 'organism', the network of people who occupy the landscape of healthcare, including us the patients, is receptive to a stimulus like this to a greater degree than ever before. There is great ambivalence in our attitude to medicine. We have already recognised that it arises from our fascination with and dependence upon the power of biomedicine to control the *mechanism* of life on the one hand, and our desire to be understood and treated as complex and unique *persons* on the other. The trend among many of those who provide healthcare, and amongst all of us on most of the occasions when we seek it, is increasingly to want the emphasis to shift towards the personal end of the spectrum. I believe this trend is sufficiently strong to make the system receptive to change. Whatever stimulus for change this book provides the effect has to be dynamic. Individuals and systems that are already responsive to it may be prompted to effect further change in some aspect of what they do or in the system within which they work, or to seek to develop and improve the ideas presented here themselves. Those who are not immediately responsive to them may be provoked to the deep-seated reflection recommended by David Greaves, and may then be prompted to contribute to the evolution of the model. In other words, the remodelling proposed in this book is intended to stir things up but does not pretend to offer a complete prescription. It is inevitably transitional – representing the passage or change from one state to another. I believe it offers a transition to a better state.

What sort of model?

The themes and arguments set out in these opening pages will of course be explored fully in the chapters that follow. And the rationale and the design principles for a new model will emerge. But what sort of model might we look for? What might we expect, or at least hope to come of the remodelling process?

It is worth recalling the summary answer to this question in the Introduction:

> A new model of medicine will not be composed of any new parts. All the necessary elements are already there. But it will comprise familiar elements in a new structure, a new order. And its key components will be two well recognised but too little valued elements of healthcare. These are that a fully effective response to illness and disease must take account of the person as a whole, and not be focused exclusively on the affected parts; must take account of the whole narrative of the illness, and not just the immediate event. Secondly, an effective response will mobilise and maximise the self-regulating self-healing potential of the patient. This is in any case a component of all medical care, and can be encouraged by a variety of subtle stimulus, including the all important placebo or 'contextual healing' effect.
>
> These two core elements of healthcare are not at all least controversial. But to promote them as primary goals of medical culture, education and practice will require a very considerable effort of will and imagination. It will require a redeployment of resources and some restructuring of the process of care. It will also require some humility on the part of all who have a vested interest in maintaining the status quo, the intellectual, clinical, political or commercial power that the structure of the existing model confers.

There are three broad domains occupied by medicine within the landscape of healthcare, that I have designated Clinical Practice, the Process of Care, and the Context of Care (Box 3.1). It does not occupy them alone, of course. Alongside the people actively engaged in the provision of medical services they are populated by many other groups: politicians, for example, environmental agencies, and patients (that's all of us) above all. Nor are the three areas entirely separate from one another. They overlap and are interdependent. Concepts of disease and illness, of health, well-being and healing, are obviously central to all three.

Clinical Practice is the transaction between the clinician and the patient. It includes the work of all members of clinical teams that have face-to-face encounters with patients, and with their families, friends and carers. It also includes the backroom scientists and technicians, medically qualified or not, whose skills provide the information and make possible the interventions that support or implement diagnosis and treatment. Clinical practice includes the work of GPs, neurosurgeons, occupational therapists, pharmacists, clinical biochemists and radiographers. It is a fact of present day health care that the broad domain of clinical medicine also includes complementary practitioners.

BOX 3.1 *Clinical Practice, the Process of Care and the Context of Care*

Clinical Practice

- The transaction between clinician and patient.
- Clinical method.
- Knowledge, skill and attitudes.
- The relationship.
- The focus of the diagnostic process.
- The focus of the treatment.
- Concepts of disease and illness; of health, well-being and healing.
- Expectations of outcome.
- Decision making and choice.

The Process of Care

- The organization, delivery and management of healthcare services.
- Evidence, targets and guidelines.
- Audit.
- Access and availability.
- Special needs provision – age, disability.
- Social v. medical care.
- Medical education.
- Medical research.

The Context of Care

- Cultural and social attitudes and expectations.
- Environment – physical and social; deprivation; inverse care law.
- Politics and law; economics.
- Private and public provision.
- Public information and education: government, media, professions, the internet.

The Process of Care is the organisation and management of healthcare services. It determines the availability of medical care and access to it. It includes the education, training and regulation of healthcare professionals.

It includes the setting of targets and the provision of incentives to encourage the pursuit of particular medical priorities. It includes public health measures that impact upon clinical practice. And it includes the research effort that underpins these activities as well as clinical practice.

The Context of Care is the cultural, social, economic, political and environmental milieu that determines so much of the process of care and the nature of clinical practice.

Any model of medicine, and certainly any remodelling process that aspires to be at all comprehensive and effective, must relate to all of these three areas. It must inform, guide, redirect, possibly inspire the progress of medicine in all three. It must be beneficial and above all useful in all three. It must identify and promote certain principles of common purpose and common achievement in all three. This of course, is a tall order. There are other considerations and other models at work in all these areas. But the implementation of the biomedical model is a primary and highly visible focus of most aspects of Practice and Process, and while constrained by Context issues, is highly influential in shaping them.

The biomedical model provides awe-inspiring insight into the structure and function of the human organism, and the medical progress that it has made possible is an achievement to be celebrated. But its dominant influence in all three of these domains of medicine is a problem.

BOX 3.2 *Words associated with aspects of medical practice and patient care*

Biomedical words	Whole person words
Objective	Subjective
Science	Art
Analyse, dissect	Synthesise, cohere
Dissociate, isolate	Comprehend, relate
Circumscribe, reduce	Compose, complete
Abstract, generalise	Constitute, individualise
Disease	Illness
Pathology, investigation	Person, narrative
Expertise	Trust
Technology, accuracy	Insight, empathy
Efficacy	Effectiveness
Drug	Placebo
Compliance	Autonomy
Control, manipulate, manage	Enable, facilitate, empower

Box 3.2 shows two lists of words associated with aspects of medical practice and patient care. The left hand column includes lists of words most likely to be associated with the biomedical approach. The other list includes words representing other aspects of health, healing and well-being that should, perhaps, be featured more strongly in our model of medicine.

There are words in the left-hand column that are sometimes used of biomedicine in a deprecatory sense by its more outspoken critics. That is a travesty. We would not possess the ability to take over and control the failing organ systems of a patient with a heart attack, or to identify and remedy serious risk factors in childbirth, or help a premature baby to survive, without the analytical and reductionist physiological insights of the biomedical model. And the two columns and the words in them are not, of course, mutually exclusive. We want accuracy *and* empathy from our doctor, science and art. Hearing the narrative of the illness, the story of sickness, is a form of investigation. Expertise encourages trust. And so on.

At the same time we all know that the biomedical focus of medical activity often neglects, sometimes ignores, and frequently has no time for the ingredients of illness and the aids to recovery and healing that have to do with the words in the right hand column. These words define what Dixon and Sweeney call "the human face of medicine". In their book entitled *The Human Effect in Medicine* they challenge the dogma of modern technological medicine that ignores the therapeutic effect of the doctor and the self-healing powers of the patient.[16]

The aim of the remodelling process will be to resolve this tension. It will require that we reconcile more effectively the focus on the pathology with the focus on the person; the focus on the immediate agent of *disease* with our understanding of the *dis-ease* – the circumstances that predispose to or compound the illness. It will require that we comprehend the scope not only for interventions that act directly upon the *dis-order*, but also for interventions that act, perhaps subtly, to encourage *order*, physiological, interpersonal, social, or whatever.

This sort of model will have a few key principles that determine what happens in the three domains of the medical landscape. For example, consider two juxtaposed words in the columns in Box 3.2, 'control' and 'enable'. A key design principle for the remodelling process will be the shift of emphasis from methods that control to methods that enable. To apply this principle the key question in any situation will of course be, 'How?' In *Practice*, in acute medicine where immediate biomedical intervention may be vital, the answer might simply be 'Calm, compassionate presence'; a physiologically and emotionally effective therapeutic tool, sometimes in short supply, as much through force of circumstances as from any lack in the carer. Or in a treatment regime the answer might be, 'Enhance contextual healing'. begging again the supplementary clinical and research question, 'How?' In *Process*, the answer might be, 'Enable the clinician to be most effective'; for which the resource might be 'appropriate evidence', or 'time to listen'. ("How can the doctor himself, as a therapeutic agent, be refined and polished to make of him a more potent agent?" WB Houston.[17]) In *Context*, the answers would be, and to an extent already are enable healthy life style, allow informed choice, encourage social cohesion, alleviate poverty, improve education – elements of what has been called salutogenesis.

One way of presenting the controlling/enabling contrast is in the dichotomy of aims for health care that general practitioner David Misselbrook describes in *Listening to Patients*.[18] He sets out alternative but not incompatible options, abbreviated and slightly paraphrased here:

> *Option 1*: Healthcare exists in order to maintain biomedical parameters within the normal range. This involves controlling any aspects of patients' lives that threaten these normative measurements. (And) necessitates continuous surveillance of the population for possible biomedical abnormalities.
>
> *Option 2*: Health care exists to enable patients to live the lives that they choose, as much as possible unencumbered by, or despite, disability – to reduce suffering – and to prevent premature death – always where compatible with the patient's goals. Aspects of option 1 will be used only when they serve these principles.

Of course, every such proposition begs a range of related questions, whose answers may require common sense or sophisticated research, and will certainly provoke debate. What is very likely is that the first step to developing the 'enabling' principle in any situation will be to listen carefully to the people on the ground, pay attention to what they say, take it seriously, and be prepared to trust their judgement. Not to the exclusion of putting it to the test, but willing to respect the informed empiricism, personal knowledge and motivated belief (of all of which, more later), of the people engaged in the activity we seek to enable.

The goal of the model

Remodelling Medicine proposes that the longstanding unease about the limits of modern Western medicine, and the evolutionary trends that I describe in Chapter 2, have reached a critical point at which the remodelling of medicine, already to an extent a work in progress, must be given fresh momentum. And it suggests the design principles on which that remodelling process should be based (Chapter 12). The aim is to focus attention more acutely on the challenges that are in many people's minds and an everyday ingredient of clinical experience; to reinvigorate debate about the way we understand and manage the dynamics of health and illness, disease processes and healing processes.

The many books and papers represented in the references demonstrate how pervasive these concerns are. The focus of my own work has been direct patient care. I have been deeply immersed in listening to people's 'stories of sickness', in the habit attributed to Thomas Sydenham of "listening intently and observing minutely the march of events in the development of disease".[19] The misgivings described in Chapter 1, have persisted and been refined throughout my career, stimulating the research and reflection that have resulted in this book. The debate itself has rumbled on, but has never sufficiently held the attention of all the protagonists.

Unhappily preoccupied with health

Ironically, this is not to say that we don't talk about health enough, or give it sufficient political priority. Health is a popular preoccupation and the target of sometimes almost feverish policy making. The point is that we seem to have got it wrong, out of perspective. Targets are being met, life expectancy is increasing and lives are being saved, blood pressure and cholesterol levels are coming down and so on. But is our well-being increasing? Is medicine making people truly well? Is medicine helping people to be more whole? (See Chapter 7, 'Medicine and Healing', and Chapter 12, 'Design principles.) At the beginning of the introduction to his masterly and comprehensive history of medicine, published in 1997, the late Roy Porter writes, "In myriad ways, medicine continues to advance, new treatments appear, surgery works marvels, and (partly as a result) people live longer. Yet few people today feel confident, either about their personal health or about doctors, healthcare delivery and the medical profession in general".[20] Or as James le Fanu writes, in *The Rise and Fall of Modern Medicine*,[21] "The paradox of modern medicine that requires explanation is why its spectacular success over the past 50 years has had such perverse consequences – leaving doctors less fulfilled and the public more neurotic about their health".

The vocation of medicine is to care for people; to enrich people's lives, however modestly. Every patient, who at some time will be you and I, should emerge from any experience of medical care feeling valued and valuable; enabled, even just a little bit, to make more of the opportunities of our lives. Every aspect of the practice of medicine, even in a laboratory remote from the patient, should be an act of 'worth-ship'. This is not a partisan point of view. An editorial in the Journal of the Royal College of Physicians in 2003 advised, "The good consultation should always leave a patient with an increase in self-esteem".[22] The question at the heart of this book is still, I suppose, the question I posed in 1976 – 'Medicine and healing: a broken marriage?'[23] Is medicine a healing vocation? If so, is the model divorced from the vocation? And if so, what can be done about it? Can we evolve a model that unites medicine and healing more effectively? This book tries to work out whether and how it can be done.

References

1 Cassell E. *The Nature of Suffering and the Goals of Medicine*. New York: Oxford University Press; 2004.
2 Marshall G. *A Dictionary of Sociology*. Oxford: Oxford University Press; 1998.
3 Marcum J. Biomechanical and phenomenological models of the body, the meaning of illness and quality of care. *Medicine, Health Care and Phlosophy* 2004; 7(3):311–320.
4 Kennedy I. *Unmasking medicine*. London: George Allen and Unwin; 1981.
5 Toon P. Occasional Paper 78. *Towards a Philosophy of General Practice* London: Royal College of General Practitioners; 1999.
6 Barbour A. *Caring for patients: a critique of the medical model*. Stanford: Stanford University Press; 1995.
7 Midgeley M. *Science as Salvation*. London: Routledge; 1992.
8 Godlee F. Editor's choice: Reclaiming the placebo effect. *Br Med J*. 2008; 336:doi:10.1136/bmj.39567.551181.47.
9 Spiegel D, Harrington A. What is placebo worth? *Br Med J*. 2008; 336:967–968.
10 Wartofsky M. Editorial. *J Med Philos*. 1978; 3:265–272.
11 Greaves D. *Mystery in Western Medicine*. Aldershot: Avebury; 1996.
12 Shakespeare, W. *Hamlet*, III, I, 56.
13 Engel G. The need for a new medical model. *Science* 1977; 196:129–136.
14 Ernst E. Complementary/alternative medicine: engulfed in post-modernism, anti-science and regressive thinking. *Br J Gen Pract*. 2009; 59(561):298–301.
15 College of Medicine Policy Document; 2010. Available from the College of Medicine. 19, Buckingham Street, London WC2N 6EF and online at www.collegeofmedicine.org.uk
16 Dixon M, Sweeney K. *The Human Effect in Medicine*. Oxford: Radcliffe; 2000.
17 Spiro H. *The Power of Hope*. New Haven & London: Yale University Press; 1998.
18 Misselbrook D. *Listening to Patients*. Newbury: Petroc Press; 2001.

19 Marinker M. The Chameleon, the Judas goat and the cuckoo. *J R Coll Gen Pract.* 1987; 28:199–206.
20 Porter R. *The Greatest Benefit to Mankind.* London: Fontana; 1997.
21 le Fanu J. *The rise and fall of modern medicine.* London: Abacus; 2000.
22 Editorial. *Clinical Medicine* 2003; 3(5):397–398.
23 Swayne J. Medicine and healing: A broken marriage? *New Society* 1976 September 2nd; 491–492.

part 2

PERSPECTIVES

PROLOGUE

Summary

- Ivan Illich's three 'torts' – clinical, social and structural iatrogenesis – still present a relevant critique of 'the limitations of medicine'.
- The paradox: "Medicine's unrest derives from a growing awareness among many physicians of the contradiction between the excellence of their biomedical background on the one hand, and the weakness of their qualifications in certain attributes essential for good patient care on the other".
- "At least some doctors are passionately concerned about what is happening. Many share Illich's concerns. But they are ignored by their colleagues and their plaints fall on deaf ears."
- "Understanding the cause of so many doctors' discontent is important, because those unhappy with their trade may lack the passion necessary to practise it well."

The aim of the chapters in this part of the book is to examine aspects of the present state of Western medicine as exemplified by medicine in the U.K. in the light of criticisms and anxieties about the dominance of the biomedical model that have been discussed in previous chapters. There are six topics, all obviously interwoven in the fabric of health care. Broadly they are:

- Medicine and society.
- Medicine and the individual.
- Medicine and science.
- Medicine and healing.
- The patient's perspective.
- Medicine in crisis?

'Medical Nemesis'?

In his provocative and stimulating, if flawed critique of medicine some 35 years ago, Ivan Illich identified three manifestations of medicine's allegedly unhealthy influence; three kinds of iatrogenesis, sickness caused by doctors.[1] These were clinical, social, and structural. The first concerned what doctors or other healthcare professionals do to patients. The second concerned the relationship between medicine and society. The third concerned attitudes to health and well-being, disease and death, and to personal responsibility for coping with these. These three domains of medical influence on people's lives obviously overlap and are inter-related.

The flaw in Illich's argument is his tendency to exaggerate some of the harms he identified in medicine, and to neglect or misrepresent some of its real achievements, and its contribution to public health policies whose outcome may have been social but which were stimulated by medical insights.

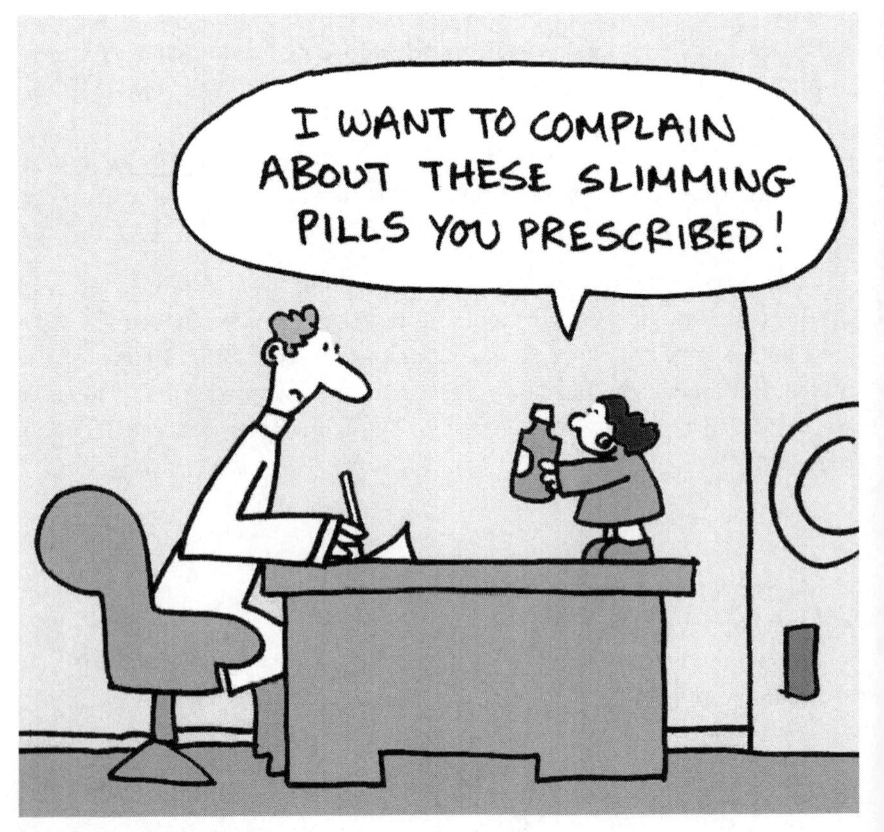

Figure P2.1 *Clinical iatrogenesis.*

Nevertheless, together with *Medical Hubris*, the most comprehensive of the responses to *Medical Nemesis*, written shortly after its publication by David Horrobin,[2] Illich's book still provides a convenient point of reference for considering the present state of modern Western medicine. The six themes listed above, together with much of 'Being a patient' in Chapter 8, represent a broader appraisal of medicine than Illich's three torts but encompass their key criticisms.

The paradox

First, we need to acknowledge the paradox at the heart of modern medicine.

> The paradox is that medical mystery thrives throughout medicine, but within a system which seeks to deny it. (David Greaves[3])

There is a paradox running through the history of scientific medicine, possibly the whole history of medicine. It is summed up neatly in a letter from a family doctor some years ago in the *British Medical Journal*: "Treating the patient as a whole is a perennial issue in medicine. Wanting to engage with the whole patient is one thing. Being able to do so is quite another . . . (it is) a pretty tall order".[4]

The paradox lies in the contradiction between the individual clinician's commitment to the biomedical model and the imperative (shared by the patient) to do something, and the desire to respond more faithfully to the patient as an individual and to the story, or bigger picture of the illness. It is beautifully exemplified in the *Oxford Handbook of Clinical Medicine*, which I quote from time to time.[5] This superb 841 page *vade mecum* of clinical practice is a treasury of biomedical knowledge and skills, but it begins with a heart-warming 20 page section called 'Thinking about Medicine'. This is all about achieving whole-person patient-centred care within "our stainless-steel universe of organised health care".

From the beginning I have acknowledged that the dis-ease within medicine arises from exactly this contradiction. In his classic 1977 critique of the biomedical model, Engel was quite clear about this. He says, "Medicine's unrest derives from a growing awareness among many physicians of the contradiction between the excellence of their biomedical background on the one hand, and the weakness of their qualifications in certain attributes essential for good patient care on the other. Many recognise that these cannot be improved by working within the biomedical model alone".[6] That is no longer a quite accurate account of present day medicine because changes in medical education have at least provided the opportunity for doctors to learn about what Lyng calls the 'meta-organic' factors that influence disease processes and healing processes.[7] The attributes essential for good patient care are recognised and represented, to some extent at least, in the medical curriculum. The problem is the opportunity to apply those attributes in the medical encounter when the biomedical agenda is so pressing and time is so short.

The contradiction has always had the following four elements:

- Contradiction between doctors' attitudes to the patient as a person and to their biomedical condition.
- Contradiction between patients' desire for a quick fix and their fascination with medical science and technology, and their desire to be seen, and listened to, as a person with a story of sickness.
- Contradiction between the attitude of individual doctors and the formal position of their profession on best practice, evidence, and professional development.
- Contradiction between personal medicine and public health.

These contradictions influence what actually happens.

> The Medical Scientific Model as an ideal type . . . diverges from the reality of modern medical practice in some important ways. The actual behaviour of patients, physicians, and other health care workers is influenced by a variety of ideational factors even in a system in which one medical paradigm is (dominant).[7]

This comment by Stephen Lyng is followed later in his book by the reflection that,

> From the 1920s . . . formal training structured by the medical scientific model – has not meant that physicians have always practised in strict accordance with the formal model. . . . The discrepancy between medical scientific theory and actual practice has been a crucial force in shaping the character of the health care system of the twentieth century.

Referring to the present day interest in complementary and alternative medicine (CAM), Cant and Sharma point out the disjunction between the views of many ordinary GPs and (the) spokespersons of their profession in regard to CAM.[8] They identify a community of GPs that is as sensitive to demands posed by changing attitudes to CAM among the public at large as to the demands of science; resulting in a tension between the *collective* interests of the profession and the interests of the *individual* doctor.

This paradox colours everything in this book. It is as striking a feature of the present state of Western medicine as it ever was. And, of course, it is a major factor in the impetus towards a remodelling process.

Without explicitly using the word 'paradox', David Horrobin clearly describes this continuing unease in the medical conscience when he reproaches Illich for his 'refusal to recognise that most of the critical material he has assembled comes from medical sources'.[2] He says, "Illich seems to be ignorant of much of the more reflective writing in medicine", pointing out that, "one of the strongest themes running through the writings of doctors from the early 19th century to our own time is the need to treat patients as whole people who happen to have a particular disease, and not just as cases of that disease". He quotes a 1938 paper by Professor John MacMurray, entitled 'A Philosopher's View of Modern Psychology': "The patient as a person requiring help is the focus of all problems in medicine. If medicine treats diseases, then a classification of diseases into bodily and mental will arise in which the unity of the person is lost sight of."

Horrobin says, the fact that there has been so much writing along these lines (to which there are many references in this book) indicates: "that the profession itself saw the danger very early on and has constantly striven to counteract it," but, he adds, "though by no means always with success. Most of the evidence on which Illich's polemic is based has . . . been gathered by doctors concerned about the problems of their own profession and anxious to improve the situation, (and) in a manner characteristic of no other profession, at least some doctors are both aware of and passionately concerned about what is happening. While the evidence has not been suppressed it has certainly been ignored by most doctors. . . . Many doctors share Illich's concerns but there is little doubt that they are ignored by many of their colleagues or that their plaints fall on many deaf ears".

Eric Cassell, who is one of these critics, writing many years after Illich but still expressing these concerns, describes and explains the paradox like this: "Practising physicians, because of their perception and their reasoning, cannot completely isolate their knowledge of facts about patients' parts from their knowledge of whole patients living in a real world. If that is the case, a sceptic might ask, why do they so often seem to pay no attention to the whole sick person, much less the world in which the patient lives? It is because their theories of disease and the science on which modern medicine is based pull them away from their natural inclination".[10]

It is high time for the voices that proclaim this paradox to be more vociferous and to be heard; and for the remodelling of medicine that their 'plaints' require to be effected.

In the introduction to his book *The Rise and Fall of Modern Medicine,* James le Fanu also points to a paradox in the present state of medicine.[11] He sees it from a slightly different perspective but one that in each particular corresponds to the themes of this book. He describes a four-layered paradox, comprising disillusionment amongst doctors (the proportion expressing 'regrets' about their choice of career quadrupled in 20 years), a similar increase in the proportion of the population 'concerned about their health' (the worried well), the soaring popularity of alternative medicine that the success of orthodox medicine might have been expected to render redundant, and the spiralling cost of healthcare that suggests that increased investment does not make health care more effective. In summary, he says, what needs to be explained is why the spectacular success of modern medicine over the past fifty years has had such apparently perverse consequences, leaving doctors less professionally fulfilled, the public more concerned about its health, alternative medicine in the ascendancy and an unaccounted-for explosion in health service costs. And he makes the extremely pertinent observation that understanding the cause of so many doctors' discontent is important, because "those unhappy with their trade may lack the passion necessary to practise it well".

References

1 Illich I. *Limits to medicine: medical nemesis, the expropriation of health.* London: Boyars; 1976.
2 Horrobin D. *Medical Hubris – A reply to Ivan Illich.* Edinburgh: Churchill Livingstone; 1978.
3 Greaves D. *Mystery in Western Medicine.* Aldershot: Avebury; 1996.
4 Woolfson T. Integrated medicine: orthodox meets alternative. Challenge of making holism work. *Br Med J.* 2001; 322:168.
5 Longmore M W. *Oxford Handbook of Clinical Medicine.* Seventh edition. Oxford: Oxford University Press; 2007.
6 Engel G. The need for a new medical model. *Science 1977*; 196: 4286; 129–136.
7 Lyng S. *Holistic Health and Biomedical Medicine.* New York: State University of New York Press; 1990.
8 Cant S, Sharma U. *A New Medical Pluralism: Alternative medicine, doctors, patients and the state.* London: UCL Press; 1999.
9 MacMurray J. A Philosopher's View of Modern Psychology. *Br Med J.* 1938; 2: 750.

10 Cassell E. *The Nature of Suffering and the Goals of Medicine*. New York: Oxford University Press; 2004.

11 le Fanu J. *The Rise and Fall of Modern Medicine*. London: Abacus; 1999.

4

MEDICINE AND SOCIETY

Summary

- Unrealistic expectations, fed by the power of medicine and the expertise of doctors, generate costly and debilitating demand and dependence within society.
- The circumstances affecting the health needs of the population vary greatly. One of the strengths of the biomedical model is that it seeks to provide the perceived best practice in response to particular disease states (the repertoire of investigations, drugs and procedures), whatever the circumstances.
- But, "Great health care, technically delimited, cannot alone produce great health".
- The remodelling of medicine must take account of the politics of medicine and healthcare delivery – the organisation of the health service. Most healthcare professionals would complain that for many years the problem has been constant 'redisorganisation'.
- The experience of health care comprises a balance between the excellence, or otherwise, of the people providing it and of the system within which they work, and the expectations, demands and behaviour of those who use it.
- An outstanding example of failure in healthcare that has been recognised for a long time is the inequality that exists in the UK.
- Promoting healthy lives is a complex challenge involving various permutations of legislation, social and political change, education, culture, fashion and material aspirations, individuals' sense of personal responsibility, and sometimes influences almost or completely beyond our control.
- The balance of responsibility towards the individual and towards society in the work of medicine can sometimes be difficult to judge. Is it right that "The commitment of the physician is not just primarily to the patient, it is fully patient-centred. Considering the common good is not an add-on; it is morally wrong"?

The medicalisation of life

> If medicine is fundamentally a social activity, and the nature of medical activity partially determines what we call sickness, then sickness is, in part, socially defined. (Howard Brody[1])

> (Certain) aspects of medicalisation make doctors miserable: old age, death, pain, and handicap are thrust on doctors to keep families and society from facing them. Some of them are an integral part of medicine, and accepted as such. But there is a boundary beyond which medicine has only a small role. When doctors are forced to go beyond that role they do not gain power or control: they suffer. (Leibovic and Lièvre[2])

> The more time, toil and sacrifice spent by a population in producing medicine as a commodity, the larger will be the by-product, namely the fallacy that society has a supply of health locked away which can be mined and marketed. (Ivan Illich[3])

> Health is a manifestation of the way society is organised and to get to the bottom of health you have to examine society. (Michael Marmot, paraphrased) (Kmietowicz 2010[4])

Illich's broad philosophical critique of society in the developed world was that a number of its key functions had become 'industrialised'. Organisations and institutions had expropriated the freedom, independence and responsibility of people to care for themselves and manage their affairs. Medicine was a case in point.

He summarised the causes of medicine's nemesis, arising when, "A professional and physician based health care system – has grown beyond tolerable bounds (and) is sickening (because) it must produce clinical damages which outweigh its potential benefits; it cannot but obscure the political conditions which render society unhealthy; and it tends to expropriate the power of the individual to heal himself and to shape his or her environment".[3] These words provoked lively debate when they were written, and we would be foolish if we were not prepared to ask to what extent they are true now.

Illich's argument was that medicine medicalises life. There are two aspects to this. Firstly that medicine creates expectations and dependency that are inappropriate and unhealthy, to which it overreacts with harmful consequences. (See 'The risks of being a patient' in Chapter 8.) In other words, it creates a vicious circle of inappropriate expectation and demand and potentially damaging supply. *The Health Care Dilemma*, written at the same time as *Medical Nemesis* put it like this: "The encouragement of unrealistic expectations of well-being and the consequent continuous extension of reported morbidity has come together with an explosive increase in the scope for seeking physical or biochemical 'explanations' for patients' symptoms. On top of this, the professional medical expertise of doctors and the absolute power which this has conferred on them to pronounce the presence or absence of disease has led irrationally to a situation in which the public increasingly turn to them with other problems also'.[5] Illich suggests that this vicious circle results primarily from the behaviour of the medical profession, but nevertheless becomes entangled with social and political tendencies that serve to reinforce it. The suggestion that doctors are *primarily* responsible for this, as David Horrobin pointed out (Prologue Part 2) is largely incorrect and unfair.[6] But a charge of collusion, at least, does need to be answered. And the vicious circle becomes a vicious spiral when the funding of health care is included. "Doctors and their organisations understandably argue for increased spending – because they are otherwise left paying a personal price, trying to cope with increasing demand with inadequate resources. Indeed this is one of the sources of worldwide unhappiness among doctors."[7]

Illich claims that medicine has served political and social tendencies that are in themselves unhealthy. He relates these tendencies to what he sees as the many ills of the industrialised society. You may recall from Chapter 2 Lyng's account of the support given to scientific medicine in America by big corporations aware of its potential for 'medicalising' social problems in the workplace.[8] Ian Kennedy describes a similar kind of collusion between medicine and industry; how as a result of the influence of the Flexner report (Chapter 2), medicine became interventionist and pharmacological, and medical education "was massively funded by foundations whose money came form pharmacological and petrochemical products. The aim was to indoctrinate the student, particularly in the use of drugs".[9]

Janet McKee made the same point even more forcefully, claiming that scientific medicine, becoming dominant at the end of the nineteenth century, "replaced the prior emphasis on social and environmental determinants of illness with a bioreductionist model".[10] She quotes another author, Berliner's view that "scientific medicine became a rationalisation for not dealing with . . . (occupational and environmental) causes of illness in a manner that would be dysfunctional (i.e. costly) to capitalist growth". An example of medicine's tendency 'to obscure the political conditions which render society unhealthy' closer to home, and which could be extended to other occupations, would be medical collusion in maintaining an unhealthy education system by accommodating the sick role of teachers made understandably ill by the system (i.e. reacting like normal human beings to stress and provocation).

Medicine, politics and economics: what to treat and what not to treat

Henry Miller's comment in the preface to his book, *Medicine and Society*, written in 1973, was certainly prophetic: "Medicine has changed more in the last forty years than in the previous four hundred. However, the political problems contingent on this change have yet to be faced. They are too important to be left to the necessarily empirical judgement of the medical profession. The aim of this book is to contribute to the dialogue that is a necessary prelude to inescapable decisions of public policy."[11]

Well, many contingent political problems have certainly been faced since then, and inescapable decisions have certainly been wrested from the medical profession. An example of this entanglement of medicine with politics is the repeated reorganisation of general practice in the NHS, the coercion of doctors into certain patterns of behaviour by financial incentives, and the setting of targets for screening and clinical outcomes. The irony is the present outcry for the running of the health service now to be taken back out of the hands of the politicians.

This political entanglement has compounded the social iatrogenesis that Illich described. And the medical profession has colluded in a process of which both it and its patients have been victims; or certainly in many respects perceive themselves as victims, whatever waiting list statistics and patient-satisfaction surveys may say.

An analysis relevant to this theme in the *British Medical Journal* concerns quality measurement from the patient's perspective. It begins, "Modern health care is recognising, albeit with difficulty, that it is a service industry and has to pay more attention to those who use it".[12] Later it says, "We therefore need to influence how patients choose to use health services, especially when treatments are ineffective or potentially harmful. It would be better, for example, if some self-limiting illnesses – such as some musculo-skeletal problems, many viral infections, and situational reactions to stresses – were less medicalised, with less drug treatment".

Doctor and patient education and charging patients for treatments of limited clinical value, are mentioned as remedies. It seems that Engel's comment in 1977 remains true, "The boundaries between health and disease, between well and sick, are far from clear and never will be clear, for they are diffused by cultural, social and psychological considerations".[13]

The social and clinical implications of political and economic management are exemplified by the invention of QALYs. Quality Adjusted Life Years (QALYs) have been devised to provide a basis for allocating limited resources according to the relative benefit likely to be gained by different patients. They are computed from the gain in life expectancy and the quality of life gained. Tentative costs per QALY (one year of 'quality adjusted' life) quoted in the Oxford Handbook of Clinical Medicine are, for example – Preventing stroke by treating blood pressure = £940 (€1,065, $1,500); Heart transplant = £7,840 (€8,887, $12,500).[14] This is a social and political solution, a 'utilitarian approach'[15] that subordinates the individual to the collective good. It may demand an uncomfortable compromise of the personal physician. In *The Mystery of General Practice*, Iona Heath refers to a quotation by Edmund Pellegrino reported in a book *Justice in Health Care*: "It is not just that Hippocratic professional ethics lacks a theory of just distribution; it is rather that it is committed to the proposition that societal goods do not count ethically. The commitment of the physician is not just primarily to the patient, it is fully patient-centred. Considering the common good is not an add-on; it is morally wrong."[16] In *The Virtues in Medical Practice*, Pellegrino and Thomasma are forthright in asserting the extent to which medicine has lost its moral compass (to borrow a phrase from contemporary British politics), as a result of various social and political compromises such as this.[17]

Eating habits, food and weight provide an example of the complex involvement of medical, social and political issues in health. The United Kingdom has a problem with eating disorders (anorexia, bulimia), often influenced by the way that the female figure is 'modelled'. Even when it does not reach this extreme, preoccupation with weight and figure is common. Diets are recommended weekly in papers and magazines, and programmes for weight loss are widespread. Nevertheless, obesity is epidemic, chiefly the consequence of overeating or poor choice of food, sometimes attributed to poverty. In January 2008 it was announced on the one hand that the prescription of anti-obesity drugs had risen eight-fold in eight years, and on the other that the government was considering paying obese patients to lose weight. Some hospitals and Trusts have debated withholding certain surgical procedures from people who are overweight.

We might paraphrase Engel's comment to read, 'The boundaries between what to treat and what not to treat, between the good of the individual and the good of society, between medicine and the state, are far from clear and never will be clear, for they are diffused by cultural, social, political and psychological considerations'.[13]

The context of care

A powerful attraction of the biomedical model, with its focus on specific, targeted interventions for precisely defined disease processes, is that it can be readily generalised to different contexts in which the disease process presents. The context may affect access to medical care – numbers and availability of healthcare professionals, geography, transport, etc. It may affect what can be done – cost and availability of drugs, investigations, surgical procedures, hospital beds, etc. It may affect the incidence or prevalence of various diseases – due to poverty, environment, diet etc. It may affect awareness of medical risk or medical need and the uptake of medical services – relating to attitudes, education, beliefs, etc. The context of medical care is widely diverse and will affect what medicine can achieve for different patients and different patient populations. But what the biomedical model provides, or seeks to provide – the perceived best practice in response to particular disease states, the repertoire of investigations, drugs and procedures – is highly standardised; increasingly subject to guidelines, in fact. The diagnostic and treatment possibilities will be the same, resources permitting, for any particular disease process in whatever context it arises; determined by the analytical and interventionist concepts and methods of the biomedical model.

That is one of the great strengths of the model. By its ability to turn illness into disease and do something about it, it can legitimately claim to be powerful and effective, and is seen to be powerful and effective. Its power and effectiveness may be limited by contextual factors that limit the resources needed to do a proper job, the healthcare budget for example. But its potential to do the job, to control disease states and manipulate body functions, is undisputed.

This capability of the biomedical model to operate effectively in response to the diseases that it recognises and equips its practitioners to treat, in whatever context the disease presents, is also one of its great weaknesses; because no disease, and certainly no illness, is independent of the context out of which it arises. The model has no answer to the contextual, 'meta-organic' factors that so powerfully determine the course of events in the health history of the patient. "Great health care, technically delimited, cannot alone produce great health."[18]

That is not to say that *practitioners* whose primary working method may be the biomedical model have no influence on the context. In relation to individual patients and communities, they provide education, counsel and advice to change or improve the circumstances that predispose to illness. And they and the scientists whose work is to investigate the causes and predisposing factors, the epidemiology, can exert invaluable influence on public health policy, and on government policy that seeks to make factors such as access and resourcing better and more equitable. It was one of the major flaws in Illich's thesis, as David Horrobin pointed out, that he failed to acknowledge the contribution of doctors and medical scientists to improvements in social welfare that were ultimately responsible for improvements in health.[6]

So it is important to emphasise this essentially holistic aspect of medicine – its concern with the context of disease within the broader pattern of patients' lives. Medicine recognises that while its favoured remedy for the *consequences* is biomedical, the all-important remedy for the *causes* often lies elsewhere.

The contrasting effect of 'context' factors to influence the outcome of treatment within the therapeutic encounter is described in Chapter 12 in the section 'Natural medicine and natural healing.'

The National Health Service is unwell

A major influence on the context of care in the UK is, of course, the National Health Service; although, since the devolution of certain parliamentary responsibilities we now have to distinguish between different organisational structures and policy initiatives in Scotland, Wales and England. These differences will have significantly different impact on the relationship between medicine and society in the three countries. The emphasis on market forces and the 'sub-contracted' private provision of healthcare, currently the policy in England but rejected in Scotland, is an obvious case in point. In July 2008, we 'celebrated' the 60th birthday of the NHS. The word 'celebrated' has to be in inverted commas, because it is a troubled institution. Here are the titles of some articles from various medical journals and the press during the weeks surrounding this event:

'Sixty years old: time to grow up.'
'The NHS at 60: time to end the fairy tale.'
'A fairly happy birthday.'
'The state of general practice – not all for the better.'
'The NHS is sick, but is it terminal?'

Much of this dis-ease has to do with the same dis-ease that has been the recurring theme of this book – the problem of providing the healthcare most appropriate to people's needs and the circumstances out of which those needs arise. In this case the dis-ease only relates to the biomedical model inasmuch as that is the product that predominately the health service sets out to deliver and consequently that its methods of delivery, the process of care, is designed to serve. There is more that the NHS sets out to do of course that is not focused on biomedical interventions. Public health medicine and some aspects of public health policy, though essentially informed by biomedical science, have goals (changes in life-style and behaviour, for example) and methods (education, media rhetoric) that do not involve biomedical control or manipulation of the problem they set out to solve.

The remodelling of medicine must obviously take account of the politics of medicine and healthcare delivery, which in the UK means the organisation of the health service. Most healthcare professionals would complain that for many years the problem has been too much remodelling – too much and too frequent reorganisation, representing different models of healthcare delivery favoured by successive governments and ministers and their advisers. The process is described by Donald Light, as "the continued and costly pattern of 'redisorganisation' caused by too many changes not well thought out"[19] and elsewhere attributed to a problem inherent in the familiar pattern of fluctuating government policies known as 'dynamic inconsistency'.[20] In his analysis Donald Berwick, suggests that, "this is not mere restlessness; it is accountability at work through the maddening, majestic machinery of politics".[18] But in a plea to the policy makers to stop restructuring, he adds, "In good faith and with sound logic, the leaders of the NHS and government have sorted and resorted local, regional, and national structures into a continual parade of new aggregates and agencies. Each change made sense, but the parade doesn't make sense. It drains energy and confidence from the workforce, which learns not to take risks but to hold its breath and wait for the next change". A parallel complaint, familiar from the media, is the proportionately greater increase in the numbers of administrators than in the number of clinicians, and the increase in bureaucracy at the expense of direct individual patient care.

Quality of care

In considering how the context of care and process (delivery) of care fit into the medical model, the challenge is to achieve a context and a process that do deliver and do not inhibit optimum care; and to be sure what we mean by 'care' in the first place. There can surely be no question that compassion is an essential ingredient, but in a paper for the NHS Federation Robin Youngson argues that "The traditional approach of metrics and targets hardly seem to fit this agenda".[21] In suggesting that compassion ('the humane quality of understanding suffering in others and wanting to do something about it') is the missing dimension of healthcare reform, and suggesting steps to be taken to strengthen this 'heart of healthcare', he accepts that measurement will be needed to evaluate the benefits that he claims for them (increased efficiency, safety and patient satisfaction), but it will need to be designed to ensure that it does not destroy the very thing we are trying to nurture. (See Chapter 8, 'Compassion, empathy and enablement'.)

At the heart of recent government policy in the UK has been the Quality and Outcomes Framework (QOF), an initiative to achieve certain clearly defined health care targets through financial incentives to general practitioners. This title provides three keywords that should help us to work out how context and process, the framework, could truly deliver care. That is obviously and undoubtedly the intention of the policy, which is supported by the establishment of the Care Quality Commission. But, of course, it all depends on what we mean by quality, and on what are the outcomes we are seeking, and on whether we are really talking about care or control. The QOF is not, for example, comprehensive. David Oliver, a doctor specialising in the care of the elderly lists a number of serious causes of distress and disability among the elderly that are omitted – urinary incontinence, falls and osteoporotic fractures, dementia, and increased prescribing in the over-65s despite the high level of illness related to multiple prescriptions and the prevalence of adverse drug reactions. He concludes, "An entrepreneurial model with a performance framework based on what is easily measurable and prioritising conditions affecting young and middle aged people does nothing to improve the care of old people – the principle users of the service".[22]

Reviewing some of the commentaries on the state of the National Health Service as it reaches its 60th birthday may provide pointers to the possible redesign of the context and process parts of the model. First of all the good news: "For example, after 10 years of reinvestment and redesign, the NHS has more evidence based care; lower death rates for major disease groups; lower waiting times for hospital, outpatient and cancer care; more staff and technologies available; in some places better community mental health care; and falling rates of hospital infection."[18] There is a high level of expressed satisfaction amongst patients: some 80% express themselves satisfied with the service, and despite suggestions to the contrary, measures of satisfaction reported by the Healthcare Commission have risen. And financial incentives for achieving targets for the treatment of common chronic diseases have, again despite some expectations to the contrary,

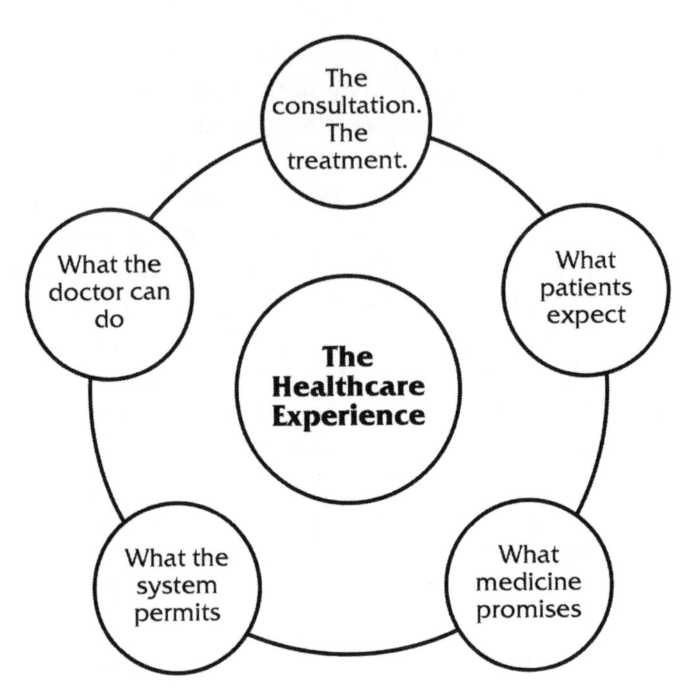

Figure 4.1 *The healthcare experience.*

shown greater benefits in areas of greatest deprivation compared with areas of least deprivation.[23]

Tales of prompt, skilful and compassionate care in a clinical environment conducive to well-being abound alongside those that tell a very different story. Access to community services and care in the community can be very good, but it can be poor. Integration of community and primary care services and specialist services, and between medical and social services, and the communication necessary to achieve it, can be excellent, or it can be shocking. In other words, the health service is like the proverbial Curate's Egg – good, indeed very good, in parts. Sometimes the difference between good and bad quality care, judged on these points, may depend on the availability of resources, and of course the wise or wasteful deployment of resources. To a great degree it will depend on the skill, attitudes and personal attributes of health service personnel – healthcare professionals, support staff and administrators, and the personnel of organisations to which health service activities, are (in England increasingly) sub-contracted.

As in all personal services the experience of health care comprises a balance between the excellence, or otherwise, of the people providing it and the excellence, or otherwise, of the system within which they work.

But even in the presence of excellence, a service is always to an extent subject to the expectations, demands and behaviour of those who use it; bearing in mind that there is a circular relationship between the attributes of a service and the expectations it engenders and the attitudes and behaviour of its users (see Figure 4.1). In health care, where these dynamics often involve the most intimate, sensitive and often distressing details of our lives and at the same time represent perhaps the most challenging expression of our desire to serve one another, a model that perfectly meets all expectations and needs will be impossible to achieve. As my senior partner used to say when my youthful idealism met with disappointment, "That's life. And there is no cure for life".

But this chastening fact does not absolve us from seeking to learn lessons from the failure of our idealism that may inform the remodelling of context and process.

Inequality

Perhaps the outstanding example of a failure that has been recognised for a long time is the inequality of health care that exists in the UK (DHSS, 1980) (much less in some other European countries, but worse in the USA). This has been called 'the inverse care law',[24] which describes the lack of health care where it is most needed. It is a failure which reflects the failure of our society and its political representatives to get to grips not just with the provision of appropriate and adequate health care, but with the social circumstances (poverty, unemployment, poor education, hopelessness) that are known to generate illness by their physiological effects as well as their effects on mental health, life-style, diet, etc., and that make health care so difficult to provide and health promotion so difficult to implement.

In situations like this, where there is a great deal of established disease, the interventions made possible by the biomedical model are badly needed but will not in themselves reduce the continuing level of sickness in the community. Medicine has a responsibility for advocacy on behalf of its patients to promote change in the social circumstances that create illness. It also has a responsibility for compassionate care of its individual patients, whether sick through their own destructive behaviour, or as a result of circumstances, or both. But this must also encourage as far as possible a sense of personal responsibility in the individual for their well-being. Medicine is at the heart of the social dilemma reflected in "the premise that we are all responsible for each other and the premise that we are each responsible for ourselves".[18]

These situations poignantly illustrate the need for a kind of 'integrated' medicine that has nothing to do with the availability of different therapeutic methods. It has to do with medicine's long-established commitment to the integrated provision of personal care, scientific knowledge, professional skill and social and political advocacy. This is an integrated model of health care that, when it works is also truly 'integrative', because it relates the well-being of the individual to the well-being of society. Ideally, it works towards what Julian Tudor-Hart, who first coined the phrase term 'inverse care law', describes as "a kinder, more imaginative, more generous world".[25] Medicine can make an important contribution to this, but it is only a contribution – to a challenge that Graham Watt, echoing Tudor Hart's words, identified as "... a challenge, not only to our generosity as a society, but also to our ability to imagine structural solutions to the inverse care law".[26]

A leader in the *British Medical Journal*, responding to the forthright 2008 WHO report on the social determinants of health, concludes "... health professionals have clear and plentiful work to do within the many systems within which we work. By placing health equity as a crucial goal and as the standard for accountability, and by recognising that social justice is the foundation of public health, we stand a better chance at rectifying current inequities and playing our part in a more just and sustainable world".[27]

These issues are explored further in Chapter 17.

In the commentary quoted earlier, however, Light suggests that policy initiatives to improve quality that are responsive to patient choice and demand will not necessarily reduce inequality and remedy the inverse care law: "Politicised choice and patient led go together to cater to demand and move further away from meeting the needs of people from minority groups or on low incomes. *Patient centred* differs profoundly and focuses on real need. The choice agenda here is likely to decrease overall quality as it increases variation."[19] (My italics.)

I have mentioned instances of medicine's unhealthily collusive relationship with society, but of course there are many instances where medicine has worked with society to its great benefit. In this instance, the failure to remedy inequalities in health care represents a failure of society, but also of medicine's integrative role in society; a role that any evolving model must reflect.

Health care policy

The relationship between medicine and society (shown in Figure 4.2), determines the context and process of care. In the UK this relationship is represented by the National Health Service, which is constantly confronted by the prospect of further reorganisation and reform. One of the recent aims has been to promote healthy lives through a greater emphasis on prevention, to improve quality of care by refining the Quality and Outcomes Framework, and to increase choice and give patients a greater role in shaping services. Taken at face value these are good intentions, but they beg a multitude of questions whose answers depend upon a complex set of factors, such as: What is the vision of health care we are trying to model? What is meant by 'quality'? What 'outcomes' are we seeking, bearing in mind that, "not all that is measured is of value, and not all that is of value can be measured"?[28] What is the legitimate and practical scope of political influence on the health-related behaviour of the population on the one hand, and on the practice of medicine on the other? To what extent will patient choice be more than 'Hobson's choice' – no choice at all or choice between a limited number of predetermined options?

Promoting healthy lives can in some instances, where the evidence is sufficiently compelling, be advanced by legislation (smoking, seat belts in cars, the sale of alcohol, etc.). In some instances it can and must be advanced through social and political change (to alleviate poverty, for example). In some instances it depends, with variable success, on education. In some instances it is powerfully influenced by culture, fashion, material aspirations. Very often it depends ultimately on individuals' sense of personal responsibility for their own lives and the lives of others in their

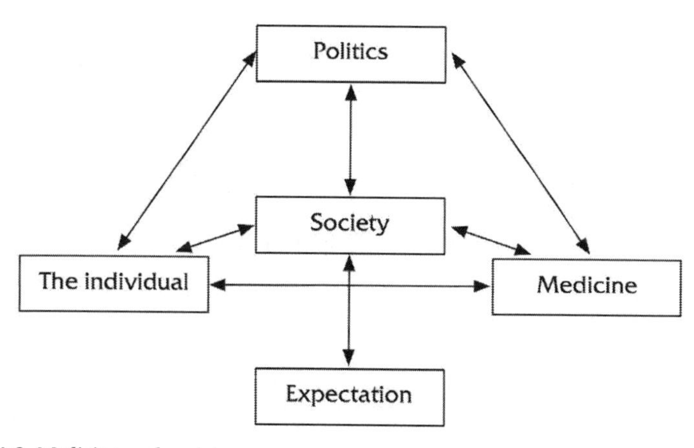

Figure 4.2 *Medicine and society.*

care. But sometimes healthy living is subject to influences almost or completely beyond our control (climate, global commodity prices, and so on). These considerations illustrate the difficulty of implementing just this one of the aims of recent healthcare strategy.

The context and process of care are the vehicles that will determine much of the appropriateness and effectiveness of whatever model of medicine and healthcare we design. They will determine what goes on in the large-scale provision of health care, and what goes on at the intimate level of the relationship between practitioner and patient. This complex interplay between medicine and society, context and process, large-scale provision and personal care can be neatly illustrated by four policy proposals or dictats (July 2008): provision to be made to make it increasingly possible for the terminally ill to die at home if they wish to do so; general practitioners exhorted to be more attentive to the personal needs, wishes and circumstances associated with their patients' medical condition; GPs instructed not to prescribe antibiotics to patients with commonplace upper respiratory and ear, nose and throat conditions; and a proposal for performance related pay for surgeons.

Providing resources for the dying to be cared for at home in future instead of in hospital if that is their wish, which in a less sophisticated medical past would have been the norm, offers patients a real choice that really matters; provided that the resources really are provided – a good policy to meet a well-recognised need for compassionate whole person care. Guidelines that discourage the prescribing of antibiotics for viral conditions in which they are not effective and that will increase the threat of resistance to antibiotics in more virulent and dangerous organisms, is also good policy to remedy a well-recognised need. Here, however, the problem is not so much a matter of responding to patient choice, but of resisting patient expectation and demand, which doctors are tempted to satisfy with a prescription they know to be inappropriate (a kind of 'placebo' in fact), because it saves time and trouble; the time and trouble involve providing the reassurance, education and advice that would be the appropriate treatment to an unhappy and possibly argumentative patient, probably one of many in the waiting room that day. Just one commonplace example of a healthcare dilemma arising from false expectations of biomedical methods that has been generated by the success of those methods; now needing correction by an instruction to doctors who, by and large, have always known better anyway but have themselves become victims of the model.

And how galling for general practitioners to be instructed to be more personally attentive to their patients. For it is the Department of Health that has made that very task, the natural concern for the 'metaorganic' context of the illness that is the essence of general practice, exceedingly difficult to fulfil by the time-consuming pursuit and documentation of biomedical, and securely evidence based 'targets'. Surgeons, too, were not surprisingly unhappy at the proposal that their pay should be related to the success rate of their operations. Nor is the implication that surgeons must be paid more as an incentive for better results particularly reassuring for patients.

These examples are not intended to belittle the aims of government health policy; there may be poorly performing surgeons and general practitioners who are uncritical or perhaps lazy in their prescribing habits, or lack empathy towards their patients. They are all examples of health service management, striving to achieve uniformly high standards. They are simply intended to reflect the complexity of the relationship between the state and healthcare practitioners, and the difficulty of implementing change in such a way that the process and context of care do not become an obstacle to the delivery of care, rather than an assurance of good quality care (see Figure 4.2).

A particular instance of this danger is described by Nigel Rawlinson, a consultant in an inner city accident and emergency department, in a recent Personal View in the *British Medical Journal*.[29] The target in question is the requirement to discharge patients from the department, or transfer them to other wards or units, within four hours. The department engaged with the policy philosophically and conscientiously. Indeed, there was little choice, "We had to engage with the targets that had been set, and use them to attract the resources we needed to treat patients faster". The philosophy required finding solutions rather than identifying problems, and "The phrase 'I treat patients not targets' was consigned to the past. Good staff, when made to work flat out to meet a deadline, will treat the clock rather than the patient". The pressure to move patients on within the deadline is reflected in the fact that most leave the department within the last 20 minutes of the four hour target period. Several sorts of harm resulting from this pressure are identified. First, the direct clinical risk that serious conditions that might have been better stabilised if the patient had stayed longer in the department will, for example, require more intensive care subsequently than would otherwise be the case. Then there are other, more subtle but important consequences:

- A patient's history has changed from one that seeks to be holistic to one that is problem solving.
- The ability to listen is undermined.

- Vulnerable, frightened, inarticulate patients become objects of annoyance rather than subjects of care.
- Open questions designed to help patients tell their story are replaced by closed questions that categorise them into a convenient group.
- The opportunity for more subtle assessment of 'the story behind the story', and to involve social and community services in solving the problem underlying the clinical presentation in the 'integrative' fashion I referred to earlier, is lost.
- Astute diagnosis of more subtle clinical conditions is compromised.

Targets, "while achieving a great deal in terms of resource and timeliness, have done this at the expense of holistic patient care (and) detract from the pursuit of clinical excellence". Not only that, the health economists' claim that those gains have improved patient care for the majority is a totalitarian argument that compromises the doctor's ability to be the advocate of the individual patient. To sacrifice this personal commitment for the sake of the majority, Rawlinson argues, is poor patient care. And in this he echoes the earlier reference to the quotation from Edmund Pellegrino which concludes, "The commitment of the physician is not just primarily to the patient, it is fully patient-centred. Considering the common good is not an add-on; it is morally wrong".

References

1 Brody H. *Stories of Sickness*. New Haven: Yale University Press; 1987.
2 Leibovic L, Lièvre M. Medicalisation: peering from inside medicine. *Br Med J.* 2002; 324:866.
3 Illich I. *Limits to medicine: medical nemesis, the expropriation of health*; London: Boyars; 1976.
4 Kmietowicz Z. Great expectations. *Br Med J.* 2010; 340 b5558:340–341.
5 OHE. *The Health Care Dilemma*. London: Office of Health Economics; 1975.
6 Horrobin D. *Medical Hubris – A reply to Ivan Illich*. Edinburgh: Churchill Livingstone; 1978.
7 Moynihan R, Smith R. Too much medicine? *Br Med J.* 2002; 324:859–60.
8 Lyng S. *Holistic Health and Biomedical Medicine*. New York: State University of New York Press; 1990.
9 Kennedy I. *Unmasking medicine*. London: George Allen and Unwin; 1981.
10 McKee J. Holistic health and the critique of western medicine. *Soc Sci Med.* 1988; 26:8;775–784
11 Miller H. *Medicine and Society*. Oxford: Oxford University Press; 1973.
12 Elwyn G, Buetow S, Hibbard J, Wensing M. Respecting the subjective: quality measurement from the patient's perspective. *Br Med J.* 2007; 335:1021–2.

13 Engel G. The need for a new medical model. *Science 1977*; 196:4286;129–136.
14 Longmore M, Wilkinson I, Turmezei T, Cheung C K. *Oxford Handbook of Clinical Medicine*. Oxford: Oxford University Press; 2007.
15 Toon P. Occasional Paper 78. *Towards a Philosophy of General Practice*. London: Royal College of General Practitioners; 1999.
16 Heath I. *The Mystery of General Practice*. London: Nuffield Provincial Hospitals Trust; 1995.
17 Pellegrino E, Thomasma D. *The Virtues in Medical Practice*. Oxford: Oxford University Press; 1993.
18 Berwick D. A transatlantic review of the NHS at 60. *Br Med J*. 2009; 337:212–14.
19 Light D. Will the NHS strategic plan benefit patients? *Br Med J*. 2008; 337:210–12.
20 Vaithianathan R, Lewis G. Operational independence for the NHS. *Br Med J*. 2008; 337 a497:380–382.
21 Youngson R. *Compassion in healthcare*. London: NHS Confederation Publications; 2008.
22 Oliver D. QOF and public health priorities don't improve care in the aging. *Br Med J*. 2008; 337 a1403.
23 Health Care Commission. *National Survey of Local Health Services 2008*. Available online at www.healthcarecommission.org.uk.
24 Tudor Hart J. The Inverse Care Law. *Lancet* 1971; 297(7696):405–412.
25 Tudor Hart J. (2008). Sixty years old: time to grow up. *RCGP News* 2008 July; 7.
26 Watt, G. (2008). The NHS at 60: time to end the fairy tale. *Br J Gen Pract*. 2008; 8(552):459–460.
27 Davey Smith G, Krieger N. Tackling health inequalities. *Br Med J*. 2008; 337:a152.
28 Bradley F, Field J. Evidence based medicine. *Lancet* 1995; 346:838–839.
29 Rawlinson N. Harm of target driven. *Br Med J*. 2008; 337 a885:237.

5

MEDICINE AND THE INDIVIDUAL

Summary

- "The crippling flaw of the (medical) model is that it does not include the patient and his attributes as a person, a human being."
- Time is a big issue. The progress of science has eroded the time available to pay attention to the person as an individual.
- The importance of the doctor's role in mediating "the experience of the patient within the revealed context of their shared humanity" is *discouraged* in the formation of the doctor's professional persona.
- Despite the importance of personal responsibility and autonomy in managing our health, there is a point at which we may legitimately surrender ourselves totally into the care of the professionals.
- There may be conflict between our personal autonomy and the best interests of others that is difficult to resolve.
- Medicine is inextricably bound up with the mystery of human nature and the fate of each unique person.
- Medicine's role requires hubris that dares to engage with this mystery, expressed in the experience of health, illness and healing. But this must be a 'humble hubris'.

Neglect of the person

> The crippling flaw of the (medical) model is that it does not include the patient and his attributes as a person, a human being. Yet in the everyday work of the physician the prime object of study is a person. (George Engel[1])

This quotation sums up much of the dis-ease in modern medicine, experienced by health care professionals and patients alike. It is a product of many factors in healthcare:

The reductionist approach

Many interventions are focused on a specific disorder in a specific part, which becomes the whole problem.

Targets

Much health care in hospital and the community is governed by targets determined by cost and efficiency or statistical norms, which marginalise personal care, and undermine the motivation of medical staff to care, and their freedom to do so.

Medicine is able to do so much

Because medicine is able to do so much, the expectation that something should be done affects patient and healthcare provider alike, and the time and effort committed to doing it often preclude the kind of enquiry, attention and reflection that would enable a better understanding and resolution of the problem in terms of the patient's personal predicament. The imperative to gather information and take action pre-empts the knowledge of the person that makes possible the wisdom that a real solution to the problem requires.

The biomedical focus

The biomedical focus also reduces the scope for those ingredients of the therapeutic relationship that are responsible for its all-important 'contextual' benefits. In his paper, 'Who Cares?', David Haslam warns, "There is a risk that we are creating a form of general practice that will not permit the placebo effect to work".[2]

These non-specific, contextual, 'placebo' effects, which will be discussed again in Chapter 12, are dependent in large part on the personal quality of the medical encounter.

Population-based medicine

Concerning the population health agenda, John Howie and two other emeritus professors of general practice (primary care) write the following: "Governments are bound to see healthcare as population based, whether in terms of preventing disease or in managing long term illness and disability. Population medicine is, however, not principally concerned with the agendas of individual patients consulting their doctors. Integrating the public health agenda into routine general practice means that the reasons for patients wishing to consult their GP are in danger of being relegated in favour of an agenda to which patients may not give priority".[3]

Much of our healthcare experience is population based rather than personal. Public Health measures such as screening and health education or promotion campaigns have reduced morbidity and saved lives. They rightly emphasise personal responsibility for aspects of health care. But they also induce a sense of herd identity, of regimentation. We become a member of a statistical target population, 'partial patients'.[4] We find ourselves in an ambiguous state of personal responsibility but collective conformity (and of course personal guilt or reproach if we do not conform).

This confusion is exacerbated by all forms of health related journalism. Much health related advice in newspapers, magazines and commercial advertising promotes trends and fashions rather than better health, alongside material that promotes or celebrates lifestyles and values that are anything but healthy. Even the public health advice that is based on medical research changes, sometimes frequently, or is subject to disagreement between medical authorities, or between medical authorities and politicians, because the research data are ambiguous or superseded by later research.

The population-based issue is indeed a healthcare dilemma. The "avalanche of public health rhetoric" as Iona Heath calls it,[5] pursues worthy goals but prejudices personal care and the autonomy of the individual. It produces measurable, statistically significant health gains, but is it, in another sense, in the context of Illich's critique of medicine and society,[6] 'sickening'?

Reinstating the individual

"The patient as a person requiring help is the focus of all problems in Medicine", wrote John MacMurray in 1938 in the quotation in the Prologue. This undoubtedly is a principle that all health care professionals have 'constantly striven' to maintain. But it remains a struggle, and often an unavailing struggle. This is because the biomedical model requires a different focus.

Ideals

The principles are clearly enshrined in the introductory section in the *Oxford Handbook of Clinical Medicine* that I have already mentioned.[7] In the words of one devotee, it "teaches how to be a well-rounded doctor – one of culture, patience, reflection, and, above all, humility".[8] There is much wise counsel here, from which several aphorisms could be extracted and framed to hang on the walls of medical school seminar rooms and consulting rooms. For example, from *A New Hippocratic Oath*:

- Patients are my first concern. I will listen to them and provide the best care I can. I will be honest, respectful and compassionate towards all.
- I will not provide treatments that are pointless or harmful.
- I will answer as truthfully as I can, and respect patients' decisions.

And under the heading 'Ideals':

- Decision and intervention are the essence of action; reflection and conjecture are the essence of thought; the essence of medicine is combining these realms in the service of others.
- Treat the whole patient, not the disease.
- Give the patient (and yourself) time: time for questions, to reflect, to allow healing, and time to gain autonomy.

Time

Time is, of course, a big issue. (See also Chapters 8 and 14.) Lyng points out how the progress of scientific medicine eroded the time available to pay attention to the person as an individual. The promise of what medicine can achieve, the expectations that promise has aroused, and the biomedical focus of the enquiry have led to an increase in the volume of work, which means less time with each individual. This violated the standards of good practice of the older physicians because it limited their ability to collect information about other aspects of their patients' lives. But it was consistent with medical scientific standards of good practice, because "to spend extra time relating to patients as people contributes nothing to resolving their health problems . . . an approach to patient care in which physicians make maximum use of their time by narrowing attention to the data needed for diagnosing disease".[9] How sadly commonplace are patients' complaints about just that tendency. It is ironic that doctors who dismiss the benefits of some complementary medicine practices that involve longer consultations often do so on the basis that, 'if I could afford to spend that amount of time with my patients, I could get the same results.' Neglect of the patient as an individual is at the heart of *The Health Care Dilemma*.[10] "Clearly . . . the patient must be treated as a 'whole person' whether in general practice or in hospital. His work, his family, his status and his satisfactions may be just as potent an influence on the state of his health as any bacteria or inherent idiosyncrasies in his metabolism or physiology.... Medical research, and more especially the advice to practitioners from pundits, also needs to take account of the whole person concept of medicine."

Susceptibility

These quotations introduce another issue that *The Health Care Dilemma* addresses and that is fundamental to the understanding of disease processes and healing processes, and generally neglected, which is the *susceptibility* of individuals to illness. The influences mentioned in the previous paragraph will affect this susceptibility, and the response to illness and the ability to recover. Of course, there are many such influences, which range from genetic and congenital factors, through environmental factors and past life events and experiences to current psychosocial problems. Not all of these will be susceptible to change, but unless they are known, the full nature of the illness, its prognosis, and the prospects for future health will not be understood. In most cases they will not be known unless the personal narrative is allowed and encouraged to unfold. And that permission and encouragement must accommodate attitudes and idiosyncratic beliefs, especially when they have no 'scientific validity'.[11] They may make little sense to the doctor, but they may be powerful influences on the individual's well-being.

The embodied individual

The quotation from John MacMurray speaks of the 'unity of the person' that is threatened by a classification of mental and physical disease. This is echoed by Howard Brody when he writes, "*Persons*, not minds and bodies, are real entities that exist in the world; mind and body simply exist as abstractions from the more fundamental unity of the person". This unity is challenged within our own experience when we are ill, and part of the responsibility of the doctor must be to recognise that state of alienation, and to seek to reconcile it and help to restore the sense of unity, the sense of personhood that has experienced an unpleasant break or split and that ought to be felt as a whole or complete. "When sick I become a *different* person in that there has been a major break or change in my story, a break in continuity. But I am the *same* person, nevertheless, in that the story remains the story of my one, single life."[12]

The attitude and behaviour of the doctor can heal (make whole) this breakdown in the unity of the person or exacerbate it. James Marcum

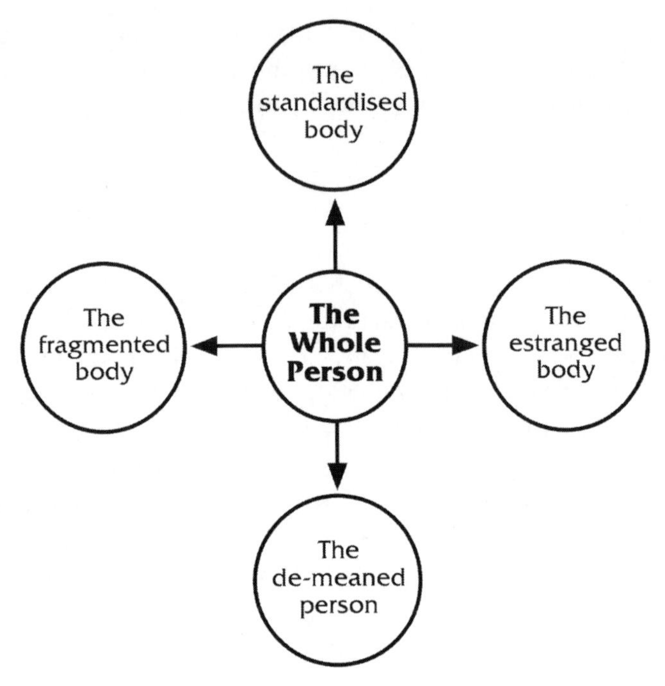

Figure 5.1 *The misdirected focus is 'de-meaning'.*

describes how the misdirected focus of the medical encounter can exacerbate the breakdown of a person's sense of completeness.[13] (Figure 5.1) It does so when it presents the image of a *fragmented body,* reduced to its disordered component parts, a *standardised body* to which the patient's body must be encouraged to conform, and an *estranged body,* alienated from the self, from the lived context of the illness, and from other people.

Marcum refers to a chapter entitled 'The Body as Territory and Wonder' in a book by A.W. Frank, in which the author describes his experience as a cancer patient. The title of the chapter relates to the medical perception of the body as a territory that becomes the property of the medical profession, colonised by physicians ("*This* will have to be investigated"). As the physicians took over, "the person within my body was sent out into the audience to watch passively". The solution to this problem of alienation is for both doctor and patient to retain a sense of wonder at the body. The patient is unlikely to achieve this whole-making sense of wonder and worth-ship if it is not in the mind and heart of the doctor.

Self-esteem

This sense of worth-ship, that embraces the body, is one important aspect of the more general self-esteem that is necessary to the patient's well-being, and which the earlier quotation from the Royal College of Physicians journal commends us to respect. And it has to be remembered that lack of self-esteem, possibly severely damaged self-esteem may be a potent influence on the person's state of health.

As patients we are vulnerable and inevitably to some degree dependent. When we are ill our self-esteem is fragile. How our vulnerability, dependence and self-esteem are handled will affect the healing process for better or for worse. The attitude and behaviour of those responsible for our care will be powerfully influential to this. But so will the way in which our illness is construed and treated. A comment in the *British Medical Journal* in March 2008 about recently published research on the over prescribing of antidepressants points out first that this 'medicalisation of mood' was originally initiated by evidence based advice to prescribe antidepressants. Then in his comment, Des Spence, a Glasgow GP, asks "How much harm have we done (by obeying this advice)? Plenty. We have accepted under-reported but common withdrawal symptoms and possible dependence issues. But worst of all we have neutered a generation of patients, making them doctor dependent, denying them the opportunity to develop coping strategies, and eroding their self-esteem".[14]

Another instance of this problem is described in Chapter 8, the capacity of medicine to create illness by extending the range of diagnostic possibilities that can be applied to patients resulting in 'epidemics' of false diagnosis of mental health problems. London GP Mike Fitzpatrick attributes the same consequence to a recommendation by the 'happiness Tsar' to provide easy access to psychological therapies to the one third of the population alleged to be in need of them. He doubts the relevance and validity of the scanty evidence for this proposal, and says, "It is immediately apparent that these rates of diagnosis can only be achieved by the dramatic inflation of familiar diagnostic categories and the expansion of the scope of psychiatric labelling from small minority of sufferers to a substantial portion of the population".[15]

Shared humanity

Iona Heath makes a supremely important point when she refers to the doctor mediating "the experience of the patient within the revealed context of their shared humanity".[5] If I understand her correctly, she is referring to an attitude which, essential though I wholeheartedly agree it is, and difficult to incorporate in the protocol of the doctor-patient relationship, is actually *discouraged* in the formation of the doctor's professional persona. The concept of the 'wounded healer' is well recognised and valued; but the revealed context of our shared humanity, including our woundedness? That powerful ingredient of a healing relationship and a component of all-important empathy must be a scarce commodity within our present day medical culture. It is, nevertheless, indispensable if we are fully to acknowledge and reinforce patients' sense of their own individual humanity, the individual and unique meaning and value of their lives.

In one of the papers that I published after my early years in general practice, while trying to resolve these issues in my own mind, and anticipating Iona Heath's remark I wrote, "We do not always have to use science in our professional role, indeed often we must not. We need only to have the courage simply to be imperfect but compassionate human beings. The problem is will our professional role permit it?"[16] I challenged the suggestion of a respected colleague, that "The general practitioner must learn to feel unafraid in that no-man's-land between the 'private lives' of his patients and the 'performance' of the consultation".[17] I suggested that on the contrary the GP would be more effective if less protectively costumed for his professional role and public performance, and that the general practitioner *must* always have the courage to feel afraid in the no-man's-land that inevitably exists between his patient's and his own deeply personal humanity. I was writing for general practitioners, but this attitude is perhaps more important, and more difficult, for specialists whose repertoire is more explicitly biomedical. This fear is, in part, a sense of awe at the inexplicable and wonderful that is always an element of our patients' lives. Doctors have to learn to tolerate uncertainty; but to be unafraid in no-man's-land is inhuman. To be human is to go fearfully on across no-man's-land in order to touch the person on the other side, who may be helped more by our compassionate fearfulness, than by a superior fearlessness.

The ability to enter into a relationship of shared humanity is a necessary attribute if we are fully to respect and enhance the patient's sense of valued individuality. This does not require huge psychological sophistication so much as simple sensitivity towards the patient and honest awareness of oneself. But I do not pretend that these qualities come easily. And they come even harder if they are do not survive the mind-bending journey through what Marshall Marinker called 'the hidden curriculum' of medical education.[18] That was his phrase to refer to the curriculum of the biomedical model that I am discussing in this book. The curriculum has changed in the 35 years since Marinker wrote those words and he had no little influence in changing it, but the hidden curriculum still to a great extent prevails; despite changes that have provided organised learning experience to nourish those all-important human attributes that are usually part of the motivation to a career in health care.

Writing in 2007, Kathi Kemper notes that there have been enormous efforts to enhance the teaching of humanism and professionalism in medicine over the past 20 years, but "in mainstream medicine, biomedical knowledge and being able to practise specific measurable skills are highly valued (and) there is less emphasis on . . . learning and evaluating (the) ability to be present with patients and relieve suffering with compassionate intentionality. Students quickly learn that courses devoted to the humanities and professionalism do not count as heavily as courses emphasising the memorisation of facts and physiologic pathways".[19]

The limits of personal competence

Having said all this about the centrality of the individual in healthcare, the importance of affirming the value of the individual, and of respecting personal autonomy, there is a point at which we, the patient, may legitimately wish, or indeed have to surrender ourselves totally into the care of the professionals. And there will be occasions when, by virtue of the superior knowledge or expertise essential to our care we will expect the professional to take charge. "To assume the value of personal responsibility for health is not to ignore the fact that under some conditions one must relinquish the responsibility for dealing with dysfunction to someone else."[9] Many of us will thankfully have relinquished our responsibility for ourselves, or for someone for whom we have been caring, in that way. But that only increases the responsibility of the professional for worth-ship.

Autonomy

Respect for personal autonomy, the individual's right to manage their own affairs, is promoted as a general virtue in health care. But it is an ambiguous virtue. A practitioner may be responsible for the care of one person whose autonomous choice in respect of their own life-style or health care may prejudice the well-being of another, a family member perhaps, also in the care of the same practitioner. In this sense, and in terms of the consequences of the individual's autonomous decision on the wider society, the allocation of resources for example, or the establishment of some ethical principle, autonomy may conflict with another virtue – justice. This may be a very difficult matter to resolve; sometimes for society as a whole; often for the individual practitioner who has to come to an understanding with their patient, and help the patient to come to an understanding with themselves.

Medical hubris and individual responsibility

In his reply to Illich's complaint that medicine's hubris in expropriating the power of the individual to heal himself and to shape his or her environment is 'sickening',[6] David Horrobin argues that on the contrary, the western industrialised model for the provision of goods and services has so undermined the desire of the majority for autonomy (we might say self-sufficiency), that those with influence and power, such as governments or the medical profession, will actually need to take decisions that require people to do things for their own good that they would not have chosen to do for themselves.[20] In other words, he was suggesting that the exertions of 'the nanny state' in collusion with the medical profession, which are such a conspicuous feature of life in the UK today, are a right and proper consequence of the majority of people's self-indulgent attitudes and behaviour, rather than a denial of their self-sufficient and unselfish better nature – human nature being what it is. The epidemic of obesity and its complications, a problem of both rich and poor sections of society, is one example of many. The response to climate change is an example on a grand scale. It is largely the product of industrialisation. It is requiring regulation of the behaviour of individuals and societies, on both a local and global scale, by those with influence and power. But the better behaviour that is being imposed by regulation is the way we should behave if we were wiser anyway.

One of the persistent flaws in Illich's argument is that the unhealthy state of affairs that he describes is the fault of the providers of 'industrialised' products and services; that they are solely responsible for the betrayal of everyone's better nature. We cannot deny that certain agents of industrial society such as the media and commercial advertising do encourage bad behaviour. But to what extent are these forces feeding, rather than creating the appetite for these products? Quite apart from biomedical issues, any new model of medicine that emerges will need to be concerned with medicine's role in addressing the seemingly intractable susceptibility of human nature to self-induced illness. This is another aspect of medicine's wider responsibility towards the well-being of humanity that was touched on in the section on inequality in Chapter 4, and that will be discussed again in Part 5.

But this is the extraordinary fascination, privilege and responsibility of medicine. The study and practice of medicine as a whole, in its most personal and intimate functions, in its most sophisticated scientific and technological activities, and in its philosophical and ethical implications, is absolutely central to our understanding of the human condition. Because it operates at the interface between society and the individual, and because it engages with people in the most intimate and often formative and potentially creative moments of their lives, it is inextricably bound up with the mystery of human nature and the fate of each unique person. Horrobin argues that medicine's role *requires* hubris, and in this sense his argument has particular force. Medicine must have the hubris that dares to engage with the mystery of human nature as it is expressed in the experience of health, illness and healing. But, although it is a contradiction in terms, it must do so with the utmost humility. One of the questions that this book poses is whether the model of medicine by which we operate is conducive to this particular blend of 'humble hubris'.

There is no doubt that the front line of medicine's response to the human predicament is the personal quality of the encounter between the healthcare professional and the patient. The greater consensus seems to be that our current medical model, including aspects of the context and process of care discussed in the last section, puts this key component of the medical endeavour seriously at risk.

References

1 Engel G. The clinical application of the biosocial model. *Am J Psychiat.* 1980; 137:5, 535–544.
2 Haslam D. Who cares? *Br J Gen Pract.* 2007; 57(545):987–993.
3 Howie J, Metcalfe D, Wallker J. The state of general practice – not all for the better. *Br Med J.* 2008; 336:1310–311.
4 Greaves D. *The Healing Tradition.* Oxford: Radcliffe Publishing; 2004.
5 Heath I. *The Mystery of General Practice.* London: Nuffield Provincial Hospitals Trust; 1995.
6 Illich I. *Limits to medicine: medical nemesis, the expropriation of health.* London: Boyars; 1976.
7 Longmore M, Wilkinson I, Turmezei T, Cheung C K. *Oxford Handbook of Clinical Medicine.* Oxford: Oxford University Press; 2007.
8 Warriner D. Medical Classics: The Oxford Handbook of Clinical Medicine. *Br Med J.* 2008; 336:393.
9 Lyng S. *Holistic Health and Biomedical Medicine.* New York: State University of New York Press; 1990.
10 OHE. *The Health Care Dilemma.* London: Office of Health Economics; 1975.
11 Dixon M, Sweeney K. *The Human Effect in Medicine.* Oxford: Radcliffe; 2000.
12 Brody H. *Stories of Sickness.* New Haven: Yale University Press; 1997.

13 Marcum J. Biomechanical and phenomenological models of the body, the meaning of illness and quality of care. *Med Health Care Phlosoph.* 2004; 7:311–320.
14 Spence, D. From the front line: Bitter sweets. *Br Med J.* 2008; 336:562.
15 Fitzpatrick M. The fallacy of Van Helmont's tree. *Br J Gen Pract.* 2010; 60(574):381.
16 Swayne J. On our best behaviour. *J R Coll Gen Pract.* 1976; 26:560–564.
17 Marinker M. *Mims Magazine* 1975; 22.
18 Marinker M. Medical education and human values. *J R Coll Gen Pract.* 1974; 24:445–462.
19 Kemper K. The Yin and Yang of Integrated Clinical Care. *Explore* 2007; 3:37–41.
20 Horrobin D. *Medical Hubris – A reply to Ivan Illich.* Edinburgh: Churchill Livingstone; 1978.

6

MEDICINE AND SCIENCE

Summary

- "The scientific attitude can permit no restrictions as to the category of natural phenomena investigated."
- The narrowness of the biomedical model, and the paradigm on which it is based, devalue and denature science and diminish medicine.
- Science makes it possible to identify markers of latent disease and causes of disease in people's life-style or environment, and develop remedies for them. But these advantages are accompanied by risks.
- Measurements of body functions and body states define 'normality', on the basis of statistical probability and significance. These definitions do not allow for the diversity and complexity of the human condition.
- They are inevitably, and necessarily, an abstraction from real life. They allow useful things to be done, but obscure the physician's view of the sick person.
- "We do not need to esteem science less. What we need is to esteem it in the right way. Especially we need to stop isolating it from the rest of life."

The scientific attitude

> The scientific attitude can permit no restrictions as to the category of natural phenomena investigated. The scientist's first obligation is to his data, wherever or however it may appear. (George Engel[1])

It should be readily apparent from earlier remarks that this book is not a complaint against science. Advanced level science was a struggle for me because my natural intellectual bent was towards the classics and the humanities, but a 'scientific passion' of a more general kind, a desire to know, to explore reality by disciplined enquiry, was instilled by incidental aspects of a good education at a young age. For example, investigating the design of mediaeval monastic architecture, or learning the periphrastic tense in Latin as the product of a metaphorical factory. In medicine, at a similarly early age it was stimulated by a book called *The Microbe Hunters* about the pioneers of the germ theory and microbiology that I found quite thrilling. Similarly exciting while working for a physiology degree was the pioneering work of Dale and others on the discovery of neurotransmitters. I am wholly committed to the enrichment by science of the totality of the human experience. Nor is this book about relegating biomedical science to a subordinate place in the medical model. We simply need to understand its proper place in the model.

The complaint is that the narrowness of the biomedical, biomechanical, bioreductionist, anatamo-clinical model, as it is variously described, and the paradigm on which it is based, devalue and denature science and diminish medicine. Lyng characterises the approach in words which demonstrate both its strengths and its limitations: "What is most noteworthy about the anatamo-clinical approach to disease classification is not the kind of evidence included in the designation of disease but, rather, that which is *excluded* (my italics).... Control of organic dysfunction that excludes direct use of subjective factors (is) the preferred method for dealing with dysfunction in the anatamo-clinical system. As with any other naturally occurring phenomenon, disease can be made the subject of rational, systematic inquiry leading to a system of verifiable knowledge about the disease process. The assumption that all disease-related phenomena can be reduced to an essential micro-level condition makes such knowledge about disease possible.... Assuming that the subject of analysis consists of discrete entities serves as an essential prerequisite for the development of a knowledge system made up of discrete categories that are universally applicable to those objective entities".[2]

The trouble is that you and I ('the subject') are not so discretely constituted. As Ian Kennedy says, "What is wrong with the concept of disease is not that there is no malfunctioning part. There may be. Rather, it is that medicine has come to concentrate on it to the exclusion of all else ... a sort of medical tunnel vision. What is not seen ... is the sick person in all his wholeness and variability".[3]

Alan Barbour warns, "When we stick too close to the disease model without appreciating the human situation we often bring to bear: the wrong diagnosis, inappropriate diagnostic procedures, ineffective therapy, unnecessary hospitalisation, increased cost, prolonged disability.... An iatrogenic illness results from the covert substitution of medical diagnoses and treatments for personal understanding and possible change.... Clearly the disease model ... is critical and life-saving when there is a disease, but when an illness is caused primarily by disturbances in the human condition, the results can be disastrous.... In our earnest quest for a disease to explain the symptoms, what happens when we find one? We are very likely to terminate the quest and explain the illness by the disease".[4]

Here are the health care dilemma and the paradox again. In medicine we have painted ourselves into a corner. As David Haslam says, 'we use the medical model because the medical model is what we use, even though it may not always be appropriate'.[5]

Screening

Screening for diseases that have not yet produced symptoms, or whose symptoms have not yet caused concern, or have not been reported, has also been called 'surveillance medicine'. It identifies what has been called the clinical iceberg, a mass of unmet medical need lying beneath the surface, invisible to the medical eye. Science makes screening possible because it learns to identify markers of latent disease and develops technology to detect them. It also, of course, seeks the means of prevention or early treatment. It saves lives and permits diseases that cannot be eradicated to be managed more effectively. It is not yet the case that all diseases that can be detected, or whose warning signs can be detected, can be treated or avoided.

It is the goal of research to find solutions to those problems; research that now often depends upon investigation and manipulation of the smallest components of our bodies, molecules, genes and cells. Research at this level invokes serious ethical controversy, as surrounded the proposed creation of 'hybrid embryos' (now abandoned). These controversies, and other ethical dilemmas in health care which relate to the definition and starting point of human life, of personhood, confront us with the metaphysical issues 'queuing at medicine's back door' (see Chapter 7). Ironically, these extreme successes of reductionist science, implicate us in the mystery of human nature, human wholeness, and healing in its widest sense.

Science also seeks to identify, and does successfully identify causes of disease in people's life-style or environment, as well as in their genes. The demonstration of the ill effects of smoking and the eventual legislation to control it, is perhaps the most familiar and most dramatic example of the success of this kind of applied science. The consequent constraints on people's life-style (the ban on smoking in public places), are resented by many who see them as an unwarranted curtailing of individual freedom, despite the huge reduction in smoking related deaths and sickness.

The extent to which screening constitutes one of the risks of being a patient is discussed in Chapter 8.

Normality and significance

The definition of disease and of the risk of disease depends to a great extent on the statistical concept of 'the normal range'. This is the range of measurements of a particular physical or physiological attribute that is judged to be consistent with normal good health and bodily function. The body-mass index defines obesity. The haemoglobin level defines anaemia. The level, and relative level of 'good' and 'bad' cholesterol (in relation to other factors) help to define the risk of heart attack or stroke. The top and bottom of the normal range are the measurements above or below which people are significantly more likely to experience the ill effects of a higher or lower level of whatever is being measured. Some people whose measurements are outside the normal range (too high or too low) will have no problem. Some whose measurements are within the normal range but towards the top or bottom will have problems. The normal range does not define normal health or well-being. It does not absolutely predict who will or will not have problems. It says that there is a certain probability that certain measurements indicate the presence or future possibility of problems.

Significance and probability determine the scientific judgement of normality, and of the justification for taking action to modify an 'abnormality'. They are based on statistics; calculations from standard mathematical formulae. Significance defines what matters and what needs to be taken seriously. Probability has to do with cause and effect. It predicts statistically whether a measurement or observation is likely to be the 'real' effect of a particular event, circumstance or activity, or whether the relationship is a matter of chance. It does not predict that the effect *will be* caused by it. Probability only relates directly to cause and effect. It does not relate to 'association'.

Causation and association are very different but often confused. An event or condition that is associated with a particular behaviour, for example, is not necessarily caused by it. Raised levels of cholesterol are strongly associated with coronary heart disease, but are not in themselves or alone the cause. Other factors come into play. Similarly, factors such as age affect the probability of an event and the calculation of the benefit of a particular treatment, so that the benefit in one age group or in one life situation may be quite different in another.

Another confusion is between the concepts of 'relative' and 'absolute' significance or risk. Significance may be exaggerated if it is presented as 'relative' rather than 'absolute'. An improvement from 1 in 1000 to 2 in 1000 in the risk of an event affecting the population (an act of nature, an accident, a disease), is a large relative improvement – 100% in fact. But it is still only an absolute improvement of 1 in 1000.

A tidy example is the trial of a drug for the prevention of fractures in women with bone mineral density significantly below the normal range (osteoporosis). The incidence (frequency of occurrence) of fractures of the vertebrae confirmed by X-ray was 3.8% in the group taking placebo (an inactive copy of the drug) and 2.1% in the group taking the drug itself. This represents a relative reduction in risk of 44%, but an absolute reduction in the number of women actually suffering fractures of 1.7%. And although reduced bone density is associated with fractures, it is not a sufficiently accurate predictor of an individual's risk of fracture to be used as a definitive guide to therapy.[6]

In everyday life, if we are asked to judge whether something is significant (matters, needs to be taken seriously), we might at first say, "It all depends". In everyday experience significance is dependent on other factors that impinge upon whatever it is that we are considering. In everyday life, the probability that something will happen, or that A is related to B, will similarly depend upon other factors that influence the turn of events. In everyday life every experience is multifaceted (there are several aspects to the experience), and multifactorial (several factors have combined to make the experience what it is). In real life every illness (the subjective experience of disorder), and the course of every disease (the onset, manifestation, progress and resolution of a pathological process), is also multifaceted and multifactorial.

But the prevailing scientific paradigm and the medical model cannot accommodate this diversity of human experience. In order to establish clear parameters for clinical decision making it has to assume a clear-cut distinction between normal and abnormal, significant and insignificant, probable and improbable. And in order to calculate those parameters it has to exclude the 'confounding variables', those facets of the problem and those factors that impinge upon it, which might complicate or confuse the assessment of the relationship between cause A and effect B. The evidence provided to practising clinicians on which in turn to base their decisions or interventions, is based on the clear-cut definitions of normality, significance and probability arrived at in this way. The scientific paradigm and the medical model cannot accommodate 'the sick person in all his wholeness and variability.'

Clinical epidemiology: a basic science for clinical medicine by David Sackett and others,[7] the so called 'bible of evidence based medicine', offers six definitions of normal in common clinical use:

- Distribution of diagnostic test results has a certain shape (pattern on a graph).
- (The observation) lies within a pre-set percentile (percentage range) of previous diagnostic test results.
- (It) carries no additional risk of morbidity or mortality.
- (The state) is socially or politically aspired to (regarded as desirable).
- (The observation represents a) range of test results beyond which a specific disease is, with known probability present or absent.
- (It represents a) range of test results beyond which treatment does more good than harm.

Bearing in mind the intention of those pioneers of evidence based medicine that the use of evidence should be weighed against individual clinical experience and expertise, these are observations that help us to decide whether to treat or not to treat; and to guard against the dangers I have mentioned of using relative risk as a measure of effect. But as we have seen, they may sometimes be given undue weight.

The great majority of medical research is directed to:

- The analysis of those 'discrete entities' mentioned earlier and the correction of their abnormalities.
- The quantitative assessment (that is measurable, as opposed to descriptive or qualitative) of the anatomical or physiological indicators of disorder.
- The efficacy of the methods (pharmacological or otherwise) introduced or already used to correct them. 'Efficacy' is the measure of whether something does what it is intended to do for a clearly defined population (group of patients) in ideal circumstances; that is with all the confounding variables controlled. Data from this research provide medicine's evidence base (see Chapter 10, Truth, Proof and Evidence).

These data (usually measurements) are inevitably, and necessarily, an abstraction from real life. They allow a lot of very useful things to be done, for which we can be grateful. But they do exclude the sick person, in all his or her wholeness and variability, from the physicians gaze. And that is one of the limitations of medicine. It is the reason for Engel's remark, "The enormous existing and planned investment in diagnostic and therapeutic technology alone strongly favours approaches to clinical study and care of patients that emphasise the impersonal and the mechanical";[8] an observation that still rings true. This is that part of the crisis in medicine (see Chapter 9) that he alleges, "derives from – the adherence to a model of disease no longer adequate for the scientific tasks of medicine".

The goal of science

There is no question that medicine needs the science that we already have. The argument is that it is inadequate, that its focus is too narrow. That it is pursuing increasingly sophisticated answers to some of the wrong questions. That science needs to rediscover its true breadth and eclecticism of enquiry, and to be more open to the allegedly improbable and implausible, if it is truly to enhance human healing.[9]

The goal of science is truth through knowledge. But there is an inescapable, essential and creative relationship between truth and uncertainty/doubt. As Schumacher warns in the quotation in the Introduction, "certainty can be the enemy of truth".[10] The strength of the scientific method is the forging of knowledge out of ideas and information by rigorous testing. But it can never finally determine the legitimate pathways of enquiry, nor the absolute criteria of certainty. To assume its competence to do so is, ironically, to take a philosophical and metaphysical position. It is also a position that sets bounds to further progress. It is the state of paradigm paralysis described earlier. As the quotation from Engel at the beginning of this section says, "The scientific attitude permits no such restrictions". We can have no absolute certainty about what constitutes human nature in all its amazing subtlety, nor about all that determines the course of illness and healing in any individual. The scientific vocation is to explore constantly and courageously the penumbra of uncertainty that surrounds our presumed and precarious certainties.

In summary, modern medical science is one of the glories of mankind, and it will become even more glorious when its reductionist focus is complemented by an expansionist vision, and its mechanistic skills by a humanist versatility.

The full quotation from *Science as Salvation* by the philosopher Mary Midgeley that I referred to earlier reads: "All human beings need some kind of mental map to show them the structure of the world. And we in the west have placed particular confidence in mapping it through methodical, detailed study . . . in general, methodical study has become increasingly divided and depersonalised, which is bound to make it less usable for each individual's understanding of life. The maps are being made to different standards. More and more, they are required to show fine detail correctly, less and less are they designed to show the whole territory needed for actual journeys. . . . We do not need to esteem science less. What we need is to esteem it in the right way. Especially we need to stop isolating it from the rest of life."[11]

References

1 Engel G. A unified concept of health and disease. *Perspect Biol Med.* 1960; 3:459–485.
2 Lyng S. *Holistic Health and Biomedical Medicine.* New York: State University of New York Press; 1990.
3 Kennedy I. *Unmasking medicine.* London: George Allen and Unwin; 1981.
4 Barbour A. *Caring for patients: a critique of the medical model.* Stanford: Stanford University Press; 1995.
5 Haslam D. Who cares? *Br J Gen Pract.* 2007; 57(545):987–993.
6 Moynihan R, Heath I, Henry D. Selling sickness: the pharmaceutical industry and disease mongering. *Br Med J.* 2002; 324:886–890.
7 Sackett DL, Haynes RB, Tugwell P. *Clinical Epidemiology: a basic science for clinical medicine.* Boston: Little Brown; 1985.
8 Engel G. The need for a new medical model. *Science* 1977; 196(4286);129–136.
9 Reilly D. Enhancing human healing. *Br Med J.* 2001; 322:120–121.
10 Schumacher E. *A Guide for the Perplexed.* London: Sphere; 1978.
11 Midgeley M. *Science as Salvation.* London: Routledge; 1992.

7

MEDICINE AND HEALING

Summary

- Medicine has always traditionally been associated with healing – with the biological process of recovery, repair and compensation, and the more comprehensive process that honours a wholeness of the person that transcends the bodily form.
- This wider perspective of healing is not an optional extra for medicine. It is medicine's *raison d'être.*
- Medicine's responsibilities vis-à-vis healing are: to support self-regulation and self-healing; to promote self-care; to intervene skilfully and compassionately when these fail; to enhance quality of life and quality of living – the value and meaning of life, including its transcendent aspect – whatever the prospect of cure.
- Medicine will fulfil its vocation and be more effective when it learns to use science in the service of healing. This is as much a matter of attitude as of practice.
- Medicine needs to distinguish between cure and healing (and treatment and healing) while it seeks to serve both.

The concept of healing is discussed in detail in Chapter 12, 'Design principles'. Here we are concerned with broader issues of the relationship between medicine and healing.

> The relationship between modern medicine and healing resembles a problem marriage. Medicine is a profession, a science and an art. Healing is an expression of a philosophy: a life force, biological and/or spiritual, whichever way you want to look at it and a process of reconciliation, which can also have a biological and spiritual meaning. The two are traditionally united by vocation, but medicine is losing touch with healing, and as in a precarious marriage, feelings and ideals are being forgotten, and becoming overlaid by false expectations and tactical problems. The failure to understand its relationship with healing, is, I believe, the true malaise of modern medicine.[1]

Medicine's responsibility for healing

Medicine has always been traditionally associated with healing. At the beginning of the book I pointed out the obvious fact that the capacity of organisms to heal spontaneously has been an evolutionary imperative. The goal of medicine has been to assist this biological process as far as possible and to take control when it fails, or to take control until the natural healing process can reassert itself. In Greek Mythology Asclepius was the god of healing, himself representing the more active interventionist approach, bringing external forces to bear to overcome the disorder and bring the individual back to an ordered state of health. His daughter Hygeia represents the more conservative health maintenance approach. In that tradition, health depends on a state of inner equilibrium and balance, and treatment aims to maintain or restore this equilibrium and encourage balance, not only between the individual's physical, emotional and spiritual aspects, but between the person and their environment. These two traditions are still represented in medicine today, of course. They reflect different paradigms of health and healing, and different models of health care. The other daughter of Asclepius, Panacea, remains sought after but unattainable.

This mythical and religious aspect of ancient medicine, and the association of medicine with religion over the centuries, emphasises that it was once concerned always with the whole person, body, mind and soul, or spirit. In some cultures and philosophies, indeed, for many health care professionals in our present day Western culture, it still is. Peter Morrell points out, "Ancient medicine was always integrated – a mind-body medicine rooted in a social and religious matrix of a culturally defined people with a definite belief system. . . . Much of the metaphysical element that was ejected from medicine centuries ago now queues at medicine's backdoor".[2] And so, the word 'healing', both historically and today has two senses: the biological process of recovery, repair and compensation by which organisms overcome or cope with defects, damage and disorder; and a more comprehensive process that honours a wholeness of the person that transcends the bodily form. A healing profession has traditionally been implicated in assisting and enabling both; until more secular, materialist and scientific times, that is. The fact that the personal and metaphysical dimensions of health and illness have been ejected from much mainstream medicine explains the great interest shown by many people in models of health care that do acknowledge and seek to respond to this subtle but indestructible aspect of human nature.

If medicine is to serve healing it has five responsibilities:

- To support the natural capacity of the body to regulate and heal itself
  - by encouraging a healthy life-style;
  - by enabling those self-healing and self-regulating processes;
  - by helping to avoid or remedy situations that are detrimental to those processes.
- To teach people to understand and manage distress and disorder that is within their personal competence for self-care or for the care of one another.
- To intervene, but only as far as and for as long as is necessary, in ways that relieve suffering and control disorder when those natural resources are impaired and until they are sufficiently recovered; or where that personal competence is too limited to cope.
- To respect the unique value of each individual, and to act in such a way as to enhance their quality of life (or as I shall suggest later, their quality of 'living'), regardless of the prospect of 'cure', the meaning and value of their life, their well-being or 'whole-being'. This will sometimes, and should more often, involve recognition of, and support for the patient's sense of the sacred and transcendent.

Right relationship

> If the distinguishing mark of clinical medicine is the healing relationship then it becomes central to the function of all physicians as physicians (Edmund Pellegrino[3])

It has been suggested that medicine needs to recover its 'soul'.[4] This means its expression of concern for the individual, for the personal experience, narrative and meaning of the illness, and for the enrichment of that individual's life that in however modest a way medicine can bring. I have expressed my regret that the relationship between medicine and healing resembles a broken marriage. As in so many failed relationships, the two partners have stopped talking to each other. Or perhaps that is not quite the case; rather that one partner, the biomedical partner long ago stopped listening. An essential goal of any remodelling process must be that the intimacy of this relationship should be restored.

The relationship actually exists intact in many encounters between patients and doctors, but it is under strain. The ideals described in the previous section, 'Medicine and the Individual', have not been abandoned. Essential to the healing relationship is trust. A key 'aphorism' in the *Oxford Handbook of Clinical Medicine* is, 'Where there is no trust there is little healing',[5] and in *The Human Effect in Medicine* Dixon and Sweeney list trustworthiness, together with self-discipline, humility, tolerance and patience as tools necessary to any clinical activity. But they make the point that these attributes are not to be separated from the use of scientific knowledge but are the context for its use.[6]

Medicine will fulfil its vocation, and be more effective, when it learns to use its science in the service of healing. This requires more than the ability to analyse, control and manipulate body functions and disease processes that is the supreme achievement of medical science. It does not require a major revolution, simply that it directs more of its attention to those things that it knows perfectly well are fundamental to its purpose – the integrity of the person who is its patient, and the natural healing resources that he or she, to some degree even in conditions of most severe damage and disability, possesses.

This is as much a matter of attitude as of practice. It is our attitude to one-another, in any relationship let alone a therapeutic relationship that confers meaning and value on the other person; a theme that will recur later. James Marcum quotes from a contributor to the book *Changing Values in Medicine* who argues that 'by reducing the body to a collection of parts, the patient as a person vanishes before the physician's gaze.'[7] That is literally *de-meaning,* and it does happen. Marcum himself asserts that, "The meaning that a patient attaches to illness and suffering, especially in chronic or fatal illness, is critical for the healing process – and that meaning is accessible through the patient's illness story"; if the opportunity is provided for it to be told. That quotation includes the intriguing and important, but apparently contradictory reference to a healing process as part even of a fatal illness.

Healing, treatment and cure

Medicine fails in its broader healing goal because of its narrow biomedical focus in a number of ways. Engel put it bluntly in his paper, saying 'Rational treatment directed only at the biochemical abnormality does not necessarily restore the patient to health, even in the face of documented correction or major alleviation of the abnormality'.[8] Alan Barbour, who was a hospital clinician, makes a similar point, elaborating it as an account of the various misconceptions and false starts that the clinical process can pursue:[9]

> "The disease is not the cause of the illness."
> "The disease itself results entirely or partly from the life situation, but the treatment is purely biomedical."

"Personal distress unrelated to the disease is superimposed (upon it). Compounding the problem of diagnosis and treatment."
"The disease is caused by multiple factors, but the medical model focuses on one particular cause or treatment."
"(The disease is a substantial primary problem, but) it is a *person* . . . who needs to surmount the illness with new value and meaning."

Howard Brody reflects the last point in particular in the description of the several possible levels of resolution of an illness:[10]

"I simply recover completely and return to the status quo."
"I make an accommodation with my rebellious body and resign myself to a different way of functioning."
"I come to listen more sympathetically to my body, to see it as a source of values that legitimately should play a role in how I live my life, and not simply as having value only when it carries out the wishes of other aspects of the self."

That last level represents a new experience of self-affirmation and self-respect; a new and better way of loving ourselves that is quite different from egotism. This is essential to the healing goal of medicine; the proper kind of self-esteem.

Medicine needs to distinguish between cure and healing (and treatment and healing) while it seeks to serve both. Alan Barbour explains it in this way: "Whereas curing and treatment refer primarily to what is done *to the patient,* healing includes, in addition to the treatment, all forces that combine to restore and foster health – the biologic mechanisms of defence and repair; the personal qualities of the doctor, the patient and their relationship; the overall understanding engendered; the social unit in which the patient lives; and the patient's ultimate propensity, latent in everyone, to restore, strengthen, and enhance physical, emotional, social, and spiritual health."[9]

This wider perspective of healing is not an optional extra for medicine, not a luxury to be afforded when time permits. It is medicine's *raison d'être.* Nor is it merely a somewhat academic philosophical and ethical context for the practice of medicine. Nor is there any discontinuity between the principles that govern the physical mechanisms of bodily healing, and the principles that govern healing on other levels of the person and of the disordered circumstances of that person's life that are implicated in the illness (see Chapter 12, 'Healing'). The condition of our bodies, the quality, meaning and value of our personal lives, our contribution to the lives of others and our relationships with one another, and our role in society, even when that is a dependent role, and even our interaction with our physical environment, are inextricably interconnected. No one health care professional can offer help on all these levels, and of course they are not necessarily implicated in meeting needs on all these levels. But no medical intervention is unaffected by what is happening on those other levels that are not the direct and immediate focus of its attention; nor fails to affect them.

The realisation of this may be peripheral to a doctor's consciousness of the task in hand, but it is not irrelevant, and should be part of the 'tacit' knowledge of his or her role. That is the kind of knowledge (described by Michael Polanyi) that is not part of the formal and conscious protocol by which we perform a task, but that subtly informs and influences its performance.[11] This more diffuse knowledge or insight not only enhances the performance of a task but also the personal satisfaction we gain from it. In a medical context it enhances patient and doctor satisfaction.

Awareness of this broader healing perspective for medical activity has two advantages. First it encourages us to recognise that there are certain basic principles that are common to healing processes on different levels. And second, it changes the expectations we may have of what medicine can or should achieve.

Healing is not a matter of remedying defects, relieving symptoms, or modifying pathological changes. These things may be a part of the process or a result of the process, but they are not in themselves the process or the purpose of healing; and healing is not necessarily the same as cure. Such narrowness will also blind us to the possibility that disease or illness may not actually be the antagonist of healing, but also the agent, drawing attention, if well handled, to the adverse circumstances that caused or predisposed us to the illness, and creating the opportunity for change. Whether or not you accept that particular concept, we may agree that understanding and change are often important ingredients of healing. We would I'm sure agree that understanding and change are often difficult and painful to achieve, for both doctor and patient. That is why they will both settle for second best as often as not, and choose a palliative prescription instead.

As Kafka remarks in his short story *A Country Doctor*, "To write a prescription is easy, but to come to an understanding with people is hard".[12] To help them to come to an understanding with themselves is harder still.

Healing is a universal quality and a universal process. We all possess natural powers of healing in our own body, mind, and spirit. We all have access to personal qualities which can assist healing in other people. There are many techniques of treatment, from wart charming to neurosurgery.

These are contributions towards healing which only specialists can make. But any person may contribute compassion, empathy, and insight. Healing is not bestowed upon people by doctors. Indeed, I do not think any individual, practitioner or therapist, conventional, complementary or religious, should assume the title 'healer'.

Doctors and others do not *make* people better; they help them to get better. And so do friends, neighbours, comedians, poets, and the makers of Guinness.[13]

References

1 Swayne J. Medicine and healing: A broken marriage? *New Society* 1976; 491–492.

2 Morrell P. Integrated medicine: orthodox meets alternative. Integrated medicine is not new. (Letter). *Br Med J.* 2001; 322:168–169.

3 Pellegrino E. The healing relationship: the architectonics of clinical medicine. In: Shelp E. *The Clinical Encounter: the moral fabric of the patient-physician relationship.* Dordrecht: Reidel Publishing; 1983.

4 Smith R. Editor's choice: Restoring the soul of medicine. *Br Med J.* 2001; 322. Available online at http://tinyurl.com/3hjkvxb

5 Longmore MW. *Oxford Handbook of Clinical Medicine.* 7th edition. Oxford: Oxford University Press; 2007.

6 Dixon M, Sweeney K. *The Human Effect in Medicine.* Oxford: Radcliffe; 2004.

7 Marcum J. Biomechanical and phenomenological models of the body, the meaning of illness and quality of care. *Medicine, Health Care and Philosophy* 2004; 311–320.

8 Engel G. The need for a new medical model. *Science* 1977; 196:129–136.

9 Barbour A. *Caring for patients: a critique of the medical model.* Stanford: Stanford University Press; 1995.

10 Brody H. *Stories of Sickness.* New Haven: Yale University Press; 1987.

11 Polanyi M. *Personal Knowledge.* London: Routledge; 2002.

12 Kafka F. *A Country Doctor, in the Penal Settlement.* London: Secker and Warburg; 1949.

13 Swayne J. On our best behaviour. *J R Coll Gen Pract.* 1976; 26:560–564.

8

THE PATIENT'S PERSPECTIVE

Summary

- The experience of being a patient is at the heart of medicine. And it is the *quality* of this experience that will have a great deal to do with the outcome.
- Illness, sickness, diagnosis, disease and suffering are distinctively different experiences, and present different challenges.
- 'The health care dilemma' is medicine's capacity to heal and to harm.
- Precise biomedical analysis of disorder is like the precision of digital sound reproduction, with the proviso that something may be lost in the digital transcription.
- The more a society spends on health the more likely are its inhabitants to regard themselves as sick. Medicine can create illness by the way that problems are construed and treated. Our surgeries and clinics are home to many 'partial patients'.
- "When health becomes the goal of human endeavour it acquires an oppressive influence over the life of the individual."
- Respondents to a *British Medical Journal* debate about what makes a good doctor identify personal qualities more prominently than proficiency in knowledge and technical skills.
- Key determinants of the patient's perspective are the use of time, patient-centredness, the management of expectations, the degree of trust, compassion and empathy, and continuity of care.

Being a patient

> This first person perspective became important to me. I felt that during my frequent dealings with the medical and healthcare professionals it was neglected. No one asked me what had changed in my life or what I had I had to give up because of my illness. Overlooking the lived experience of illness is a mistake because there is so much important knowledge to be gleaned from it – for example, that the most effective intervention might be helping the patient to

> regain their everyday life despite their illness. The ultimate aim of medicine is to help those who are ill regain their life, habits and activities. But it is impossible to do this without knowing about the patient's usual life and how it has been affected by illness. (Havi Carel[1])

The experience of being a patient is at the heart of medicine. It is perhaps the one life experience we will all share apart from birth and death (both of which in Western medicine are likely to involve us in the patient role). And it is the *quality* of this experience that will have a great deal to do with the outcome. But nowadays the experience is not limited to encounters with doctors or other healthcare professionals when we feel ill, or are born or die. Health is a cultural preoccupation. And health awareness, and consequently our perception of ourselves as in some sense patients, is stimulated by an array of influences from popular magazines to government edicts, regardless of how our bodies are behaving.

Illness, Sickness, Diagnosis, Disease and Suffering

Wonder drug stole my memory was the title of a newspaper article telling the tale of the journalist's misfortunes following the prescription of a statin, a drug to lower his blood cholesterol level.[2] The story is a nice example of what we mean by the words that provide the title of this section; words that we use to describe the experience of being a patient. And it is a nice example of medicine's responsibility for health and illness – that is, medicine's responsibility to keep us well, *and* medicine's responsibility for sometimes making us ill, known as iatrogenesis (created by doctors) – the healthcare dilemma.[3]

Mr Hudson, whose medical history is summarised in figure 8.1, was pretty healthy, except for moderately high cholesterol, but he became a patient when that moderately high cholesterol was detected, perhaps by routine screening. Raised cholesterol is a risk factor for heart disease. It is not necessarily a cause of heart disease. It may do no harm at all. But there is an increased risk of heart disease if the cholesterol level is raised. Statins significantly reduce the incidence of heart disease in people at high risk by lowering the cholesterol level. Other factors adding to a high risk of heart disease are a family history of heart trouble, particularly at a young age, raised blood pressure,

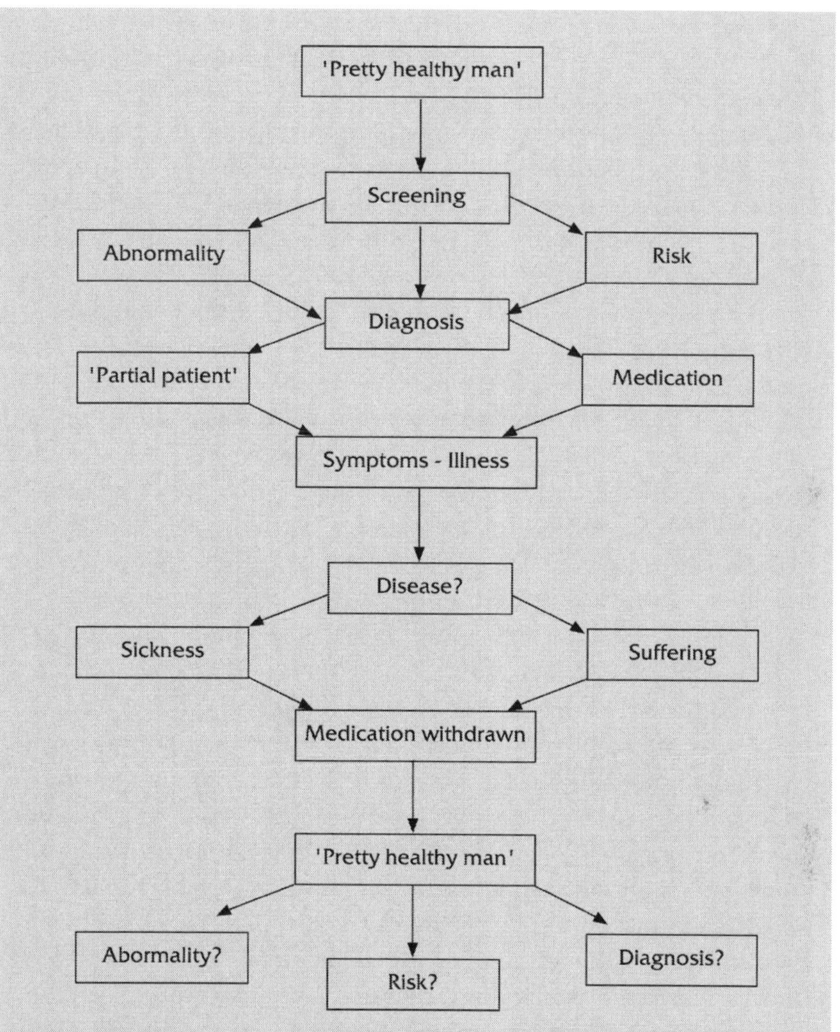

Figure 8.1 Mr Hudson's medical history.

smoking, overweight, and a sedentary life style; and certain other co-existing conditions such as diabetes. But because GPs are required to screen for raised cholesterol, many people who feel well and consider themselves to be in normal health, and who will never have a heart attack, will be detected with raised cholesterol. They find they are not in 'normal' health after all. They have become patients, or at least 'partial patients',[4] and may be put on medication. They have acquired a diagnosis – hypercholesterolaemia (or hyperlipidaemia), too much cholesterol (or fat) in the blood. They do not have a disease exactly

– or do they? There may be no pathological changes in their body, but they are not quite 'normal' are they?

Becoming a patient and having a diagnosis changes us, to a greater or lesser degree, depending on the circumstances and our personality. We have all experienced this. We see ourselves slightly differently. We may feel slightly different. Being a patient is a role. We are not just a (lower case) patient, someone who goes to a doctor. We are also a (upper case) Patient, someone with a new status, new responsibilities or needs perhaps, a new routine in life. This is obviously true if we feel there is something wrong with us and want something done about it. But it is also true if we feel well but have acquired a diagnosis and now wear the label 'Patient'. Which is what happens when routine screening reveals a risk factor, or more worryingly early signs of an actual disease. And it is the fact that becoming a Patient is likely to affect us 'worryingly' when we previously felt well that may be a cause of illness.

Illness is a feeling that all is not well (obviously); that something is wrong with us; that something, even the common cold, is interfering with our normal equilibrium, the familiar emotional or physical pattern of our life. We develop symptoms. A change like this may be so trivial or commonplace (exam nerves, for example) that we would not, and should not regard it as illness. But our individual tolerance of such things varies greatly. The common cold and nervousness cause symptoms – changes in our physical or emotional state. But symptoms that may be a normal and acceptable reaction to events for one person may amount to a disability for another. Becoming labelled with a diagnosis when we previously felt well is likely to cause symptoms – negligible and taken for granted for some, but distressing for others, making them ill.

We do not know whether the discovery of his raised cholesterol adversely affected the journalist in question in this way. He may have taken it in his stride. But after a time he developed symptoms. He did not associate these with the treatment of his hypercholesterolaemia at first, but his memory was increasingly impaired, and he also developed poor circulation in his fingers and toes. All was not well. Because he did not attribute the symptoms to the treatment he considered other explanations – some kind of incipient dementia for the memory loss, perhaps; the repetitive strain of his furious two-finger typing for the poor circulation in his fingers. The memory loss and its association with dementia caused what sounds like a sense of dread – "a gripping sensation around the heart." It was an unhappy time for both him and his wife who said, "I thought that this was how life was going to be for the next 30 years." Not only did he have specific and distressing symptoms, but they were both evidently ill with anxiety. He also became unusually reclusive for fear of making a fool of himself in public. His symptoms interfered with his golf and his tennis, and his use of words, the tools of his trade. He became a sick man, in the sense that his illness compromised his ability to be himself and take his usual place in the world.

He was also suffering. He was distressed in a variety of ways. He was embarrassed, fearful; even at times, reading between the lines, humiliated. He suffered loss of integrity, in the sense of being a less integrated person; and of meaning, in the sense of following his vocation and enjoying his relationships. Technically he also had a disease in that his condition involved pathological, though ultimately reversible, changes in the brain and his extremities due to the known put poorly understood effects of some statins in some people.

This story has a happy ending because the symptoms resolved when Mr Hudson eventually discovered their possible association with the drug, and stopped taking it. I am grateful to him for sharing his experience publicly for a number of reasons. Firstly, it is a helpful illustration:

- Of the nature of illness: a subjective state in which we experience symptoms which disturb the normal equilibrium of our life, causing discomfort or inconvenience.
- Of the concept of disease: observable disorder of body tissues or functions.
- Of sickness: a state in which illness or disease interfere with our normal social functions and relationships.
- Of suffering: distress compounded of physical and/or emotional symptoms with loss of our sense of meaning and integrity as a person.
- Of the part played by diagnosis in establishing the patient state, or role, regardless of the presence or absence of underlying disease.

The second reason for gratitude is that it illustrates 'the health care dilemma'. This is its ambiguous character – its capacity to heal and to harm. The direct risk of adverse effects, and the indirect risk of turning well people into patients, the so called 'medicalisation of life'; both with the admirable aim of saving lives and reducing disability.

The story's illustration of the health care dilemma also highlights two related issues mentioned in Chapter 6. One is the difference between cause and association: raised cholesterol is not in itself a cause of disease although it is associated with increased risk of disease. The other is the difference between relative risk and absolute risk: an apparently large reduction in the relative risk of a particular event as a result of treatment may translate into a very small reduction in the absolute number of people who suffer the event. The health care dilemma lies in 'penalising' the many people ('partial patients') who show an associated risk factor for the sake of the (relatively) few for whom it represents a serious risk, by instituting health-care regimes on the basis of statistics of relative risk, when the absolute benefits affect a far smaller number.

The third reason to value this story is that it is a story. Through its narrative it brings to life this person's predicament, this couple's predicament in all its complexity. In fact it must implicate their friends and colleagues, too, who would have been touched to some extent by their predicament. It is a story of a non-disease with a happy ending, but it has many of the ingredients of all stories of sickness.

And finally a key reason for including it in this chapter – the story illustrates medicine's responsibility towards the individual, as against its responsibility towards society. It emerges as the consequence of a public health campaign based on good science and with admirable aims. But it concerns the unique and personal predicament of a particular individual, as does every episode of illness, disease, sickness and suffering.

The 'Digital' patient

> The demands on a doctor are less complicated when the problem that confronts him or her is one of straightforward, exclusively physical illness. Unfortunately there is no such thing. Any illness involves some degree of fear, pain, embarrassment, uncertainty, shame or guilt – as well as loss of status, earnings, independence or confidence.[5]

The prevailing model of clinical practice has already been characterised as being based on our increasing ability to control and manipulate body function and disease processes and engineer solutions to hitherto intractable problems. These skills depend upon a range of other advances in science and technology that provide increasingly sophisticated diagnostic and surgical techniques and pharmacological interventions. They include for example developments in genetic and stem cell research, drugs precisely targeted on cancer cells, and non-invasive surgical techniques. The power of developments such as these to modify disease processes and defects is immense. So of course is the cost.

Medicine is driven by science through the insights and influence of many different disciplines, and by the technological possibilities they give rise to. The dominant medical model is called a mechanistic model, often pejoratively by its critics, because it treats the human organism rather like a faulty machine, or a machine that can be predicted to develop a fault. It is called a reductionist model because, in increasingly minute detail, it reduces the machine to an assemblage of separate, or sometimes to a limited extent interactive component parts, and analyses and addresses its faults in those terms.

This analysis can now be achieved with great precision. It has been likened to the precision of sound reproduction that digital technology provides, but with the proviso that something may be lost in the digital transcription. David Haslam believes that for people who are as passionate about music and electronic gadgetry as he is, something very special may be lost in digital as opposed to analogue recording, and fears that there is an analogy here to patient care; that, "our digital templated world poses a risk of missing the analogue subtlety of our patients' lives".[6] In a *British Medical Journal* editorial, 'Enhancing human healing', David Reilly uses the same metaphor when he writes, "Creative medical caring might – require balancing short term, analytical, quick fix thinking with analogic holistic processing".[7]

But it would be very surprising if anyone reading this has not benefited from some medical intervention that has emerged from this 'digital' model, and is not extremely glad of it. We would be very reluctant to forego any of its benefits, as the heated arguments about rationing of healthcare and the availability of sophisticated but costly treatments demonstrate. It may be a relatively small minority of patients who will need the increasingly sophisticated and increasingly costly investigations and treatments that are continuously being developed, but no one wishes to be denied them, by dictat of the National Institute for Clinical Excellence (NICE) or by the 'post code lottery' of local budgeting policy. So was Illich's prediction that progress in the medical 'industry' would yield diminishing returns, and unaffordable returns at that, misplaced? That question still requires a thoughtful answer.

The risks of being a patient

> Treating blood pressure is one of the least satisfying activities in the whole of medicine, turning people who feel well and have no idea that there is anything 'wrong' with them into life-long tablet takers who often experience side effects of one type or another. (James Willis, General Practitioner)[8]

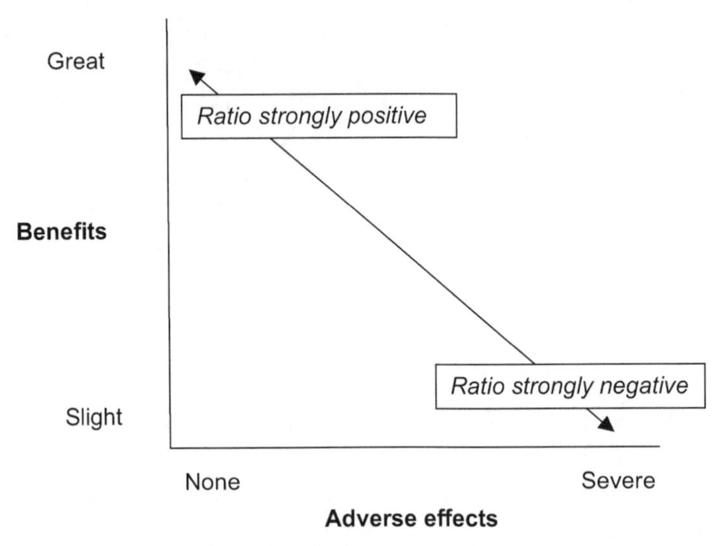

Figure 8.2 *The therapeutic ratio of medical care.*

Ivan Illich's critique of medicine highlighted clinical iatrogenesis, the burden of clinical damage caused by modern medicine, which he predicted would come to outweigh the clinical benefits.[9] Contemporary doctors share this concern. The first leader in a themed edition of the *British Medical Journal* addressing readers concerns about 'the medicalisation of life' carried the title, 'Too much medicine? Almost certainly'. Commenting, "... presumably few would agree with Ivan Illich that 'The medical establishment has become a major threat to health'. Many might, however, accept the concept ... that increasing medical inputs will at some point become counterproductive and produce more harm than good".[10] And they quoted the editorial that followed giving an analysis of data revealing that the more a society spends on health care the more likely are its inhabitants to regard themselves as sick.[11]

The 'therapeutic ratio' is a calculation of the balance between the advantages and disadvantages of a particular procedure in a particular individual (see Figure 8.2). Amputation of a leg that is the site of a sarcoma (a particularly vicious cancer) will result in disability but may save a life. The therapeutic ratio is positive. The therapeutic ratio for a drug that might cause adverse effects to a patient found to have raised blood pressure, who is feeling well but is *statistically* at risk of developing a stroke or heart attack but may never do so, is less easy to assess and may be negative. Judging the therapeutic ratio for an individual should be an automatic discipline whenever a medical intervention is planned. *All* medical interventions carry risks, and the potential for direct risk is a factor in any decision to intervene.

But Illich is suggesting that the therapeutic ratio for the whole of medicine, the cumulative consequences of all medical interventions including investigations and prophylaxis, is already or will inevitably become negative. Medicine as we know it, he argues, is bound to do more harm than good. He includes in this assessment not only treatments that although undoubtedly of potential benefit cause adverse effects, but also unnecessary investigations that may be undertaken for the 'worried well', or the antibiotics still prescribed for self-limiting infections to meet patient expectations for something to be done. He also includes treatments and investigations ordered to avoid any possible suit for malpractice on the basis that not everything had been done that might have been done.

The alarmingly high levels of illness and death resulting directly from medical interventions are well recognised and deplored. Audit of such events is required and corrective measures are proposed. The same is true of the harmful consequences of medical care that are not the direct effect of medical interventions but the consequence of being caught up in the medical system, such as hospital acquired infections.

Illich also includes in this category of iatrogenic harm the psychological effects of screening and predictive diagnostic procedures. These have increased in number and sophistication since he wrote, and their capacity to cause anxiety, and to swell the population of the worried well is recognised. So too is the burden of unnecessary medication resulting from them. In his paper 'Who cares?', David Haslam writes, "I sometimes wonder whether our obsession with screening for disease has had the side effect of creating illness".[5] This idea that medicine creates illness has been echoed by others since Illich, too. The problem is explored at length in 'The Tyranny of Diagnosis', by Charles Rosenberg.[12] *The Health Care Dilemma*[2] expressed it in terms of the "authority of doctors to decide whether or not to confer a disease on their patient". In his 1981 BBC Reith Lectures, *Unmasking Medicine,* Ian Kennedy accused medicine of creating illness by the way that distress arising from causes that are not primarily pathological but personal and social, is construed and treated.[13] And although Howard Brody also wrote about the value of a diagnosis itself as treatment, he was equally clear that when physicians diagnose a condition they may be creating illness "just as a lawmaker creates crime".[14] A perfect example of this is presented in an editorial in the *British Medical Journal* expressing concern about the development of a new version of an established classification of mental illness that is widely used around the world – the *Diagnostic and Statistical Manual of Mental Disorders (DSM).*[15] The new draft version under discussion, scheduled to appear in 2013, is the fifth of its kind, DSM-V, and the author's concern is that it will multiply the unwitting contribution of its predecessor, DSM-IV, to the creation of "epidemics" of false positive diagnoses of mental illness. That is, a marked increase in the attribution of certain diagnoses to patients whose condition did not actually warrant them, on the basis of the indications listed for those diagnoses in the Manual. The author identifies three of these epidemics, and fears that the new classification could potentially set off eight more, "In their (well meaning) efforts to innovate, (the proposals) could expand the territory of mental disorder and thin the ranks of the normal. . . . Because the suggested changes all occur at the boundary between mental disorder and normality, they could create vast numbers of misdiagnosed new patients." Remember, too, the similar problem described by Mike Fitzpatrick, which I outlined in Chapter 5.

The story quoted at the beginning of this chapter is another eloquent example of this problem – the use of the cholesterol-lowering group of drugs called statins, often quoted in the face of their increasingly widespread use as one kind of illness creation. Hundreds of patients at risk need to be identified and treated (the number needed to treat), and so labelled as potentially ill, to avoid a handful of serious cardio-vascular problems. It is good news for the few individuals in whom the problem will be avoided; although of course neither they nor anyone else will ever know exactly who it is that, thankfully, is saved by it. But it is not such good news for the hundreds who do not need the drug because they are not that statistically predictable but anonymous few. Statins have other preventive benefits as well, which will reduce the number needed to treat in proportion to the smaller number who actually benefit, but the point is clear. Cholesterol levels are one measurement that has statistical significance in the assessment of risk. They are important to the unidentified few who would fall victim to that risk without treatment. But they are a burden to the similarly unidentified many who would not – the 'partial patients'.

One of the editorials in the themed 'medicalisation of medicine' edition of the *British Medical Journal* in 2002, focusing on the unaffordable cost of increasing medicalisation, takes statins as a case in point. Emphasising their modest impact on major morbidity and mortality (disease and death), and the staggering cost of achieving these benefits for the minority of patients who avoid serious events, the authors comment that, "Extending therapy to a non-diseased population may also have important ethical implications, as treatment with statins may lead to perceptions of illness".[16]

And the problem has not gone away. A 2008 editorial 'Strategies for prescribing Statins' in the same journal details the lack of clarity and certainty in research data. It does not inspire confidence in the benefits of the sort of widespread programme of treatment that is being advocated. It concludes, "Despite the results of recent high dose statin trials, it is unclear whether possible benefit really translates into clinical practice. All we can say is that everyone at *high* risk of cardiovascular complications (and anyone with manifest disease) should be offered a standard dose of statin".[17] (My italics) Nevertheless, although the benefits of the 'treat to target' approach are particularly questionable, the UK Quality and Outcomes Framework emphasises the importance of measuring cholesterol and having targets. This is particularly ironic in relation to the many debilitating, but of course less measurable, conditions that it does not encompass (see David Oliver's remarks in Chapter 4).

In this context we may have some sympathy with Illich's comment that, "With this first measurement (the specific gravity of urine), doctors began to read diagnostic and curative meaning into any new measurement they learned to perform".[9] David Haslam reflects, "I believe it is now well accepted that our state of well being as humans is derived from cultural and social influences rather than simply absence of disease. But when we get someone through our door, we now feel a duty – driven by a complex mix of ethical, altruistic, legal and financial reasons – to screen them for conditions they didn't know about, and offer lifelong treatments for something that may never have happened".[6] It is reported that the American Academy of Pediatrics and the American Heart Association have recommended treating children as young as 8 who present risk factors for cardiovascular disease with statins, and even from the age of 2 where there are major risks; preventative treatment that would be lifelong.

It seems we are moving away from the wise precept that, "Clinical practice requires the establishment of agreed cut off points to identify disease and separate people for whom treatment should be beneficial from other patients for whom the risks of diagnosis or treatment might outweigh the benefits".[18]

The January 12th 2008 edition of the *British Medical Journal* carried a review of a book about medicine in the United States that began, "Yet another book about the healthcare 'system' everyone loves to hate". The title of the book, by Shannon Brownlee, is *Overtreated: Why too much medicine is making us sicker and poorer.*[19] Elsewhere in the same edition of the *British Medical Journal*, an analysis paper titled 'On the trail of quality and safety in health care', begins with the sentence, "Despite many years of effort and numerous programmes to improve the quality and safety of health care, major problems persist".[20] Successive episodes of the BBC Radio 4 medical programme *Case Notes* (Jan 29th and Feb 5th, 2008) addressed, respectively, the problem of adverse drug reactions, and the problem of hospital acquired infections. Within the same seven days the BBC Radio 4 programme *The Moral Maze* tackled the clinical, ethical and political implications of the increasing unaffordability of modern medicine, and the morality of rationing. Some of Illich's pronouncements seem to have been more prophetic than he was given credit for at the time.

As far as I know there is no research that quantifies the *cumulative* therapeutic ratio of all medical interventions – the total sum of the distress, illness and death they cause weighed against the total sum of improved quality of life they achieve. We would like to believe that the ratio is strongly positive. But unless we know for sure, Illich's pessimistic predictions must be always at the back of our minds. And whatever the actual balance, we do know that the incidence of sickness (in its broadest sense) that is the direct or indirect consequence of the practice of medicine is very high. This alone might justify the conclusion that the model is not working very well.

Awareness, participation and choice

Health awareness

"When health becomes the goal of human endeavour it acquires an oppressive influence over the life of the individual. If people's lives are ruled by measures they believe may help to prolong their existence, the quality of their lives is diminished." These warning words come from the book by Michael Fitzpatrick called *The Tyranny of Health*.[21] Its purpose is summarised as to expose the dangers of the explosion of health awareness for patients and doctors. It argues that health propaganda is having a very unhealthy affect upon the nation. Patients are made unnecessarily anxious as a result of health scares that have greatly exaggerated the risks of everyday activities. Doctors are encouraged by government to tell people how to live more and more aspects of their lives. NHS reforms push doctors into playing a wider role in regulating their patients' behaviour and rationing the allocation of resources. There is a need to establish a clear boundary between the worlds of medicine and politics, so that doctors can concentrate on treating the sick – and leave the well alone.

That summary expresses the core of the argument, but the book covers a lot of ground very thoroughly. For example, he discusses in detail the implications of the problem of 'the normal range' that I raised in Chapter 6, with regard to several aspects of our lives and everyday activities; implications that have generated clinical guidelines and legislation whose justification remains open to question.

The trouble is that the situation is even more complicated than the particular and deliberate focus of the book implies. In his conclusion Michael Fitzpatrick explicitly states a theme that is central to *Remodelling Medicine*, "The first responsibility of a doctor *as a doctor* is to provide medical treatment for *individual patients*". Proposing a much more restricted definition of medical practice, he says, "(this) does not mean that doctors should ignore the social determinants of illness and disease. It means distinguishing clearly between taking up these issues in a political and in a medical way". A few pages previously he has written, "We have considered two interlinked trends which have the effect of diminishing individual autonomy: the medicalisation of life and the politicisation of medicine". It is certainly true that these two trends do interact in the way he suggests. And it is true that together they do have a controlling influence that diminishes both individual freedom and individual responsibility. But the relationship is not two-way between medicalisation and politicisation, but three-way, actively involving the role of patients.

Participation and choice

> The programme aims to facilitate the telling, shaping, and preservation of the unwritten and unspoken stories of healthcare so that those who devise and implement strategy, as well as those directly involved in care, can act in a more informed, effective, compassionate and humane manner.[22]

This note from the 'Minerva' pages of the *British Medical Journal* drew attention to the programme *Patient Voices* on the website www.pilgrim projects.co.uk. produced by Pilgrim Projects. The Patient Voices rationale reads:

> The Patient Voices programme is partly an attempt to redress the balance of power between healthcare clinicians and managers and the people they serve, and partly an attempt to give decision-makers a different kind of opportunity to understand the needs of patients – other than the dry results of surveys and statistics. If patients are really to be 'at the heart of healthcare', as the Department of Health suggests they should be, then their views and their stories are of paramount importance in any attempt to reform health care services.
>
> Patient Voices are short (typically less than three minutes) digital stories combining video, audio, still images and music that reveal patients' stories in a unique way.
>
> They:
>
> - Can highlight gaps in the system.
> - Can reveal near-misses and form 'free learning opportunities'.
> - Promote healing and reconciliation.

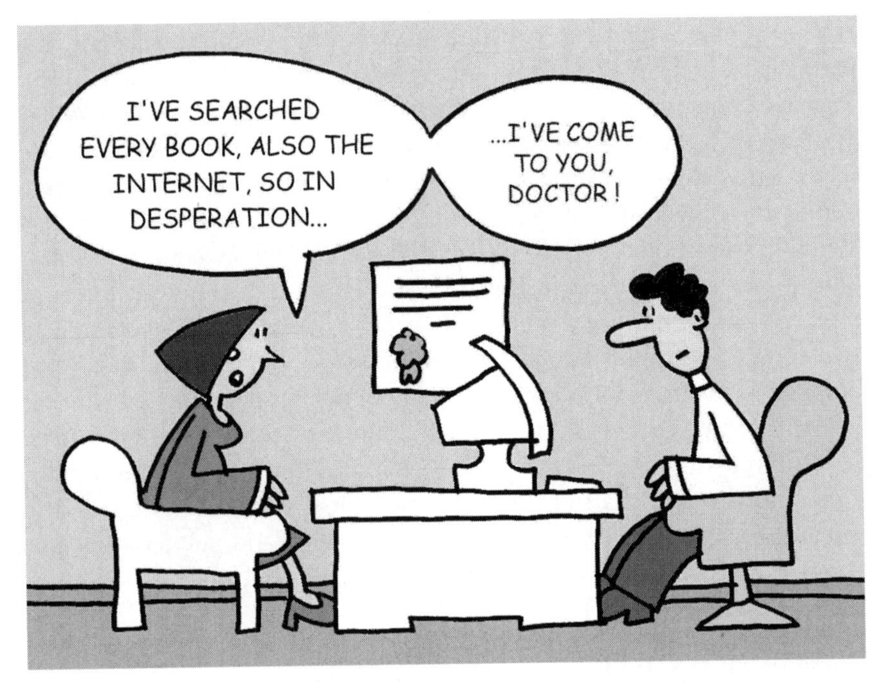

Figure 8.3 *The internet now plays a large part in healthcare.*

> - Can allow patients' and carers' (and professionals if appropriate) voices to be heard.
> - Can carry forward stories that might otherwise be lost.
> - Are created in a spirit of collaboration and partnership.
> - Are intended to touch hearts, thereby reinforcing the notion of patients at the heart of care.
>
> The Patient Voices programme aims to capture some of the unwritten and unspoken stories of ordinary people so that those who devise and implement strategy, as well as clinicians directly involved in care, may carry out their duties in a more informed and compassionate manner.

I warmly recommend that you visit the website and listen to the stories, and learn about the workshops in which they are collected.

The existence of this programme (as well as the www.healthtalkonline.org site already mentioned), its aim and its content, tell us or remind us of a number of things: that the internet now plays a large part in healthcare; that for all the surveys demonstrating patient satisfaction there are still unmet patient needs that are primarily personal rather than biomedical; and that it should lie within the human resources of a health service to meet; and that patients' voices, our voices, are increasingly to be heard and represented in healthcare planning and provision – if planners and providers are willing to listen. The patient perspective is achieving increasing recognition and importance – at least, in theory.

This rapidly accelerating trend towards patient participation in healthcare, and access to information from many sources, including the internet, is *SWOT*-laden (if you know that piece of project planning jargon). In other words, it has many *Strengths*, and not a few *Weaknesses*. It offers great *Opportunities*, and carries real *Threats*. The dilemma lies in achieving a truly healthy balance between the benefits of better information, greater knowledge, participation and choice on the one hand, and the risks of confusion, exploitation and the medicalisation of life on the other.

Relationship

> I remember the time Shipman gave to my Dad. He would come round at the drop of a hat. He was a marvellous GP apart from the fact that he killed my father. (Christopher Rudol[23])

'What's a good doctor and how do you make one?'

This was the title of a themed edition of the *British Medical Journal* in 2002 whose first leader was headed by the above quotation.[24] These excerpts gleaned from a survey of opinions from patients and readers, and from several of the articles by a variety of clinicians and academics give a flavour of the discussion:

> "The most highly rated aspect of care was humaneness, followed by competence/accuracy, patients' involvement in decisions and time for care."
>
> "Readers from 24 countries responding to a *British Medical Journal* debate about what makes a good doctor allude to desirable personal qualities more prominently than proficiency in knowledge and technical skills."
>
> "When good (as an adjective) qualifies doctor, a great deal of its meaning is determined by what is meant by doctor."
>
> "A poor doctor is generally credited with good intentions but inadequate knowledge and skills."
>
> "Both interpersonal relations and technical skills are rated highly."
>
> "A good doctor is one who listens and does not hurry me."
>
> "The patient wants to be an informed and empowered consumer, but the doctor prefers a long-term relationship with a docile patient."
>
> "Patients would be better served by doctors entering Medical School after the age of 22."

> "A good doctor is simultaneously learned, honest, humble, enthusiastic, optimistic and efficient. He or she inspires total confidence in patients and daily reviews the magical relationship that by itself constitutes best treatment for any kind of ailment and the best starting point for confronting all causes of pain and suffering."[25]

> "One of the essential qualities of the clinician is interest in humanity, for the secret of the care of the patient is in caring for the patient."[26]

Provision of information and opportunities for participation feature highly as desirable characteristics in most studies.

A letter in this edition of the *British Medical Journal* is worth quoting at length. It is headed, 'We are trying to make doctors too good':[27]

> Medical training demands that doctors master at least the basics of a host of scientific disciplines-anatomy, pharmacology, molecular biology, computer science, epidemiology, nutrition and diet psychology, and so on. At the same time, they are asked to be insurance specialists, anthropologists, ethicists, marriage counsellors, small business owners, social workers, economists. . . . Doctors reel under the breadth of expertise they are supposed to master.

> As society becomes increasingly medicalised, and more and more social problems that used to be the jurisdiction of law or religion (such as drinking too much alcohol or coping with stress, street violence, or general world weariness) fall under the rubric of medical care, doctors are expected to understand more and more as they heal our social and our physical failings. Doctors simply cannot assimilate so much information, or at least they cannot assimilate it well. The truly good doctor must, of course, be technically proficient and know the craft of medicine. In addition, however, the good doctor must be able to understand patients in enough breadth to call on a community of skilled healers – nurses, social workers, insurance specialists, yoga teachers, psychotherapists, technicians, chaplains, whatever is necessary – to help restore the person to health (or perhaps, to support the person in their journey towards death).

> To do that, the doctor must be able to be touched by the patient's life as well as his or her illness. . . . Good doctors are humble doctors, willing to listen to their patients and gather together the full array of resources – medical, human, social, and spiritual – that will contribute to their patients' healing.

Time

The average patient visiting a doctor in the United States gets 22 seconds for his initial statement, then the doctor takes the lead. In a research study where patients were allowed to talk until they stopped spontaneously, the mean talking time was 92 seconds. Seven of 335 patients talked for more than five minutes. Doctors do not risk being swamped by their patients complaints if they listen until a patient indicates that his or her list of complaints is complete. Two minutes of listening should be possible and will be sufficient for nearly 80% of patients.[28]

In a research study involving patients with mild or moderate depression, an intense sense of time pressure and self-imposed rationing of time in consultations were key concerns among the patients interviewed. Their accounts often showed a mismatch between their own sense of time entitlement and the doctor's capacity to respond flexibly and constructively when more time was needed. The impression doctors gave in handling time sent strong messages about the legitimacy of the patient's illness and their decision to consult. Patients' self imposed restraint in taking up doctors' time has important consequences for the recognition and treatment of depression.[29]

The problem of consultation time is explored again in Chapter 14 ('Finding the time, and making best use of it') and in Chapter 15 ('Time, again').

Patient centredness

An analysis of patient centredness in videotaped consultations selected and submitted as part of the examination for Membership of the Royal College of General Practitioners by more than 2000 candidates revealed only limited ability to achieve patient centred outcomes. The results suggested that only a few doctors regularly use the ability fundamental to good consulting to elicit patients' ideas, concerns and expectations, to check their understanding of the problem, and involve the patient in decision making. This despite three years postgraduate training in general practice based on the precepts of the College which hold these abilities to be necessary markers of good general practice.[30] The authors do not say so, but even the best training and the best of intentions may be undermined by the biomedical constraints and expectations of routine general practice.

Expectations

Some of the quotations and references given here directly reflect the qualities patients look for in doctors. Some reflect the qualities doctors expect of themselves. And some reflect the expectations of doctors who are trainers, responsible for 'making' good doctors. Together they paint a picture that most people will recognise of the diversity of attributes we look for in doctors. And they reveal the near impossibility of finding them packaged in any one person, certainly all the time. And although we should not be surprised when we do not find them in the combination and in the measure that we personally would wish for, the package is only a *near* impossibility. They are qualities that doctors should aspire to and patients are entitled to look for, and we should at least hold them out as an ideal to reflect upon.

But of course, circumstances will affect expectations. There will be occasions when all that matters is that the doctor should be briskly efficient and technically expert, and bedside manner will be of less importance. There will be others when patient, empathic listening is precisely what we need as patients, and precisely what the doctor needs to offer if they are to get to the heart of the matter. Different medical roles require more or less of one or other of these medical 'modes'. As a letter to the *British Medical Journal* states, that not all surgeons can counsel, and fewer psychotherapists can operate. Some people have a natural ability to be more sympathetic than others, and some do not.[31] But many doctors will need to be able to switch between different modes or combine them in varying proportions at different times if they are to be really useful to the diverse population of patients, personalities and problems they serve.

This diversity is of course mirrored in the personalities of people coming into the healthcare professions. Enlightened selection and training should encourage and develop the core qualities essential in every role in addition to those most necessary in particular roles. That very diversity should encourage the various attributes that each of us possesses to rub off on one another to some extent, and enrich our own repertoire of personal qualities. (See 'Interprofessional education' in Chapter 19.) Medical education should enable individuals to find a role to which their personal attributes and vocation are best suited, and in which they are best fulfilled. And it should aim to develop whatever necessary attributes are not naturally well developed in a particular individual. Life-long learning should continuously enhance, and where necessary correct the package of attributes that an individual brings to the task.

The medical model needs to be sufficiently flexible and versatile to accommodate the diversity of needs and expectations that patients may legitimately have of their doctors and health professionals. And to match this in the repertoire of attributes of the professionals who serve us.

Trust

Trust is one of the core principles of the therapeutic encounter discussed in Chapter 14, 'Clinical Practice', and is, of course, central to the relationship that patients look for in their doctor (or any other health care practitioner). As a description of our expectations of trust in the physician I cannot improve on the account given by Edmund Pellegrino and David Thomasma in their book *The Virtues in Medical Practice*: "We expect to open the most private domains of our bodies, minds and social and family relationships to her probing gaze. Even our living and dying will engage her attention and invite her counsel. The system cannot provide the reassurance we want. (In contrast to our expectations of the work of an airline pilot, for example.) Ultimately we must place our trust in the person of the physician. We want someone who knows about us, treats us non-judgementally, and is concerned for our welfare. We want someone who will use the discretionary latitude our care requires with circumspection – neither intruding nor presuming too much nor undertaking too little. We must be able to trust her to do what she is trusted to do, that is, to serve thee healing purposes for which we have given our trust in the first place."[32]

Compassion, empathy and enablement

> Compassion is an (essential) moral virtue in medicine and in all healing . . . because the physician or nurse cannot heal, that is make whole again, without feeling and knowing the nuances of a particular patient's predicament of illness. . . . We cannot restore whatever measure of healthful harmony may be possible to the functioning of body and mind if we create an element of disharmony through the healing relationship itself. (Edmund Pellegrino and David Thomasma[32])

Two other core principles of the therapeutic encounter, compassion and empathy, are essential ingredients of the 'humaneness' that was quoted above as the most highly rated aspect of care. Sadly, and perhaps surprisingly – "Empathy is often cited as a core value in the health profession, yet its lack in modern medicine seems to be widespread".[33] Later in the same letter to the *British Medical Journal* the authors lament, "Needing to prove that compassion is not a luxury but a fundamental requirement of a healthcare system is a damning indictment of our current ways of thinking". They make these comments in the context of whole person care, and "the organisational, structural and personal limitations that general practitioners and hospital specialists face in trying to provide holistic care". They suggest that the healing power of compassion needs proving by "scientific method and focused research (if it is not) to slide from neglect to decay".

This may seem a bizarre proposition. Do we really need to go to such lengths to prove that 'humaneness' is an essential ingredient of healthcare? Yet they put their finger on a key dilemma that is a recurring theme in this book and discussed particularly in Part 5, when they refer to the limitations doctors face in trying to provide *holistic* care. What they do not say, but what is clearly implied, is that those organisational, structural and personal limitations are framed by the need to serve the biomedical culture and priorities of modern medicine. This is emphasised by the data they report from a study at the NHS outpatient clinic at Glasgow Homeopathic Hospital. The homeopathic method exemplifies a holistic approach in that it takes full account of patients' individuality and narrative (see Chapter 13). Of 200 patients, sixty six rated their consultations as 'better', and fifty two as 'much better' than their usual consultations with their general practitioners. Of those 118 patients, thirty-eight rated the consultation as 'better', and sixty one as 'much better' than consultations with other hospital specialists. The size of this group indicates how many of the 200 patients, nearly 50%, had been or still were in conventional hospital specialist care at the time of referral to the Homoeopathic Hospital.

The purpose of the study was primarily to investigate the relationship between empathy and enablement. 'Enablement' describes the effect of a clinical encounter on a patient's ability to cope with and understand his or her illness. No patient reported a high enablement score with a low empathy score, and it is significant that it was this perception of the doctor's empathy and not the length of consultation that related to better enablement. The time available for the consultations was much more than a General Practitioner would be able to provide, but comparable to other specialist out-patient departments.

The earlier section on 'Awareness, participation and choice' in this chapter touched upon other influences that equip us as patients to do more for ourselves, and it is worth considering the distinction between enablement and other aspects of autonomy. As this reference to the Glasgow Study illustrates, enablement grows out of a relationship with another person who is knowledgeable, insightful, concerned, respected and to be trusted. This applies in any sphere of life. It is, for example an aspect of good parenting and any kind of mentoring. It involves an exchange of knowledge and the building of self respect, competence, perhaps courage, certainly a positive attitude and a more hopeful awareness of possibilities. This is other than and more than may be gained from participation in exploring problems and solutions, unless the necessary quality of relationship is also present. And participation does not guarantee it. It is also different from the empowerment that may come from patient choice or from access to more information, often very sophisticated, on health matters, that is readily available today. Enablement is part of the whole-making process that should be at the heart of the medical endeavour.

'Compassion in healthcare: the missing dimension of healthcare reform?' is the title of a paper in the Future Debates series commissioned by the NHS Confederation (www.debatepapers.org and www.nhsconfed.org/publications).[34] It is written by Robin Youngson, a consultant anaesthetist and co-founder of the national Centre for Compassion in Healthcare in New Zealand. It is to an extent a personal view, not formally representing the views of the NHS Confederation. But it is certainly a view that demands to be debated, and that has obvious implications for the remodelling of medicine.

Two of his key points are that care, compassion and some aspects of basic care delivery appear under strain in health systems around the world; and, putting compassion and care back into healthcare requires action at system level, by organisational leaders, and by individuals. He defines compassion as "the humane quality of understanding suffering in others and wanting to do something about it. . .". He identifies some of the organisational, structural and personal limitations that medical staff have to face (see Box 8.1). The rapid turnover of patients in hospital to increase productivity, allows too little time to establish a trusting relationship and get to the heart of the matter (see the critique of Accident and Emergency discharge targets by Rawlinson at the end of Chapter 4); shift work and the fragmentation of responsibility (a serious concern of those who oppose the introduction of polyclinics); a critical focus on pathways, tasks, and documentation (an inevitable by-product of targets); increasing tension between evidence based nursing care with its scientific research agenda, and broader policy directions for nursing with a holistic concern for the whole patient; the fact that the Western model of medical professionalism rests on foundations of a biomedical approach, rational detachment and objectivity and that does not encourage or that may even actively discourage empathy, which is often diminished in medical students during clinical training – Marshall Marinker's 'hidden agenda' (Chapter 5).[35]

BOX 8.1 *Organisational, structural and personal threats to care*

- Productivity – bed occupancy, turnover.
- No time for trust, or 'the heart of the matter'.
- Shift work, fragmentation of responsibility.
- Pathways, tasks, documentation.
- Evidence/research v. holistic concern.
- Rational detachment, objectivity.

Although compassion is an assumed value, Youngson finds it is scarcely mentioned in any documents about healthcare strategies or aspirations. In a search of websites of all the quality-improvement organisations he was unable to find the word 'compassion' at all. And empathy is not just a matter of sentiment, it yields practical benefits. We have seen how empathy enables patients, and Youngson insists that there is compelling research to show that empathic concern and investing time up front to check a patient's needs increases efficiency and safety, as well as patient satisfaction. The reality is that we cannot afford the time NOT to listen.

In his action plan for putting compassion back into healthcare, which we might very well want to incorporate into a remodelling process, he includes: *Declare* compassion as a core value; Declare compassion as a management and leadership competence. He maintains that empathy is as much a skill as an inborn character trait, and that therefore it can be developed as a personal and leadership competence. This process requires space and opportunity safely to recognise, accept, and perhaps express one's personal vulnerability, because, 'We cannot expect health professionals to bring compassionate caring to their patients without some personal healing'.

For American Physician Harvey Chochinov, part of the essence of medicine is to avoid or mitigate the loss of dignity that is involved in becoming a patient.[36] He, too, believes that this important aspect of humaneness is put at risk because 'Kindness, humanity and respect – the core values of medical professionalism – are too often being overlooked in the time pressured culture of modern health care'. Our dignity is inevitably compromised when we become a patient:

> The word patient comes from the Latin *patiens*, meaning to endure, bear, or suffer, and refers to an acquired vulnerability and dependency imposed by changing health circumstances. Relinquishing autonomy is no small matter and can exact considerable costs. These costs are sometimes relatively minor – for example, accepting clinic schedules or hospital routines. At other times, the costs seem incompatible with life itself. When patients experience a radical unsettling of their conventional sense of self and a disintegration of personhood, suffering knows few bounds. To feel sick is one thing, but to feel that who we are is being threatened or undermined – that we are no longer the person we once were – can cause despair affecting body, mind, and soul.

Empathy and compassion are the remedy for this and the guarantors that dignity is preserved:

> Compassion refers to a deep awareness of the suffering of another coupled with the wish to relieve it. Compassion speaks to feelings that are evoked by contact with the patient and how those feelings shape our approach to care. Like empathy (identification with and understanding of another's situation, feelings,

> and motives), compassion is something that is felt, beyond simply intellectual appreciation.

He acknowledges that the habit of compassion may not come easily, but points out that it can be expressed quite simply:

> Although the process of arriving at compassion can be difficult or complex, showing compassion often flows naturally and can be as quick and as easy as a gentle look or a reassuring touch. In fact, compassion can be conveyed by any form of communication – spoken or unspoken – that shows some recognition of the human stories that accompany illness.

And he agrees that if it does not come naturally a compassionate disposition can be developed:

> Healthcare providers arrive at compassion through various channels. For some, compassion may be part of a natural disposition that intuitively informs patient care. For others, compassion slowly emerges with life experience, clinical practice, and the realisation that, like patients, each of us is vulnerable in the face of ageing and life's many uncertainties. Compassion may develop over time, and it may also be cultivated by exposure to the medical humanities, including the interdisciplinary field of humanities (literature, philosophy, ethics, history, and religion), social sciences (anthropology, cultural studies, psychology, sociology), and the arts (literature, theatre, film, and visual arts). Each of these will not speak to every healthcare provider, but they can offer insight into the human condition and the pathos and ambiguity that accompany illness.

Eric Cassell implies this, too, when he writes that the habit of 'attentive listening' can be acquired during medical education, and that the judgement of patients' values (characteristics that strongly affect their experience of illness and suffering) that attentive listening based on trained observation permits, is found to be reliable and consistent.[37]

Continuity of care

Three of the commonest complaints that patients make (problems that most of us, as patients or clinicians are likely to have encountered at some time) are:

> "He didn't have my notes."
> "No one had told her/me (what had been done, what was to be done, when to come again, etc)."
> "I see a different doctor every time."

These are common examples of the three types of failure of patient care described in an article that argues that continuity of care matters.[38] The first is a failure of continuity of information, the second of continuity of management, and the third of continuity of relationship. They result in inefficient care and impersonal care. They cause frustration for staff, waste of time and resources, and distress for patients. But they are not universal problems, and all three sorts of continuity are often achieved perfectly well.

They are, however, easily put at risk, again by organisational, structural and personal limitations. The present emphasis on improving access to medical care, particularly in primary care, and the concept of 'polyclinics' and walk-in clinics, carry this risk. Loss of continuity of information and management can theoretically be avoided by good communication, increasingly electronic. Continuity of relationship is more precarious. But it necessarily underpins the effectiveness of the other two kinds of continuity. Since there are so many opportunities for discontinuity when care crosses disciplinary and organisational boundaries, continuity in its broadest sense will always depend on individual clinicians taking responsibility for the longitudinal care of patients with whom they have on-going relationships. And it is the availability and quality of that relationship that is so important to most patients. In some circumstances and when we are fitter it may not be so important. But in others, and when we are less able and more vulnerable it certainly is. Although speed of access matters, rigid systems of triage (sorting patients according to severity of need) or walk-in care that limit choice of clinician discourage long term relationships and ultimately compromise quality of care, particularly for patients less able to negotiate personal care for themselves.

References

1 Carel H, Johnson S, Gamble L. Living with lymphangioleiomyomatosis. *Br Med J*. 2010; 340 c848:148–149,
2 Hudson C. Wonder drug stole my memory. *Daily Telegraph* 2009; 12th March.
3 OHE. *The Health Care Dilemma*. London: Office of Health Economics; 1975.
4 Greaves D. *The Healing Tradition*. Oxford: Radcliffe Publishing; 2004.
5 Swayne J. Medicine and healing: A broken marriage? *New Society* 1976; 491–492
6 Haslam D. Who cares? The James Mackenzie Lecture 2006. *Br J Gen Pract*. 2007; 57:987–993.
7 Reilly D. Enhancing human healing *Br Med J*. 2001; 322:120–1.
8 Willis J. *Friends in low places*. Abingdon: Radcliffe; 2001.
9 Illich I. *Limits to medicine: medical nemesis the expropriation of health*. London: Boyars; 1976.
10 Moynihan R, Smith R. Too much medicine *Br Med J*. 2002; 324:859–60.
11 Sen A. Editorial. *Br Med J*. 2002; 324:860–861.

12 Rosenberg C. The Tyranny of Diagnosis: Specific Entities and Individual Experience. *The Millbank Quarterly* 2002; 80(2):237–260.
13 Kennedy I. *Unmasking medicine*. London: George Allen and Unwin; 1981.
14 Brody H. *Stories of Sickness*. New Haven: Yale University Press; 1987.
15 Frances A. The first draft of DSM-V *Br Med J*. 2010; 340:c1168;492.
16 Freemantle N, Hill S. Medicalisation limits to medicine or never enough to go round *Br Med J*. 2002; 324;864–865.
17 Donner-Banzhoff N, Sonnichsen A. Strategies for prescribing statins *Br Med J*. 2008; 336:288–9
18 Melzer D, Zimmern R. Genetics and medicalisation *Br Med J*. 2002; 324:864–865.
19 Kamerov D. Review of the week: What is wrong with US health care *Br Med J*. 2008; 336:99.
20 Grol G. Berwick D. Wensing M. On the trail of quality and safety in health care. *Br Med J*. 2008; 336:74–6.
21 Fitzpatrick M. *The tyranny of health*. Abingdon: Routledge; 2001.
22 Minerva. *Br Med J*. 2008; 336:1198.
23 Rudol C. In: Barkham P. The Shipman Report. *The Times* 2002 July 20th.
24 Hurwitz B, Vass A. What's a good doctor and how can you make one? *Br Med J*. 2002; 325:667–668.
25 Sotelo J. *What's a good and how do you make one?* (Letter) *Br Med J*. 2002; 325:712.
26 Peabody FW. The Care of the Patient. *JAMA*. 1927; 88: 877–882
27 Wolpe P. We are trying to make doctors too good. *Br Med J*. 2002; 325:712.
28 Langeutitz W, Denz M, Keller A *et al*. Spontaneous talking time at start of consultation. *Br Med J*. 2002; 325: 682–683.
29 Pollock K, Grime J. Patients' perceptions of entitlement to time in general practice consultations for depression *Br Med J*. 2002; 325:687–90.
30 Campion P, Foulkes J, Neighbour R *et al*. Patient centredness in the MRCGP video examination. *Br Med J*. 2002; 325:691–692.
31 Nolan P. (Letter) *Br Med J*. 2001; 322:865.
32 Pellegrino E, Thomasma D. *The Virtues in Medical Practice*. Oxford: Oxford University Press; 1993.
33 Mercer SW, Watt GC, Reilly D. Empathy is important for enablement. *Br Med J*. 2001; 322:865.
34 Youngson R. *Compassion in healthcare*. London: NHS Confederation Publications; 2008.
35 Marinker M. Medical education and human values. *J R Coll Gen Pract*. 1974; 24:445–462.;
36 Chochinov H. Dignity and the essence of medicine: the A B C and D of dignity conserving care *Br Med J*. 2007; 335:184–187
37 Cassell E. *The Nature of Suffering and the Goals of Medicine*. New York: Oxford University Press; 2004.
38 Guthrie B, Saultz JW, Freeman GK *et al*. Continuity of care matters. *Br Med J*. 2008; 867:548–554.

9

MEDICINE IN CRISIS?

Summary

- Medicine as a health care system and as a healing vocation has reached a crisis point – a turning point, a time of decision, possibly of danger.
- The elements of the crisis include – a crisis of cost and resources, the increasing dangers of medical practice, the failure of mechanistic care to promote well-being, the loss of vocational commitment, a crisis of morale, and a crisis of morality.
- Medicine colludes in its own devaluation.
- But the crisis can be a turning point, an opportunity, if the medical professions are prepared to grasp it.

> Something has gone wrong with healthcare. Doctors tell us medicine is in crisis while nurses say they are in despair. Despite the commitment of health professionals, the good intentions of politicians and administrators and unmistakable support of the public, we face a crisis of caring, a crisis of costs and crisis of commitment. (College of Medicine Policy Document[1])

I begin this book with the words, "There is something wrong with the way we do medicine in the modern Western world". This is quite a mild statement set beside the assertion of some commentators, including some doctors, that medicine is in crisis. The NHS 60th birthday headlines quoted in Chapter 4 certainly suggest it. Crisis is a strong word, sometimes taken to mean a point of actual or impending disaster. That is probably not the case. But I have to agree that this harsher criticism is certainly true if we take crisis to mean, as it does, a turning point, a time of decision, possibly of danger. This is true of medicine in two senses: medicine as a healthcare system is in crisis, and medicine as a healing vocation is in crisis. The two kinds of crisis are of course related. The elements of both crises are already evident in earlier chapters and further evidence will emerge in later chapters. At this mid-point, here is a summary of these elements (see Box 9.1). You will recognise in some of them echoes of the predictions of Ivan Illich in *Medical Nemesis*.

BOX 9.1 *Elements of crisis*

- Cost and resources.
- Adverse effects.
- Loss of vocation.
- Loss of morale.
- Moral malaise.
- The devaluation of medicine.

A crisis of cost and resources.

The success of modern medicine, its ability to do so much, has turned into what David Peters, in an article addressing these issues calls, "a technological arms race against disease".[2] The costs of its weaponry have spiralled out of control, but magic bullets still have to be found and magic machines to elucidate our ills with ever greater precision have to be built. And everyone insists they have a right to them; both the patients who need, or believe they need them, and the doctors who need, or believe they need to use them. Clinical judgement, practical wisdom, watchful waiting, are seldom an acceptable management strategy now.

These facts recall that Engel's remark, "The enormous existing and planned investment in diagnostic and therapeutic technology alone strongly favours approaches to clinical study and care of patients that emphasise the impersonal and the mechanical". This is an observation that still rings true. This is that part of the crisis in medicine that he alleges, "derives from – the adherence to a model of disease no longer adequate for the scientific tasks of medicine".[3] It is one end of the spectrum of costly demand, rightly or wrongly perceived as medical need. At the other end are the escalating needs of chronic illness in an ageing population. Modern health care had become unaffordable before the financial crisis of 2008. That crisis has only shown up the cost crisis in medicine in high relief.

An exercise in the *British Medical Journal* to identify potential cost savings in the NHS in the light of the financial crisis is revealing. 'Experts' guide to saving money in health'[4] asked leading representatives of a dozen different medical disciplines to recommend ways of saving money in their field. It not only showed that the effect of the crisis, like the prospect of execution, does concentrate the mind, in this case to good effect in agreeing that something could be done. It also highlighted certain recurring themes. The commonest was the overuse of diagnostic tests and investigations; usually as an unnecessary routine that added little or nothing to the management of the problem where clinical knowledge and acumen should suffice; sometimes multiplying costs because tests are ordered in batches that include several that are not relevant to the solution of the problem, sometimes inducing a further 'cascade' of tests to elucidate some vague apparent abnormality in the first test. Another theme was the use of procedures of little or no real therapeutic benefit, or procedures for which better alternatives exist. Another was better integration or delegation of services, sometimes to avoid unnecessary, prolonged, harmful or costly hospital admissions.

Running through these examples is the common thread that has already emerged – the tendency to do things because they can be done and that come to be expected, rather than because they should be done. But one other common theme was the need to 'invest to disinvest' by developing or implementing procedures or processes that could avoid or replace those

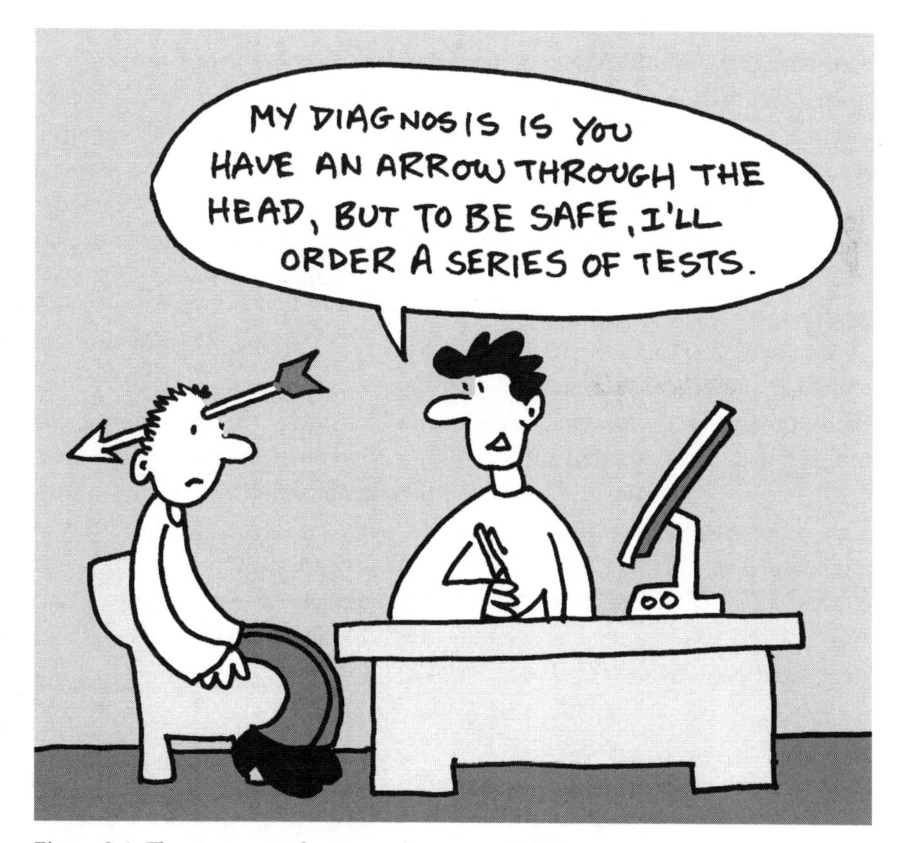

Figure 9.1 *The commonest theme was the overuse of diagnostic tests.*

that might be done away with. So the wasteful use of one sophisticated technique can sometimes be avoided by the introduction of another, possibly more sophisticated technique. It is a matter of the discerning and discriminating use of science and technology.

Modern medicine is increasingly dangerous.

Before the germ theory of disease was properly understood, before aseptic techniques were introduced and then antibiotics invented, most serious infections were lethal. And medical interventions often caused or transmitted those lethal infections. Most medical procedures, such as blood-letting, and surgical techniques often did more harm than good. Progress in medical science overcame these problems.

But now medicine has become more dangerous again. 'The risks of being a patient' in Chapter 8 discusses this. Surgery continues to get safer, but illness and death from the adverse effects of drugs is notoriously common. Hospital acquired infections cause unnecessary illness and claim lives. Numbers of hospital beds have been falling for some years, but rates of hospital admission are currently (2010) increasing by 6% a year. This means a rapid turnover in bed occupancy, which increases the risk of infection. *But* – one reason for the increase in hospital admissions is the reduced quality and accessibility of out of hours cover in primary care. *While* – the European working hours directive undermines comprehensive hospital staffing and jeopardises adequate training opportunities for hospital doctors.

Medicine is fraught with risk. Its direct risks are obvious, the adverse effects of drugs and technology, for example. Its indirect risks are sometimes obvious too, for example hospital acquired infection. But some indirect risks are not at all obvious. They include every biomedical diagnosis that misconstrues the more complex dynamics of illness and misdirects the therapeutic effort (see Alan Barbour's list of misconceptions and false starts in Chapter 7), and every medico-political manipulation of clinical practice (regulations, targets and guidelines for example) that subverts the wisdom and judgement of individual doctors on behalf of individual patients.

Mechanistic health care undermines well-being

This danger is such a recurring theme in the book that it hardly needs restating. The mechanistic vision of biomedicine seeks the control of disease but neglects the well-being of the person. It distracts attention from the 'story of sickness', that more holistic perspective which is necessary to make sense of the illness and enhance the well-being of the patient (see 'Health, well-being and quality of life', Chapter 12).

Medicine is losing its vocational commitment

The constraints and directives of biomedical priorities on the one hand, and social and political priorities on the other, are undermining the vocational satisfaction and commitment of health professionals. The mismatch of demand with resources, and of expectations with what is possible causes the frustration and unhappiness described by Moynihan and Smith[5] in Chapter 4, and the ebbing away of the vocational passion to do the job well described by James le Fanu.[6] Compassion is repeatedly acknowledged to be lacking in health care, not simply because people are incapable of it, but because often the system does not allow for it. If the motivation to become a health care professional is, at least in part, a desire to *care* for people, this lack of opportunity is frustrating and demoralising. And if the opportunity for compassionate care is denied, we should not be surprised if the well-spring of compassion sometimes runs dry.

A crisis of morale

> There is now a crisis of morale in the medical profession (that) has largely materialised since 1984 (when) medicine was the most popular career for bright school leavers and general practice was the number one career choice for British doctors. Something terrible has happened since then. Nobody wants to go into general practice any more and all the established doctors can't wait to get out. Everybody says the same thing – there is too much paperwork, we have lost our independence, and the pressures get more and more unbearable. We seem to have been taken over by the same alien culture that is spreading through the rest of modern society. (James Willis[7])

These words were written by James Willis, a GP for some 30 years at the time of their first publication in 1995, in a book called *The Paradox of Progress*. He and I were members of the same group of enthusiastic young entrants to general practice in the late 1960s who were beneficiaries of the pioneering vocational training scheme that I described in Chapter 1. In fact the displacement of education by training (which is "the sort of process you use to prepare a performing animal"), is one of the demoralising features of modern medicine for James. But the programme we joined really was a vocational *education*, opening our hearts and minds to the challenges and riches of the sort of personal patient care that had attracted us to medicine in the first place. The paradox of progress for James and for very many doctors has been "the problem of retaining respect for human values in an increasingly systematised world". His two entertaining and deeply thought provoking books *The Paradox of Progress* and *Friends in Low Places* develop this theme.[6,8]

Broadly speaking there are three strands to his argument that are also central to my own. One is that for all our desire for technical mastery of disease processes it is the complexity and mystery of the individual human experience of illness that is at the heart of medicine's healing vocation ("These human things are really the things that matter *most* in the end"); our capacity to *understand* this and respond to it effectively is being eroded in the systematised biotechnical world of modern medicine. That is demoralising.

The second strand is the entanglement of medicine with the culture of our society and medicine's collusion with its dehumanising tendencies. ("Technical hubris has brought with it nemesis for the personal aspects of life.") That is demoralising, although perhaps more insidiously so.

The third strand, which underpins the other two is that "our present course is based on a wrong paradigm, an out-dated understanding of the way in which reality operates". James describes this way of thinking in terms borrowed from Guy Claxton as the 'over-mind',[9] a dominant managerial modus operandi in which rules and regulations stifle the wisdom and insight of conscientious, resourceful, free individuals, and human complexity is subordinate to statistical norms. The over-mind is afflicted with paradigm paralysis, the McNamara fallacy (described in the next chapter), and scientific tunnel vision. For any doctor motivated at all by a healing vocation all this is deeply demoralising.

A subtle but profoundly important element of this disturbing situation that James Willis brings out in both his books is the debilitating effect of regulation on the mind. Rules, targets and protocols are designed to improve efficiency, and they can give the impression that the practitioner knows what he or she is doing. But the impression that this knowledge represents a true *understanding* of what is going on may be an illusion. The level of regulation currently imposed upon medicine devalues, displaces

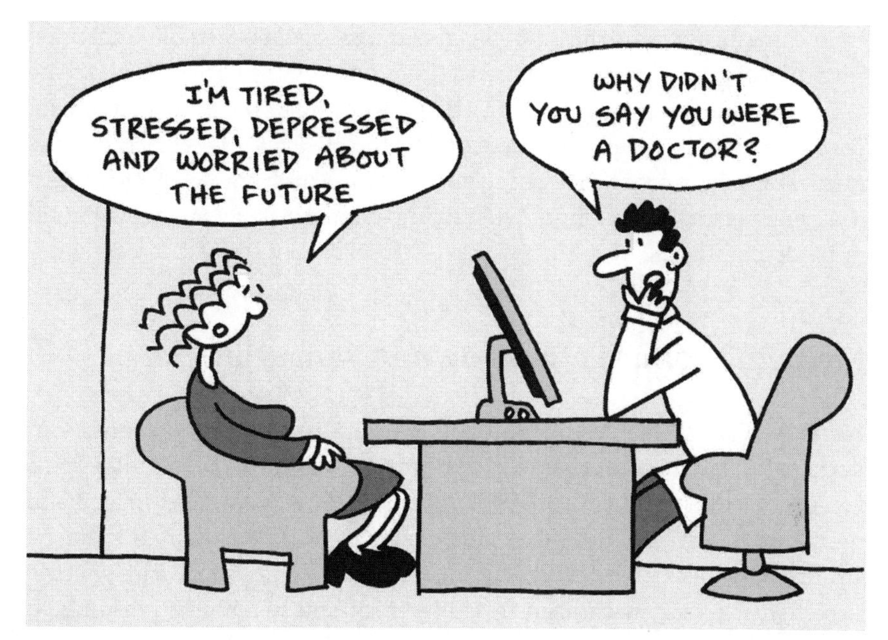

Figure 9.2 *A crisis of morale.*

and even de-skills the immensely versatile human mind. It deprives doctors of the creativity of mind that is so essential to solving *human* problems, as opposed to analysing technical ones. This 'cognitive fluidity' is the distinctive attribute of the human mind. Its application, its use in solving complexity, is what the mind is for. It is a doctor's most useful tool. The level of regulation to which it is now subjected is alien to it, and deeply demoralising.

For example, from *The Paradox of Progress*: "The idea that regulation is a good thing *per se* is an illusion. Regulation destroys humanity. It undervalues the individual human being, his mind, his motivation and his integrity. Unfortunately GPs have to some extent colluded in the process of reducing their practice to a lot of sterile formulae. They have done this because they have shared in the illusion that this is what is necessary for progress". And from *Friends in Low Places*: "Rule following is absolute. It is blind, and it produces terrible, empty certainty. Actions based on rule-following may be *indistinguishable* from actions based on understanding. But in fact they come from entirely different places. . . . We now live in a world in which it is increasingly being assumed that the application of formulae trumps the application of understanding. . . . All you have to do is in order to do medicine is to *follow the instructions*. Paint in the numbers, join up the dots, look up the rule, surf the net, print out the answer."

In other words, as earlier chapters have suggested, doctors have colluded with the plausibility construct of the day, the prevailing world view, the unhealthy culture of our society. They are working to the wrong paradigm. To quote David Haslam again, they use the medical model because the medical model is what they use, even though it may not be appropriate.[10] It all goes against the grain of what being a doctor is all about. It is bound to be demoralising.

Medicine colludes in its own devaluation

Medicine cannot blame others for its crisis. Albeit with good intentions perhaps, it has allowed itself to be seduced by science and technology to a greater extent than their achievements justify. And it has encouraged and fuelled the unreasonable expectations and excessive demand that it struggles to meet. It has been submissive to cultural, social and political expedients. It has succumbed to commercial and materialist pressures. It has allowed itself to be pushed about and manipulated. It has lost sight of its goals. Or if that is not quite true, those goals have become thoroughly confused.

A crisis of morality

> The professions are moral communities with immense moral power. If they use it well they can become paradigms of disinterested service that can raise the level of conventional morality. (Edmund Pellegrino and David Thomasma[11])

Doctors are consistently rated as the most highly esteemed of all professionals, and as such could be held to represent the health care professions as a whole. Both our vocation and our role and high profile in society impose great moral responsibility.

By writing 'our', I am deliberately identifying myself with the vocation and profession that I love and the colleagues I like and admire that share that vocation. I am deliberately associating myself with them in acknowledging that as a profession, though not necessarily as particular individuals, we are failing properly to fulfil our moral responsibility.

This is first and foremost a responsibility to the individual patient. "The principles of medical ethics are statements of the right and good that derive from helping and caring in a special kind of human relationship." That is another quotation from *The Virtues in Medical Practice*, the book by Pellegrino and Thmasma quoted at the beginning of this section. It is a chastening but at the same time inspiring book that all health care professionals, and certainly doctors, should read. It is chastening in that it sheds a harsh light on our lapses of moral responsibility, but inspiring in that it affirms the 'virtues' that lie, or should lie at the heart of our vocation and our professional role. In that second quotation they get right to the heart of the matter – our responsibility to a person in need within 'a special kind of human relationship', a very special and highly privileged relationship. Our responsibility is to do what is right and good for that person in seeking to achieve those 'ends and purposes of medical activity', which Pellegrino and Thomasma later define as "the restoration or improvement of health and, more proximately, to heal, that is to cure illness and disease, or when this is not possible to care for and help the patient to live with residual pain, discomfort or disability". We must be faithful in doing what we are trusted to do, "that is, to serve the healing purposes for which the patient has given their trust in the first place".

This is by no means an easy task. In fact it can be very difficult. It requires a substantial measure of what they call phronesis – a concept introduced by Aristotle meaning practical wisdom, moral insight, the capacity to discern what moral choice or course of action is most conducive to the good. Phronesis is the capability to consider the mode of action in order to deliver change, especially to enhance the quality of life.[12] These qualities are hard to come by. And they are not the automatic fruits of a medical education, even though they are traits of character whose formation is every bit as important as the technical education that a student certainly will receive. The responsibility to be faithful to the individual patient is made an even harder task by a health care culture in which this relationship of trust has been in many instances displaced by a contractual relationship threatened by litigation, by a policy or market driven relationship, or by a relationship in which the health care professional has become the technical servant of the patient's autonomy. True discernment of what moral choice or course of action is conducive to the good may be seriously compromised by social and cultural constraints such as these, however well-endowed with practical wisdom and moral insight we may be.

This is the crux of our moral responsibility towards our individual patient and the society we serve. Pellegrino and Thomasma are uncompromising about it: "If doctors, as a healing community really want to recapture a sense of moral integrity, the most important thing they can do is to resist and refuse to do anything that violates the promise to act in the patient's interests. . . . Were physicians to take moral leadership, the medical profession could be a model and an inspiration for others." This means we *will not* "reshape our ethical codes to conform to the ethos of the market place" or any other social or cultural influence that is demeaning to the special kind of human relationship with which we are entrusted; that we *will* "stand firm in the belief that being a physician imposes specific obligations that forbid turning oneself into an entrepreneur, a businessman, or an agent of fiscal, social, or economic policy"; or adopt any role or attitude that is less than completely faithful to the ends and purposes of our vocation.

Aspects of this moral responsibility have been implied in much that has already been said in previous chapters, and the theme will recur in later chapters too; particularly with regard to the quality of the therapeutic relationship (Chapters 12 and 15), to truthfulness in medical science (Chapters 10, 11 and 18), and with regard to the relationship between medicine, society and culture (Chapter 17). Here are some of the attributes that Pellegrino and Thomasma commend as virtues in medical practice:

- *Phronesis* – which they also describe as practical intelligence that summates the virtues and applies them to particular situations. It provides the link between the intellectual virtues – those that dispose to truth (as represented by art, science, intuitive and theoretical wisdom), and those that dispose to good character (e.g. temperance, courage, justice, generosity).
- *Prudence* – the indispensable connection between cognition of the good and the disposition to seek it in particular acts.
- *Trust* – The central importance of trust has already been emphasised in Chapter 8, and the 'ingredients' of trust are described in Chapter 15 ('The heart of the matter').
- *Justice* – the strict habit of rendering to others what is due to them. This is not always compatible with autonomy.
- *Fortitude* – the tenacity to obtain the required treatment for a patient; resistance to any pressure or temptation that will diminish the good of the patient.
- *Temperance* – self-control, discretion; the responsible use of power on behalf of patients.
- *Compassion* – the ability to feel something of the unique predicament of the patient.
- *Integrity* – a close correspondence between the integrity of the practitioner and the integrity that we are seeking to restore in our patient; between the person of integrity and the integrity of the person. The completeness, wholeness and unity we seek to restore in our patient must be reflected in ourselves and in the integrity of our values.

But these are uncontroversial moral attitudes that are quite easy to discuss in the abstract and sign up to. A more immediately affecting and shaming example of a moral failing at the practising heart of UK medicine is revealed by hospital doctor Max Pemberton, writing in the *Daily Telegraph* about his experience participating in *The Jeremy Kyle Show* on television.[13] He describes his deeply chastening realisation of the demeaning attitude of some (many?) doctors to the 'underclass' who are the show's usual guests – as he suggests the middle class 'voyeurs' of the programme are likely to regard them (gaining 'A Hogarthian glimpse into their excesses and debauched lives'). "They don't have time for the likes of me", one guest explained when he asked why she had not been to her doctor for help. "For people who are disempowered and disfranchised like her (those living on sink estates, unemployed and uneducated), doctors are distant, fearsome creatures who don't listen and don't help. They dismiss her and the problems she faces, despite the fact that she is in far greater need than the middle classes who clutter up surgery waiting rooms. . . . For those who feel marginalised and ignored by the medical profession, Jeremy Kyle (and his faultless aftercare service) is a saviour." If it is fair to generalise this insight across our society, then the crisis of morality in medicine has a personal aspect that requires a *metanoia* (change of heart and mind) of us all.

Resolving the crisis

We cannot deny the crisis described in this chapter. But this is not a point of impending disaster; it is a point of decision, a turning point, an opportunity. The momentum for change described in Chapter 3 is sufficient to exploit that opportunity. It is this book's acknowledged ambition that the analysis of the crisis and the arguments and recommendations for 'regime change' (Part 5) presented here will add to that momentum. The energy, resources and vision necessary for this evolution, this metamorphosis and remodelling, are the inherent properties of the healthcare professions – if we have the courage and determination, and the humility to realise them.

References

1 College of Medicine Policy Document 2010. Available from the College of Medicine. 19 Buckingham Street, London WC2N 6EF and online at www.collegeofmedicine.org.uk

2 Peters D. Biomedicine in crisis: cost, cure, compassion and commitment. *Journal of Holistic Healthcare* 2009; 2(1):2.
3 Engel G. The need for a new medical model. *Science* 1977; 96(4286);129–136.
4 Cook S. Experts' guide to saving money in health. *Br Med J.* 2010; 340 c1281;622–624.
5 Moynihan R, Smith, R. Too much medicine? *Br Med J.* 2002; 324:859–60.
6 le Fanu J. *The rise and fall of modern medicine.* London: Abacus; 1999.
7 Willis J. *The Paradox of Progress.* Abingdon: Radcliffe; 1998.
8 Willis J. *Friends in Low Places.* Abingdon: Radcliffe; 2001.
9 Claxton G. *Hare Brain, Tortoise Mind: Why intelligence increases when you think less.* London: FourthEstate; 1998.
10 Haslam D. Who cares? *Br J Gen Pract.* 2007; 57(545):987–993.
11 Pellegrino E, Thomasma D. *The Virtues in Medical Practice.* Oxford: Oxford University Press; 1993.
12 Wikepedia (www.wikipedia.org)
13 Pemberton, M. Don't scoff at Jeremy Kyle – to many he's a saviour. *Daily Telegraph* 2010 November 22nd.

part 3

MAINTAINING CAUSES

The central argument of this book is that the focus of medical practice and research needs to shift from diagnostic and therapeutic processes that address disorder in the parts (the disease) to those that address the dynamics of disorder in the whole (the person); and from those that permit control of the first to those that enable self-regulation in the second. Previous chapters have suggested that there is little argument that this change of emphasis is desirable and would be fruitful. That possibility is explored further in Part 4. But it is apparent that that the status quo, the predominately biomedical focus, still prevails. These next two chapters examine the reasons for this state of affairs.

10

TRUTH, PROOF AND EVIDENCE

Summary

- Evidence Based Medicine is the current orthodoxy, but there are clinicians who distrust its influence, which may not reflect the intention of its pioneering authors.
- The chapter examines the principles of knowledge, truth and meaning that are the essence of all good science and that must underpin any system of evidence.
- In real life, the value of evidence from analytical and experimental scientific methods is complemented by a variety of other ways of knowing.

Attitudes to evidence

Evidence rules; O.K?

Well, yes and no. All medical treatments and procedures applied to individuals or populations are nowadays expected to be evidence based according to the rules of the scientific paradigm. This standard is applied rigorously to any new treatment or procedure that is up for adoption into the medical repertoire, though there are some to which it is difficult to apply, particularly surgical procedures.[1] Many that are more long established have not been so rigorously tested. The proportion that has been justified by such evidence is not as great as we might expect.

Evidence Based Medicine (EBM) – the conscientious, explicit, and judicious use of current best evidence in making decisions about the care of individual patients[2] – is the current orthodoxy. But there are not a few clinicians and commentators who distrust its influence; certainly the influence that it has come to exert, and that may be somewhat removed from the original intention of the authors of the classic text that gave birth to it. Some of these critical comments will be presented later in the chapter. But the assumptions about the nature of evidence, and the concept of proof may not be as robust as many like to think. And their coercive power for the validation or otherwise of what is being proposed or tested, and of its usefulness need to be reassessed.

The nature of paradigms and the problems associated with them were explained in part two of the Introduction, but to recapitulate briefly: Any medical treatment or procedure, and particularly any innovation, has to contend for acceptance within the prevailing medical paradigm, and bear the burden of proof. In science, the concept of the paradigm was developed most cogently by Thomas Kuhn (1922–96) as an explanation of the way that scientific attitudes and beliefs, and the research and development programmes that follow from them become established, and of the difficulties involved in changing them, and of the kind of revolution required to do so.[3] A paradigm can be thought of as a kind of mind set that determines, and restricts, the direction in which scientific thinking and investigation is allowed to progress. It determines the parameters of what Kuhn called 'normal science' and is defined in Box 10.1.

BOX 10.1 *Definition of paradigm*

A paradigm is a conceptual framework, adequate for its time but not eternally true, and essentially metaphysical because it is actually a framework of ideas and values, whatever 'objectivity' it may claim.

By contrast, Karl Popper (1902–94), does not trust the scientific community to define its playing fields and position its goal posts in this way. He insists, "A genuine commitment to the truth gives scientists the courage to challenge the truth of particular theories, including the ones associated with a scientific paradigm".[4] On this basis he introduces the concept of 'falsifyability' as the necessary test of any scientific proposition. It requires that a hypothesis be stated in such a way that it can be disproved by experiment.

Popper deprecates the somewhat totalitarian vision of science promoted by Kuhn, and favours a more open and democratic approach. Scientists should put their principles to the test of experiment in the same way that politicians put their policies to the test in elections.

Popper's approach is deliberately to challenge, and through the outcome of challenge to change the minds of the scientific community, when the evidence requires it. But his principles also required justice in their application. Tests should not be biased towards a dominant theory. There must be a level playing field. "Tests must not be burdened with concerns about the costs and benefits of their outcomes, which would be tantamount to match fixing." In a book discussing the tension between the philosophies of Kuhn and Popper, Steve Fuller comments, "This metaphor reveals the remoteness of this normative ideal of science from actual scientific practice".[5] There is good reason for contemporary researchers in unorthodox fields of medicine to endorse this view.[6]

Reality, Truth and Knowledge

It is helpful to look behind the scenes of this debate at the principles of knowledge, truth and meaning that are the essence of *all* good science, and that must underpin any system of evidence.

Reality

First, some observations on 'reality', because any scientific endeavour is, surely, above all an exploration of reality, of our understanding of the way things really are. Two diametrically opposed views of the way things are will be held, for example, by a materialist like Richard Dawkins who sees no sense or value in any metaphysical interpretation of reality, and a theist like me for whom such an interpretation is inescapable. We both have 'motivated belief' for our understanding of reality,[7] but in the absence of falsifyable evidence I am willing to be guided by 'inference to the best explanation'. (See 'Ways of knowing', later in this chapter.)

Reality is the bigger picture that comprehends, makes sense of and gives value to every facet of human experience. It is intimations of reality that give meaning and direction and a passionate desire to the exploration of our experience; that arouse 'scientific passion'.[8] It is intimations of reality that give meaning and value to our individual lives.

Truth

Secondly, what do I mean by 'truth', and how is science implicated in the pursuit of truth? Scientist and Philosopher Michael Polanyi (1891–1976) offers a definition that I find helpful: "Truth lies in the achievement of a contact with reality – a contact destined to reveal itself by an indefinite range of yet unforeseen consequences."[8]

Truth reveals itself in those intimations of reality that persuade us that there is some coherent order and meaning in our experience and our existence, and that at the same time inspire us to seek that true order and meaning. They are order and meaning that transcend the accumulation of facts. It is this kind of intimation of reality that leads mathematicians to judge the validity of an equation by its 'beauty'.[9]

Another author, Keith Ward, puts it like this: "When we apprehend a truth we . . . seek by intelligent enquiry to understand something of the nature of things, of how things really are in their characters and relationships. . . . Truth always lies beyond us, in its fullness. Yet we discern something of it".[10]

Writing as a doctor, and speaking, I hope, for other healthcare practitioners, I suggest that in clinical practice we seek, or should seek as complete an understanding of our patients as we can, in order that we may respond as faithfully as possible to the truth of their unique individuality and the unique problem that they present to us; a truth which in its fullness will always lie beyond us but which is the implicit goal of our work.

The second part of Polanyi's definition is of absolute importance. It says that truth is creative. It is not simply accurate information about the situation that confronts us. In any field of enquiry or endeavour, whatever it is of the truth that we glimpse, if it is really true, makes possible consequences – new insights, opportunities, discoveries, departures – as yet unforeseen.

In clinical practice, if we respond faithfully, whether in the diagnostic process, in the management of the problem, or in the quality of the therapeutic relationship, to whatever is revealed to us of the truth of the patient's life, we are assisting a healing process whose essential nature is not just remedial but creative. It, too, involves new insight and understanding, new discovery, new growth, new ways of being; basic principles of healing, that apply on every level of experience from the physiological to the spiritual.[11]

Clinical practice requires truth of us in many senses and many ways. It does require accuracy of observation, and diligent enquiry. But ideally it also requires complete attentiveness to the patient as an individual, and to the patient's story, unprejudiced by our own well-being, attitudes, expectations, beliefs or desires. It consequently requires truthful self-knowledge, and a reflective approach to what we do. And that truth will lead in turn to new discoveries, insights and strengths in our own lives.

In evaluating our practice, clinical or scientific, exemplary truthfulness is required, in what we claim for it, in how we seek to explain it, and in the willingness and the methods with which we investigate it. And all this requires that we are motivated by the 'scientific passion' that Polanyi describes. In clinical medicine, as Conrad Harris points out, "Every patient presents us, in a sense, with a research project".[12] The immediate goal of that search for truth, and the passion that motivates us, is the well-being of the individual patient. But the pursuit of that immediate goal is also a reaching out towards a greater and more universal truth about the human condition. I suggest that we have a responsibility to think critically and imaginatively about the truth of what is revealed to us in our patients' lives, and of our response to the problem they present, for the sake of what is to be learned about it, what is to be learned from it, and what is to be communicated about it. Because it is 'a contact with reality destined to reveal itself by an indefinite range of yet unforeseen consequences'.

Knowledge

> Knowledge is an extrovert element which a doctor acquires during his long and demanding education in order that he may direct it outwards upon the patient. But wisdom is an introverted element in the doctor's psyche; it has its origin within; and it is what makes him look not at the disease but at the bearer of the disease. It is what creates the link that unites the healer with his patient and the exercise of which makes him a true physician, a true healer. It is wisdom that tells the physician how to make the patient a partner in his own cure. Knowledge may enable you to memorise the whole of *Gray's Anatomy* or *Osler's Principles and Practice of Medicine* but only wisdom can tell you what to do with what you have learned. (Robertson Davies[13])

The pursuit of truth inevitably involves a pursuit of knowledge. You may be familiar with the quotation from TS Eliot's poem – *Choruses from 'The Rock'*:

> Where is the wisdom we have lost in knowledge? Where is the knowledge we have lost in information?[14]

Placing knowledge somewhere between wisdom and information like this puts it in a helpful perspective. It is not just information. It does not of itself confer wisdom. But it embraces information, and its proper function is to develop wisdom. The acquisition of knowledge goes hand in hand with intelligence, the power of the intellect. But like all great human attributes, intelligence can be well or ill-used. The reviewer of a book by biologist and theologian Celia Deane-Drummond, draws attention to a warning that echoes those words from Eliot, and that has real resonance for modern medicine. It is that our dependence on ever increasing technical wizardry points in the direction of what Deane-Drummond calls 'transhumanism', the triumph of intelligence over humanity, and a disastrous failure of wonder and wisdom.[15]

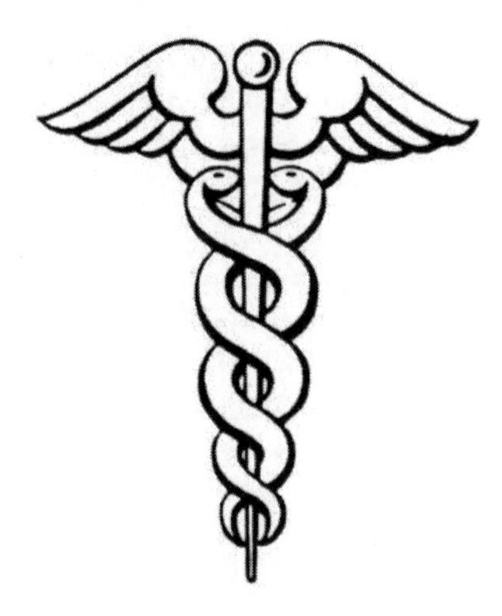

Figure 10.1 *The Caduceus*

The quotation at the beginning of this section is from a lecture by Robertson Davies called 'Can a doctor be a humanist?', which addresses the question – 'Can a doctor possibly be a humanist in a society that increasingly tempts him to be a scientist?' By 'humanist' he means a person with a deep interest in, insight into and care for human nature. He talks about the Caduceus, the familiar symbol of medicine and healing, and the identification of the two snakes coiled around the staff of Hermes with Knowledge and Wisdom (Figure 10.1). He discusses the tension between these two essential attributes of the physician's craft, the importance of keeping the right balance between the two, and the risk of allowing them to become opponents, of allowing knowledge to displace wisdom. He suggests "instead of calling them Knowledge and Wisdom let us call them Science and Humanism". I am indebted to a paper by Brendan Sweeney for introducing me to this most thought provoking lecture, and the delightful book in which it appears.[16]

So if wisdom is not to be lost in knowledge we have to treat knowledge with proper respect, but also with circumspection. All knowledge will not be true, but it must serve the truth, and must be willing to be displaced by new knowledge that is closer to the truth. It is within this perspective that we should regard the breadth of knowledge that a scientific community brings to the pursuit of truth and the exploration of reality. Popper himself writes: "The old scientific ideal of *episteme* – of absolutely certain, demonstrable knowledge – has proved to be an idol". The demand for scientific objectivity makes it inevitable that every statement must remain tentative for ever. It may indeed be corroborated, but every corroboration is relative to other statements which, again, are tentative. Only in our subjective experiences of conviction, in our subjective faith, can we be 'absolutely certain'.[7] In *Personal Knowledge* Michael Polanyi only mentions Popper in passing, but his whole thesis invokes a kind of faith in what is known – the 'tacit knowledge' by which we perform so many functions and that is not susceptible to logical analysis, and the creative tension that exists between this and formal scientific method.

In a challenging paper on 'Clinical medicine and the quest for certainty', Grant Gillett, a neurosurgeon in New Zealand, provides quotes from Hippocrates. "Even if it is not always accurate in every respect the fact that it is able to approach close to a standard of infallibility as a result of reasoning – should commend respect for the discoveries of medical science. Such discoveries are the product of good and true investigation, not chance happenings. But we also need to hearken to the critical voices that teach us about the provisional nature of knowledge when it is properly evaluated as *an evolving human endeavour* rather than an increasingly clear and bright map of biomedical reality."[1] (My italics.)

And we must remember that knowledge is more than an accumulation of facts. Eric Cassell again:

> Facts do not stand alone; they derive their meaning from their relationship to the other facts with which they form a whole; and also from that very whole of which they are a part. . . . This is of great importance to us as physicians. We elicit medical facts because of our need to understand, and what we want to understand are not isolated facts but wholes – whole kidneys, whole bodies, whole persons, and even whole communities.[17]

In other words: Knowledge = Facts + Understanding + Meaning.

Personal knowledge

My exploration of these themes has been greatly assisted by the book, *Personal Knowledge*, first published in 1958 by Michael Polanyi (1891–1976), from which I have quoted already.[8] It was introduced to me as essential reading if I was seriously interested in achieving a better understanding of the limitations of scientific proof.[18] Polanyi's working life overlapped that of Kuhn and Popper, but preceded them by some 20 years. It is an intellectually challenging but most exciting book, because it is about the kind of scientific passion that I believe is felt by many who work in medicine, whether in research or in direct patient care. Its Key themes of the book are summarised in Box 10.2.

BOX 10.2 *Key themes in Personal Knowledge*

- The ideal of detached scientific objectivity is a fiction.
- There is available to us a truer kind of objectivity that derives from our intimations of universal truth.
- This objectivity has an intuitive quality that has informed all great science.
- This glimpse of objective truth inspires 'scientific' passion'.
- Scientific passion is a heuristic passion – a passionate desire to find out or discover.
- BUT – The conclusions to which we are lead by our scientific passion are not infallible; they may be false but they are never meaningless.
- Personal knowledge is not license to speculate. It demands discipline, and rigorous discrimination of error, and discernment of its fruitfulness – the creative potential to yield unforeseen consequences.
- Scientific truth can be discovered, but not constructed.
- The methodology of proof, however, is constructed and contingent, and can never be absolute.
- Neglect of the principles of objective truth and personal knowledge will allow 'the tendency towards a universal mechanistic conception of things – completely to denature our image of man'.

Objectivity and intuition

Fifty years ago Polanyi challenged the ideal of detached scientific objectivity. He did not believe in it, and took great pains to demonstrate, by reference to various scientific methodologies, that it is a fiction. Firstly he insisted that all attempts to establish rules for scientific validity involve a measure of personal judgement, even though that judgement is collective and consensual within the scientific community. They are therefore contingent and provisional.

More radically perhaps, he proposed an altogether new meaning for the concept of objectivity. Not as a dispassionate, unbiased, value-free statement of observable fact, but as an intuition of universal truth, an intimation of reality. He writes, for example, of the theory of Relativity as, "... pure speculation, rationally intuited by Einstein ..."

Insights of this kind are of the nature of scientific discovery. Polanyi quotes Pasteur, for example, who said of his conviction, against very strong opposition, that fermentation was a function of the living cells of yeast, "If anyone should say that my conclusions go beyond the established facts I would agree, in the sense that I have taken my stand unreservedly in an order of ideas which, strictly speaking, cannot be irrefutably demonstrated".

Personal knowledge as Polanyi defines it, is not therefore a kind of subjectivity, but an objectivity that wholly subordinates the subjective to an intimation of truth that lies beyond us; that is transcendent, if you like. It is not a construct of our intellect or imagination, but a glimpse of a greater truth.

For example, mathematical physicist John Polkinghorne has stated that it is generally agreed among mathematicians that mathematics is not a process of construction, but of discovery; that mathematicians are not playing complex games of their own contriving, but exploring a pre-existing reality.[9]

Scientific passion

Many readers of this book who are involved in medicine and the sciences will already have understood, and perhaps recalled from your own experience what is meant by scientific passion, but Polanyi vividly evokes the connection between scientific discovery and scientific passion. "Personal knowledge in science is not made but discovered, and as such it claims to establish contact with reality *beyond* the clues on which it relies. It commits us, passionately, and far beyond our comprehension, to a vision of reality. Of this responsibility we cannot divest ourselves by setting up objective criteria of verifiability. Like love, to which it is akin, this commitment is a 'shirt of flame', blazing with passion, and also like love, consumed by devotion to a universal demand."

Criteria of scientific proof

Polkinghorne and Polanyi both emphasis the circularity in the relationship between theory and experimental proof, which Polanyi describes in the following way. "The rules of scientific *procedure* which we adopt, and the scientific *beliefs* and valuations which we hold, are mutually determined. For we proceed according to what we *expect* to be the case and we shape our *anticipations* in accordance with the success which our methods of *procedure* have met with." (My italics).

This warning about seeing only what we have learned to expect is echoed by Conrad Harris in the paper quoted earlier in which he encourages general practitioners to be more attentive to the, so to speak, corroborative detail of patients' stories (he calls it pathography) that does not fit the familiar clinical picture; not only for the sake of good patient care, but for the sake of fruitful research: "The observation and description of what is before one's eyes, *unconditioned by preconceived ideas,* is the starting point of all scientific research" (my italics). It requires only a shift in perspective.[12]

John Polkinghorne states, "There is an inescapable circularity in scientific argument. I think we have come to learn that the vocabulary of proof, in that strict logically coercive and inescapable sense, is actually not a very interesting category. Most things elude it. Even mathematics".[19] Doctors and medical scientists must learn to avoid, or at least to be aware of the risk of this circularity in clinical case taking and analysis, and in research, and not to pre-empt the conclusions we reach. The circularity in scientific argument may be inescapable, to an extent, but awareness of the risk will likewise prevent a pre-emptive closing of the circle. Otherwise science would never advance. Unfortunately, some doctors' and medical scientists' attitudes particularly, to unorthodox ideas, do become pre-emptive in this way. Pre-existing expectations do produce a closed circle, even occasionally a surprisingly vicious circle. And the vocabulary of proof is used coercively.

Polanyi writes, "No rule of scientific procedure is certain of finding truth and avoiding error". Perhaps the over-riding criterion should be integrity rather than proof; an integrity that accepts that the circle of knowledge is never closed, and that is always open to, and willing to give ground to the emergence of new insights, whatever we have hitherto believed or been lead to expect.

Destructive analysis

Integrity will insist that the operation of intuition, personal knowledge and scientific passion in science does not mean that anything goes. Personal knowledge is not license to speculate. It demands discipline, and rigorous discrimination of error. Despite the elusiveness of proof, rigorous experiment is necessary. As Polanyi says, "This method of criticism is indispensable – destructive analysis remains an indispensable weapon against superstition and specious practices".

But the rules and interpretation of experiment must be applied critically and with discernment. The 'mutually determining' nature of scientific theory and scientific procedures, and the risk of paradigm paralysis, must not be allowed to suppress emergent truths that do not fit. As Polanyi also says, ". . . to deny the feasibility of something, merely because we cannot understand in terms of our hitherto accepted framework how it could have been done or could have happened, may often result in explaining away quite genuine practices or experiences".

Evidence

> Evidence is a very fluid concept. If something fits our worldview and our prior probabilities and concepts, we are very happy to accept some reasoning as evidence. If something does not fit into our way of thinking, then even the best experimental evidence can be easily dismissed. Evidence is a complex beast. It is a concoction of empirical data, sprinkled over a plausible theoretical model, and fitted into the framework of a plausible worldview. (Harald Walach[19])

As these observations and the discussion of paradigms and models in part 2 of the Introduction make clear, the nature and validity of evidence is pre-empted by the paradigm that sanctions it and the model that it serves. They will strike a chord with many who are uneasy about the demands of evidence in clinical practice, which are not only imposed in the name of science but in many instances by policy makers. And they will encourage those who explicitly question its coercive power.

Gillett, whom I quoted earlier says this (referring back to the work of Kuhn and Michel Foucault):[20] "The underlying thought is that validated knowledge in an area of human inquiry is a joint product of intellectual exploration and the power structures that legitimate certain conceptualisations and modes of exploration. For instance, power is exercised in medical scholarship by authoritative bodies enforcing positivist conceptions of argument and investigation which go under the name of evidence based medicine. – An atmosphere is created whereby any views that depart from statistical methodologies based in the natural sciences are regarded as inferior or suspect".[1]

Gillett's comment quoted earlier about the provisional nature of knowledge when it is properly evaluated as an evolving human endeavour, and the discussion of reality, truth and knowledge, are echoed by Iona Heath in *The Mystery of General Practice*. Commenting on the dissonance between the biomedical model and the general practice model, she quotes Carl Rudebeck: "According to (the requirements of scientific biomechanical medicine), an answer should be numerical or it is not an answer. If on the other hand, research is looked upon as an activity adding to or changing our prevailing comprehension of reality . . . then the range of issues may be considerably widened. . . . The evaluation of the quality of research at one instant and according to strict formal criteria . . . is somewhat contradictory to the process of knowledge production itself."[21]

Controlled trials are the favoured methodology of evidence based medicine, designed to test the validity of a proposition about patient care by controlling the variables that might prevent a statistically valid answer to a specific question; usually a question about one specific intervention in one specific condition in a clearly defined population of patients. Gillett describes this methodology as "the current fundamentalism of the prospective randomised, controlled, double-blind trial". Toon, writing about the philosophy of general practice, comments, "It is a small but logically dubious jump from seeing the evidence from controlled trials as the soundest evidence on which to base clinical actions to the view that there is no other valid evidence for clinical activity".[22] Controlled trials generate evidence of interventions made under ideal test conditions. The limitations of this evidence are summarised simply and clearly in an article about the use of placebos in an edition of the *British Medical Journal* focusing on that theme: "Published evidence applies to a patient only if that patient has similar characteristics to patients in the study population. Even if this is the case, their response can rarely be accurately predicted. This is one of the problems with evidence based medicine: often its application to the individual is under less than ideal conditions."[23]

In other words, what actually happens – the *effectiveness* or clinical outcome in practice – may be different because the context is different. This effect of context on evidence is explained nicely, though in the course of examining a different issue, in a paper by Bernard Crump. He writes, "Experimental evaluation is based on an approach to the establishment of causation that can be described as successionist. The changes in outcome that occur in the experimental and control group are all that matters, and are observed externally. The context in which these changes occur is relevant only in so far as they can confirm the adequacy of the randomisation process. This failure to take account of context leads to at least two problems. Where evaluations lead to the conclusion that an intervention works, it is not known why it has worked. They are also prone to lead to the conclusion that an intervention does not work when another perspective is that the impact is place and context specific".[24] He goes on to describe by contrast 'generative' methods of evaluation used in social science that are rigorous and exacting but that emphasise the capture of evidence about the context in which interventions take place.

The dangers of over-reliance on certain kinds of evidence is amusingly illustrated by David Haslam in his lecture 'Who Cares?' which in essence is also about the limited appropriateness of the medical model to general practice.[25] He does this by quoting 'The McNamara fallacy':[26]

- The first step is to measure whatever can be easily measured. This is OK as far as it goes.
- The second step is to disregard that which can't be easily measured or to give it an arbitrary quantitative value. This is artificial and misleading.
- The third step is to presume that what can't be measured easily really isn't important. This is blindness.
- The fourth step is to say that what can't be easily measured really doesn't exist. This is suicide.

I have already referred to Iona Heath's reservations about the role of politicians and health service planners in misconstruing the nature of general practitioner care (Chapter 2). Others have regretted the use of evidence as a political tool. Evidence in the public health arena is a two edged weapon. Social structures and ideologies are interactive. Medicine and politics are no exception. Medical research fuels public health policy. Public health policy affects the organisation and delivery of health care. Medicine itself fuels 'the avalanche of public health rhetoric',[22] which in turn determines what happens in practice. The imposition of targets for clinical activity allied to financial incentives, for example, is an evidence based manipulation of both the medical profession and the patients – with the very best of intentions, but with consequences that are not necessarily always healthy, as we have seen. Nevertheless, the health gains resulting from public health policy are often beyond dispute. The banning of smoking in public places is an example of the public health triumph of good science (epidemiology) eventually driving policy. Epidemiology – the detailed observation and analysis of the march of events in the development of disease in order to understand the avoidable causes of the disease and to do something about them, has been one of the great advances of modern medicine; evidence in the service of health maintenance and disease prevention.

The trouble is that in this context, again as we have seen, the individual can become the herd. What is statistically good for the patient population detracts from the needs of individual patients, and may disregard social and cultural influences that bear heavily upon them. What is good practice for doctors in terms of performance targets may dictate and constrain the doctor–patient relationship, making care of the whole person more difficult to achieve.

Some critics see serious risks of the politicisation of evidence based medicine (EBM). Dixon and Sweeney spell this out clearly in the second chapter of their book *The Human Effect in Medicine*.[27] They argue that EBM distorts health care, and indeed the proper nature of science; that the dominant medical scientific paradigm, cannot hold a position of unassailable centrality in clinical practice; that a rational appreciation and cognitive evaluation of information is only a part of the practice and understanding of medicine; and that (the EBM approach) is based on an inadequate explanatory model, inappropriate to the complexities and constantly evolving nature of the human condition. They conclude that "the view of science currently espoused by practitioners, demanded by managers and applauded by politicians has devalued an intellectual standpoint into an ideology".

Maya Goldenberg, writing in *Social Science and Medicine*, expresses perhaps the extreme pole of discontent with the EBM movement – "an antiquated understanding of 'facts' about the world in the assumption that scientific beliefs stand or fall in the light of the evidence".[28] She offers extensive criticism of the EBM approach, but the summary proposes that, "The appeal to the authority of evidence that characterises evidence-based practices does not increase objectivity but rather obscures the subjective elements that inescapably enter all forms of human enquiry. The seeming common sense of EBM only occurs because of its assumed removal from the social context of medical practice".

A nice summary of the prevailing discomfort at the imposition of EBM is given in Marshall Marinker's editorial résumé of the relevant chapter in a book called *Sense and Sensibility in Medicine*.[29] He asks, "Why (do) so many leading GPs react in this strongly ambivalent way to what must surely be regarded as a substantial contribution to the enhancement of clinical standards. What is going on?" He suggests the following answers:

- The language of EBM somehow misses the point of the clinical encounter in primary clinical general practice.
- Fear that what begins as 'best information' on which to base a decision can easily be transformed into contractual instruments disguised to control not simply facilitate the management of the patient.
- A suspicion that clinical judgment will be supplemented with protocols and algorithms of diagnosis and treatment that will constitute (perhaps legally) the accepted and mandated response to illness.

He comments, "These may well be quite unrealistic fears (the progenitors and proponents of EBM would certainly deny such dirigiste[i] ambitions), but they are quite widely felt and expressed".

i *Dirigisme*: Policy of state direction and control in economic and social matters. (*Concise Oxford Dictionary*).

Indeed they are still quite widely felt and expressed. Twelve years later, Des Spence, a 'dissident voice' from general practice writing regularly in the *British Medical Journal*, echoes these sentiments under the heading *Medicine's living death*. He says that when evidence began to be presented systematically in the early 1990s it left some room for discretion. "Then, however, came the march of the guideline machines, and by 2000 things were getting out of hand. . . . Since then guidelines have become ever more restrictive and prescriptive. . . . Evidence is treated like solid bricks rather than the shanty corrugated iron that it is. This is the slow garrotte of medical judgement. . . . So discretion, once the cornerstone of the medical profession, is dead. It has been replaced by mass production medicine with . . . patients all treated the same with no thought to individual views or need. . . . Our job is being reduced to a mere collection of algorithms."[30]

Ninety per cent of medical encounters in the UK take place in general practice where the problems that patients present do not conform to the tidy definitions of the EBM guidelines. Many of these illnesses still elude precise biomedical diagnosis when they are referred for specialist opinion, though they may be fitted into one. But general practitioners in particular are likely to have the sceptical attitude to EBM that has been described, though they may be obliged to implement its guidelines, as Spence regretfully remarks later in his piece.

The natural approach to clinical decision making in general practice, the cornerstone as he puts it, was described to me by the late Robin Pinsent, a co-founder of the Royal College of General Practitioners Research Unit, as "informed empiricism".[31] This process of medical judgement is pragmatic, dealing with matters according to their practical significance or immediate importance, but based on a judicious blend of insight, experience, and formal evidence evaluated in the context of the individual problem. It is a harder task than the following of prescriptive guidelines and algorithms because it must take account of the variables that the analysis that provided the formal evidence excluded. It requires education and training. Informed empiricism is every bit as scientific as a strictly evidence based approach; rather more so in fact, because it acknowledges that every patient presents us, in a sense, with a research project, as Conrad Harris points out (Chapter 2).[12] It will occasionally misconstrue a problem when the metaorganic 'variables' confuse a necessary biomedical explanation, but no more so or more often than when the assumption of a biomedical explanation leads to neglect of the personal 'variables' that are the heart of the problem, and 'the disease is not the cause of the illness'; one of Alan Barbour's 'misconceptions and false starts that the clinical process can pursue'[32] (Chapter 6). This approach to clinical decision making is well recognised and respected, but is increasingly difficult to apply as EBM becomes enshrined in biomedical dogmatism and health policy targets.

This problem is described trenchantly in a book by an American doctor, Jerome Groopman, reviewed in the *British Medical Journal*:

> Doctors need to think 'outside the box' much more often. . . . Failure to do so starts early in the medical training cycle, as medical students and junior doctors all too rarely question cogently, listen carefully, or observe keenly. . . . What's partly to blame for this is today's rigid reliance on evidence based medicine and even, to an increasing extent, on highly sophisticated technology that has taken us away from the patient's story.[33]

I am fascinated by the resonance, particularly in the second sentence, with the teaching of the 17th century physician Thomas Sydenham, who has been called the father of modern clinical medicine. His reputation is said to have rested on "his empiricism . . . his determination to observe and examine each individual patient with the open mind of a natural historian'. He taught us to 'listen intently and question the patient minutely about the march of events in the development of disease".[34]

The tension between the interpretive approach to diagnosis and treatment based on the individual experience of illness and the story, and the analytical evidence based approach, is explored by Tessa Greenhalgh in 'Narrative based medicine in an evidence based world', mentioned earlier.[35] This concluding chapter from a comprehensive study of the importance of the patient's story to the understanding and management of the illness, corrects a common misconception about the original intentions of the evidence based medicine (EBM) movement. The concept of EBM was not intended to preclude clinical judgement and the application of informed empiricism. The author, Trisha Greenhalgh, quotes its pioneers: "The practice of evidence based medicine means *integrating* individual clinical expertise with the best available external clinical evidence. . . . By individual clinical expertise, we mean the proficiency and judgement that individual clinicians acquire through clinical experience and clinical practice".[2] She argues, "Genuine evidence based practice actually *presupposes* an interpretive paradigm within which the patient experiences illness and the clinician-patient encounter is enacted". The belief that the EBM approach rests upon the assumption that clinical observation is totally objective and should, like all scientific measurements, be reproducible is incorrect. Its founding fathers made no such claim to objectivity. It seems it is the followers of the EBM movement who have turned their wisdom into a rigid doctrine they did not intend. As Greenhalgh concludes, "The irrevocably case based (i.e. narrative based) nature of clinical wisdom is precisely what enables us to contextualise and individualise the problem before us. Far from obviating the need for subjectivity in the clinical encounter, the valid application of empirical evidence *requires* a solid grounding in the narrative based world".

Ways of knowing

Science is a way of knowing. The word derives from the Latin *scire,* to know. Epistemology is the theory of the method or grounds of knowledge (COD); the study of ways of knowing, we could say. One reason for distrusting the dominance of the biomedical model is that its particular analytical method restricts our ways of knowing, and there are other ways of knowing that must, and indeed in practice do belong to our medical epistemology (Box 10.3). Medicine has to deal with the reality of individual patients' lives, a reality that is expressed on different levels of experience, probably on several different levels of experience at the same time, from the molecular to the transcendental, in different individuals. "Different levels of reality may be expected to have their idiosyncratic characters, and there will not be a single epistemic rule for all." In other words, there will not be a single best way of knowing to meet all situations.

BOX 10.3 *Ways of knowing*

- Analytical/experimental scientific method.
- Motivated belief.
- Inference to the best explanation.
- Tacit knowledge.
- Intuition.
- 'Mindlines.'

Motivated belief

The quotation I have just used is from the physicist and priest John Polkinghorne, whose scientific credentials are impeccable.[7] In the same passage he writes,

> Scientists are not inclined to subscribe to an a priori concept of what is reasonable. They have found the physical world to be too surprising, too resistant to prior expectation. . . . Instead the actual character of our encounter with reality has to be allowed to shape our knowledge and thought. . . . The instinctive

> question for the scientist to ask is not 'Is it reasonable?', as if one knew beforehand the shape that rationality had to take, but 'What makes you think that might be the case?' Radical revision of expectation cannot be ruled out, but it will only be accepted if evidence is presented in support of the new point of view that is being proposed. *Science trades in motivated belief.* (My italics)

The cornerstone of much scientific research, and certainly of the science on which the biomedical model is based, is repeatable experimental confirmation, usually in controlled conditions. But many disciplines are not susceptible to this kind of investigation: many surgical procedures, for example; history; geology and the fossil record; the events recorded in astronomical observations; theories of the origin of life; many human predicaments that require a systematic solution. All these have a scientific component. In addition most other non-scientific explorations of reality also lack recourse to repeatable controlled investigation, including theology, whose relationship to science John Polkinghorne is exploring in the pages I have quoted.

The fact that a phenomenon or proposition cannot be investigated so scrupulously does not mean that the evidence that 'makes you think that might be the case' is not just as important as evidence that can be so rigorously tested. Nor does it mean that the quality of evidence should not and cannot be assessed intellectually. The evidence is essential to the motivation, and well founded motivation is essential to the belief. But motivated belief acknowledges that judgments such as these, including "the quality of a painting, the beauty of a piece of music, or the character of a friend, depend upon powers of sympathetic discernment, rather than being open to empirical demonstration". Polkinghorne implies that they are by no means subordinate ways of knowing because in fact "no form of human truth-seeking enquiry can attain absolute certainty about its conclusions".

Inference to the best explanation (abduction)

This is not far removed from the process of motivated belief, but involves choice between alternative or competing theories. The evidence can be construed in various ways, one of which is the most intellectually coherent and satisfying. It involves weighing evidence and judging probability, not proof. In a medical context a good example is what is known as 'differential diagnosis'. A doctor weighs the evidence of the available symptoms and signs, and perhaps the results of tests, and judges the probability that a particular diagnosis best explains what is going on. The differential diagnosis of a headache could be a hangover, a migraine or a sub-arachnoid haemorrhage (bleeding in the brain). Any one of those could be a correct diagnosis. But it might also be an incomplete explanation if it neglects the circumstances that predisposed to the physiological disorder; which is a possibility that is central to the problem, the healthcare dilemma that this book is exploring. On the human scale, inference to the best explanation is often the only path we can follow, but it is not unscientific. It is also a necessary path of enquiry on the largest scale. The fact of the rational intelligibility of the universe, and of the explanatory power of science to unfold it, are not themselves self-explanatory. Einstein famously commented that "The most incomprehensible thing about the universe is that it is comprehensible". This remarkable fact, "The bedrock belief upon which all intellectual enquiry is built . . . is one of the main considerations that have led thinkers of all generations to conclude that the universe itself must be the product of intelligence".[7] This is inference to the best explanation. It is also motivated belief. The evidence is clear, the reasoning logical, but the conclusion is not absolute, and in this instance never can be. Claims about evolution at the level of species (macroevolution) or molecules (microevolution) depend similarly on inference to the best explanation because they concern unrepeatable past events.

Informed Empiricism

This term, introduced to me, as mentioned, by Robin Pinsent, is his description of GPs' way of knowing. It comprises their education and training and the research evidence related to the task in hand. But it also comprises experience, and allows that the actual character of their encounter with the reality of the patient's life and predicament should shape their knowledge and their thought (to paraphrase John Polkinghorne). Informed empiricism develops clinical acumen and clinical judgement. It acknowledges targets and guidelines but is not a slave to them because it knows that they are a generalisation and an abstraction that may or may not need to be applied to the individual patient. It is true to the original spirit of evidence based medicine. Informed empiricism enables the process of inference to the best explanation, but allows that the explanation may be unique to the individual patient, and accepts, "Every patient presents us, in a sense, with a research project. Every time we intervene in patients' lives we are conducting experiments".[12] But these observations by Conrad Harris carry an injunction to the open-mindedness towards the data that should be the rule for all scientists and clinicians. We should never be content "to stop asking questions once (we) find a pattern (we) know how to deal with (for fear that) going on may lead us into uncharted waters. . . . There is always a gap between what we know and what we need to know, and if we are not constantly exploring a little of it we are in danger of forgetting that it exists". Informed empiricism must be a dynamic way of knowing. Just as, indeed, all ways of knowing must be dynamic.

Tacit Knowledge

Tacit knowledge is a concept developed by Michael Polanyi as part of his exploration of *Personal Knowledge*.[8] It describes the things we know, and things we know how to do that we cannot be taught, or that we learn without being taught; activities that we cannot precisely describe or explain to others. It is knowledge or technique that we discover by doing. A child learning to speak discovers the grammatical construction necessary to make sentences without being told how to do it. Adults may correct mistakes, and the knowledge and the skill may be refined by rules taught in later life, but the knowledge by which coherent speech begins to emerge is tacit knowledge. Similarly, we cannot describe or explain precisely what is involved in learning to ride a bicycle or hammer in a nail. There is a whole repertoire of knowledge and skill that we acquire in this informal and tacit fashion that will influence our actions, our behaviour and our interpretation of experience in many areas of life, including science.

I have already mentioned this tacit knowledge by which we perform so many functions and that is not susceptible to logical analysis, and the creative tension that exists between this and formal scientific method. It is one of the attributes of the mind whose subjugation to rules, regulations and protocols, and subsequent neglect James Willis laments in my references to his work in Chapter 9 ('A crisis of morale'). He is describing much the same thing as tacit knowledge when he writes about the 'under-mind', borrowing the concept from a book by Guy Claxton, *Hare Brain Tortoise Mind: Why intelligence increases as you think less*.[36] The book documents the evidence that it is the under-mind, or subconscious, that enables us, in Willis's words, to "operate better if we take a side-step and switch off our focused, logical, analytical, conscious approach for some of the time. And not just a bit better – we operate a *lot* better".[37] To neglect its operation in making medical judgements, he argues, can actually do harm. Tacit knowledge, the under-mind, is fed by experience, the things we learn without knowing that we are learning, or how we are learning, because the human mind is subconsciously alert to the things it needs to know. It is enfeebled if it is undernourished by over-investment in logic and lack of interest in the diversity of human experience.

Intuition

Intuition is the immediate apprehension of something. It is an attribute or faculty that enables us to grasp, to perceive, to be aware, to know something about our circumstances, our environment or another person, without conscious reasoning. It may be apprehended by the senses (we feel there is something wrong) or by the intellect (I know that person is lying). It is not the same as the process of picking up non-verbal cues that should be part of our repertoire of clinical and psychological skills in medicine, and in life for that matter. Howard Spiro discusses the role of intuition in medicine in his book *The Power of Hope*,[38] and quotes Henri Bergson's account of intuition as an inward and immediate vision of reality that contrasts with the knowledge gained by the systematic application of our intelligence in science.[39] But intuition has paved the way for the prodigious work of intelligence in science, of which Einstein's initial perception of the phenomenon of relativity is perhaps the best known example. It is an example that suggests that intuition is to an extent dependent on the openness of a prepared mind. On the other hand, psychologist Bruce Hood has argued recently in his book *Supersense* that intuition is an innate faculty that we all possess, which is perhaps our common belief.[40]

Mindlines

This diversity of ways of knowing is exemplified in clinical practice by a study of knowledge management in primary care whose objective was, "To explore in depth how primary care clinicians (general practitioners and practice nurses) derive their individual and collective healthcare decisions".[41] The authors found, "clinicians rarely accessed, appraised, and used explicit evidence directly from research or other formal sources. Instead, they relied on what we have called 'mindlines', collectively reinforced, internalised tacit guidelines, which were informed by brief reading, but mainly by their interactions with each other and with opinion leaders, patients, and pharmaceutical representatives and by other sources of largely tacit knowledge that built on their early training and their own and their colleagues' experience. The clinicians, in general, would refine their mindlines by acquiring tacit knowledge from trusted sources, mainly their colleagues". Mindlines "were grown from experience and from people who are trusted; they were 'stored in my head' but could be shared and tested and then internalised through discussion, while leaving room for individual flexibility. (They) might well be modified when applied to an individual patient after discussion and negotiation during the consultation;

at this stage patients' ideas of what is the appropriate evidence about their particular case (their own personal history, what their family has experienced, what they have read in the media, and so on) could influence the application or even the continuing development of the mindline. Further adjustment might subsequently happen during swapping stories with colleagues or in audit or critical incident meetings".

I would be very surprised if, in the midst of the inevitable uncertainty of medical practice, all clinicians do not employ these ways of managing knowledge, and the seven 'ways of knowing' that I have described, in medicine and indeed in life, and find them essential in making sense of their own and their patients' experience, and deciding what to do about it.

Conclusion

Evidence, like a paradigm, is an essential foundation for exploring reality, but it is not that reality. Evidence is information, an essential contribution to the acquisition of knowledge. But it must not be mistaken for knowledge, let alone truth. The scientific paradigm prescribes the information that fits the paradigm and the methodology that is appropriate to the research that will provide that information. The evidence acceptable to the paradigm sustains the paradigm. The relationship shows the circularity described by Polanyi and Polkinghorne, that is its danger. A paradigm that is open to information that does not fit will be a creative paradigm, open to that 'indefinite range of yet unforeseen consequences', new knowledge. One that is not will become an ideology, a victim of paradigm paralysis. Wisdom is the attribute we need to perceive both the value and the limitations of our paradigm.

The goal of our exploration of reality is truth. Evidence is an essential tool with which to dig for truth, but it is not truth. Truth is universal and indivisible. Evidence is contingent and conditional. Science, within its particular frame of reference – answering the questions 'What?' and 'How?' – is one of evolved humanity's glories, and a tributary pathway to truth. Evidence is the tool that it has fashioned and refined. But science is not the whole story. It does not, for instance, answer the question 'Why?'. There are other tributary pathways. The dialogue between science and theology, for example, although it is a dialogue of the deaf at its polarised extremes, is very fruitful where there is cross-border trade in intellectual goods between the two domains, the 'traffic in truth' that John Polkinghorne recommends.[42] In this context, the relationship between evidence and truth is nicely illustrated in an essay amongst the works of the twentieth century theologian Austin Farrer. He is questioning the proposition that a truthful scholar is one who will not go an inch beyond the support of the evidence, and asks the question, "What is the supreme motive of the truth-seeking mind? Is it to explode shams, or to acknowledge realities? And (if) there are realities . . . too intangible to be proved, will intellectual honesty discount them, or will it embrace them?" (Echoes of the quotation from Schumacher in the Introduction). In Chapter 11 we will meet Thomas Kuhn's warning that "the man who embraces a new paradigm at an early stage (the 'paradigm pioneer' we will meet in the next chapter) must often do so in defiance of the evidence"; a decision that can only be based on faith.[3] Faith is the twin of love, says Farrer. (You will remember how Polanyi asserts that scientific passion is akin to love (p.171); and how Polkinghorne tells us that mathematical truth is recognisable by its beauty (p.166)) And love, Farrer continues, "with its inexhaustible appetite for what deserves loving, sees beyond evidence . . ."; when faith, the act of will by which we determine to accept or trust what draws our love, comes into play. "But though faith and love go beyond absolute evidence, they are not blind. If we *really* love and trust . . . we do not wish to entertain a fantastic image (of the object of our love)". (My italics.) And reflecting Polanyi's account of the role of personal knowledge he says, "After all the detection of shams, the clarification of argument, and the sifting of evidence – after all criticism, all analysis – a (truth-seeker) must make up his mind what there is most worthy of love, and most binding on conduct, in the world of real existence". Medicine operates in the world of real existence. Evidence is indispensable, but we must always be willing to see beyond the evidence and beyond the boundary of the paradigm that has hitherto sustained it. I suspect that the authors of *Follies and Fallacies in Medicine,* whom I quoted in the Chapter 2, would be unsympathetic to some of the propositions in this book, but really it has a similar aim, "to reach inquisitive minds, particularly those who are still young and uncorrupted by dogma". It addresses the same sort of errors that they were concerned with, "errors of doctrine, systematic errors which are part of dogma and accepted truth, distortions which set obstacles in the path of rational thought and enquiry".[43]

References

1 Gillett G. Clinical medicine and the quest for certainty. *Soc Sci Med.* 2004; 58:727–738.

2 Sackett DL, Haynes RB, Tugwell P. *Clinical Epidemiology: a basic science for clinical medicine.* Boston: Little Brown; 1985.

3 Kuhn T. *The structure of scientific revolutions.* Chicago: University of Chicago Press; 1996.

4 Popper K. *The Logic of Scientific Discovery.* Abingdon: Routledge; 1992.

5 Fuller S. *Kuhn vs. Popper. The struggle for the soul of science.* Cambridge: Icon; 2006.

6 Whitmarsh T. The Nature of Evidence in Complementary and Alternative Medicine: Ideas from Trials of Homeopathy in Chronic Headache. In: Callahan D. *The Role of complementary and alternative medicine: accommodating pluralism* Washington DC: Georgetown University Press; 2002. pp148–162.

7 Polkinghorne J. *Theology in the Context of Science.* London: SPCK; 2008.

8 Polanyi M. *Personal Knowledge.* London: Routledge; 2002.

9 Polkinghorne J. *Exploring Reality.* London: SPCK; 2005.

10 Ward K. In: *Defence of the Soul.* Oxford: Oneworld; 1998.

11 Swayne J. Homeopathy Wholeness and Healing. *Homeopathy* 2005; 94: 37–43.

12 Harris C. Seeing sunflowers. *J R Coll Gen Pract.* 1989; 39:313–319.

13 Davies R. *The Merry Heart : Reflections on Reading Writing and the World of Books.* New York: Viking Press; 1997.

14 Eliot T. *Collected Poems 1909–1962.* London: Faber and Faber; 1963.

15 Habgood J. Review: Christ and evolution; wonder and wisdom by Celia Deane-Drummond. *Science and Christian belief* 2010; 22(1):187–188.

16 Sweeney B. The place of the humanities in the education of doctor. *Br J Gen Pract.* 1998; 48:998–1102.

17 Cassell E. *The Nature of Suffering and the Goals of Medicine.* New York: Oxford University Press; 2004.

18 Polkinghorne J. Personal communication, 2008.

19 Wallach H. The Campaign against CAM and the notion of "Evidence-Based". *J Altern Complement Med.* 2009; 15(10):1139–142.

20 Foucault M. In: Rabinow P. editor. *The Foucault Reader.* London: Penguin; 1984.

21 Heath I. *The Mystery of General Practice.* London: Nuffield Provincial Hospitals Trust; 1995.

22 Toon P. Occasional Paper 78. *Towards a Philosophy of General Practice.* London: Royal College of General Practitioners; 1999.

23 Pittrof R, Rubinstein I. The thinking doctor's guide to placebos. *Br Med J.* 2008; 336:1020.

24 Crump B. Should we use large scale healthcare interventions without clear evidence that benefits outweigh costs and harms? – Yes. *Br Med J.* 2008; 336:1276.

25 Haslam D. Who cares? *Br J Gen Pract.* 2007; 57:987–993.

26 Handy C. *The Empty Raincoat.* London: Random House; 1995.

27 Dixon M, Sweeney K. *The Human Effect in Medicine.* Oxford: Radiffe; 2000.

28 Goldenberg M. On evidence and evidence based medicine. *Sci Med*. 2006; 62:2621–2632.
29 Marinker M. Introduction. In: Marinker M. *Sense and sensibility in medicine*. London: BMJ Publishing Group; 1996.
30 Spence D. Medicine's living death. *Br Med J*. 2008; 337:a674.
31 Pinsent R. Personal communication, 1980.
32 Barbour A. *Caring for patients: a critique of the medical model*. Stanford: Stanford University Press; 1995.
33 Woods D. Review of the week: Living in a box. *Br Med J*. 2007; 334:856.
34 Marinker M. The Chameleon the Judas goat and the cuckoo. *J R Coll Gen Pract*. 1987; 28:199–206.
35 Greenhalgh T. Narrative based medicine in an evidence based world. Greenhalgh T. *Narrative Based Medicine*. London: BMJ Books; 1998.
36 Claxton G. (1998). *Hare Brain Tortoise Mind: Why intelligence increases as you think less*. London: Fourth Estate; 1998.
37 Willis J. *Friends in Low Places*. Abingdon: Radcliffe; 2001.
38 Spiro H. *The Power of Hope*. New Haven & London: Yale University Press; 1998.
39 Bergson H. *Creative Evolution*. New York: Modern Library; 1944.
40 Hood BM. *Supersense*. New York: Harper Collins; 2009.
41 Gabbay J, le May A. Evidence based guidelines or collectively constructed "mind-lines"? Ethnographic study of knowledge management in primry care. *Br Med J*. 2004; 329:1013–1017.
42 Polkinghorne J. *Traffic in Truth: Exchanges between Science and Theology*. Norwich: Canterbury Press; 2000.
43 Skrabanek P, McCormick J. *Follies and Fallacies in Medicine*. 3rd edition. Eastbourne: Tarragon Press; 1988.

11

CHANGE AND RESISTANCE TO CHANGE

Summary

- Patient preference has always been one factor in the process of change. But patients have always been in two minds about what they want – technical control of bodily ailments, or to be treated as a person rather than a disordered mechanism.
- The advance of science and the achievements of science changed the culture and heightened people's expectations of what scientific medicine could offer.
- Models and paradigms will always be in a sense experimental, never a perfect representation of reality. But they can be very resistant to change. 'Paradigm paralysis' inhibits progress. 'Paradigm pioneers' struggle to be heard.
- The achievements of science reveal a material reality that for many is completely satisfying and sufficient. But not for all.
- The word that best sums up this deficiency is 'meaning'. 'Science for understanding' has become subordinate to 'science for manipulation'.
- The 'border dispute' between the biomedical and holistic paradigms is a fruitless controversy. We need elements of both if medicine is to fulfil its healing vocation.

A Changing Scene

There is no denying that the evolutionary struggle I have described is real. Nor that it has been going on for a long time. I have described its persistence throughout the 40 years of my career in medicine, and its far longer history in Steven Lyng's account of the reluctance of family doctors in America to adopt fully the scientific ethos off the post-Flexner (post 1910) medical paradigm.[1] In fact the struggle between the emerging biomedical model and other models of health care that he describes had already been quite lively in America during the 19th century. There were three contributing factors. One was the dislike of 'heroic' medicine (Chapter 2). Another was the success of Thomsonian medicine, a well organised and widespread system of botanical medicine that offered a popular alternative to primitive scientific medicine. The third, which overlapped the Thomsonian period, was the rise of homeopathy, introduced by doctors from its original base in Europe and widely taught in dedicated medical colleges until its near demise in the aftermath of the Flexner report, whose commission it is claimed was largely motivated by the American Medical Association's determination to suppress the competition offered by homeopathic practitioners.

There are some instructive lessons about the nature of the struggle from this history, which I have drawn from Lyng's account. Firstly, it is clear that patient preference, unsurprisingly perhaps, has always been one factor in the process of change. And it is also clear that patients have always been in two minds about what they want. And patients, you and I, are still attracted by the authority, power and mystique of the medical profession, by the promise of control of bodily ailments and the 'quick fix'. At the same time we very much want to be treated as a person rather than a disordered mechanism, and for the biographical context of our illness to be understood as much as the biological substance of our disease.

In the early days, the choice was easier, because heroic medicine was so unpleasant and not conspicuously more effective, and probably expensive being in the hands of the elite, that the low-tech alternatives were obviously attractive. But fashion and income played a part, and those whose education and social status made them aware of advances in medicine were more likely to avail themselves of what it had to offer. For poorer and less well-educated patients, more 'domestic' forms of medicine were the natural choice. Patients of Thomsonian medicine were predominately in the latter group. Homeopathy's arrival established a different pattern. It shared the appeal of low-tech alternatives to heroic medicine, but was favoured by more sophisticated and wealthier patients. A significant difference, in terms both of its standing with patients and with the established profession, was that its practitioners were themselves members of the medical establishment, trained in the growing tradition of scientific medicine. This in itself constituted a greater challenge to that establishment. But the challenge was aggravated by the fact that the principles of homeopathy were so diametrically opposed to those of the increasingly dominant scientific model. Firstly they emphasised the importance of basing a treatment strategy on an appreciation of the dynamics of the illness in the whole person. Secondly they emphasised the importance of treating it as an individual illness rather than as a particular pathological state. And thirdly they invoked the self-regulating and self-healing capabilities of the body and the mind, rather than employing methods of treatment designed to control the disorder.

But Thomsonian medicine and homeopathy both gave way to the rise of modern medicine. The advance of science and the achievements of science changed the culture and heightened people's expectations of what scientific medicine could offer. Expectations create demand, and the focus of that demand shifted towards the regular, now orthodox medical profession. And that demand was now met by treatments and procedures that were increasingly effective and patient friendly. In addition Lyng attributes the decline of Thomsonian medicine and homeopathy to three other factors, dissention about treatment principles and methods amongst the practitioners, the integration of orthodox principles and methods within the unorthodox practice, and also the adoption of some of the principles and methods of unorthodox practice within regular medicine. Finally, because the outcome of the Flexner report was to close down all medical colleges that did not conform to the curriculum of scientific medicine that it recommended, other models of practice were relegated to the 'fringe', and became disreputable.

This brief history of events in America conveniently reflects trends, influences and tensions in the evolution of medicine that have been alluded to already. They include cultural and social developments, popular preferences and expectations, compromise between different paradigms, accommodation of one model by another, and the disarray of adherents to an unorthodox paradigm in the face of the hegemony (dominant leadership) of scientific orthodoxy.

This pattern of events on the ground represents the interplay of plausibility structures, paradigms and models, the exploration of reality, and the problems of truth, proof and evidence that are discussed in earlier chapters.

The problem with paradigms

Struggle and competition, even amounting to revolution as Kuhn proposes,[2] are as much in the nature of the evolution of ideas as the evolution of species. Paradigms are essential to the evolutionary process. They are 'species' of thought within which 'mutations' occur that give rise to new insights. The models that are built with the conceptual framework of the paradigm help us to explore the reality that the paradigm attempts to describe, and will always be in a sense experimental, unless we make the mistake of assuming that the paradigm and its models are perfect representations of reality. But during the life of a paradigm it will exert a very firm hold on most people for a considerable period, and inevitably, it seems, on some or many even when it reaches its 'best before' date. Its adherents may have a great deal invested in it, intellectually, psychologically, philosophically, politically or economically, so that its surrender, or even modification may not just be unwelcome but even literally unthinkable. Thus Thomas Kuhn wrote about the obdurate nature of established paradigms under the title, 'The structure of scientific *revolutions*'. Joel Barker makes this point in a rather more homely fashion as it applies to the business world: "When a paradigm shifter asks you to change, they are asking you to forsake your investment in the present paradigm. What has that investment given you?

- Your power to solve many important problems.
- Your status among your peers as a problem solver.
- Monetary remuneration (in many cases your salary is based on how well you use a paradigm).
- Perhaps even your title and the corner office that are the result of your facility in using the paradigm."[3]

It might be impolite to make too precise an analogy with the world of medical science, but, for instance, item 3 would translate into research grants. Barker says: "New paradigms put everyone practising the old paradigm at great risk, The better you are at your paradigm, the more you have invested in it, the more you have to lose by changing paradigms".

'Revolution' is an apt term for the challenge of a new paradigm because, as Kuhn points out, it is the nature of scientific authority itself that is being called into question. It considers itself self-evidently true and perceives no need to justify itself from first principles. But when scientific revolutions succeed, Kuhn suggests, they do so at first not because the adherents of the existing paradigm are persuaded of a new way of seeing things, but because other people's views (which in medicine, of course, importantly includes patients' views) start to count.

"To mount a serious challenge to the existing paradigm, a new conceptual framework will be needed to accommodate its anomalies in a way that scientists will take seriously." According to Kuhn, when these anomalies that signal a new paradigm arise, they may be invisible to the majority of normal science adherents. Further, when they are encountered, they may be ignored, suppressed or discredited.

Lyng comments, "One cannot hope to adequately perceive new dimensions of reality unless one is equipped with a system of appropriate cognitive categories. In modern Western culture, we have access to an extensive and systematic set of cognitive categories for perceiving the organic aspect of the disease process, but we possess few categories that are appropriate to the metaorganic realms".[1]

By 'metaorganic' he means those components of the illness and the 'story of sickness' that are peripheral to, and often antecedent to the organic disease process itself.

Joel Barker presents, ironically, some great examples of opinions that in retrospect reveal the lack of the necessary cognitive equipment to foresee otherwise:

> "Sensible and responsible women do not want to vote." (Grover Cleveland, 1905)
> "There is no likelihood that man can ever tap the power of the atom." (Robert Millikan, Nobel Prize winner in Physics, 1920)
> "There is no reason for any individual to have a computer in their home." (Ken Olsen, president of Digital Equipment Corporation, 1977)

Barker quotes a fascinating example of how cognitive conditioning and expectations influence what we are capable of perceiving. Groups of chess players, ranging from novices to international players were shown the layout of pieces in a partly completed, but actual chess game for five seconds, and then asked to recreate the layout as accurately as possible. The experts achieved 81% accuracy, compared with about 33% for the novices. When, however, the experiment was repeated with the pieces arranged randomly on the board by a computer, the experts' recall of the layout was actually worse than the novices'. The experts did not respond to what they saw because it did not correspond to the assumptions they had learned to make about the deployment of chess pieces. And as Conrad Harris pointed out, in clinical medicine, "What we expect to find is powerfully conditioned by what we have learned. . . . This sets the limits of what we ask our patients about and the extent to which we are prepared to ignore anything they tell us that is not required by, or does not fit, a pattern with which we are familiar".[4]

In the same vein, Michael Polanyi writes: "It is the normal practise of scientists to ignore evidence which appears incompatible with the accepted system of scientific knowledge, in the hope that it will eventually prove false or irrelevant".[5]

The prevailing paradigm may be extended to try and include the anomaly, adopting certain of the anomalous principles or practices into the orthodox framework, as mentioned in the synopsis of events in America; or as in the current tendency to explain away the response to complementary and alternative treatments as placebo effects, in many instances perhaps rightly so. In the book discussing the philosophies of Kuhn and Popper mentioned earlier, Fuller comments that scientists are not taught to be mentally flexible. Hence, he says, echoing the earlier quote from Polanyi, revolutions progress because "argumentation in science does more to sway uncommitted spectators – than to change the minds of the scientific principles themselves".[6]

Popper *does* require that people of the prevailing mind-set *are* persuaded of a new way of seeing things *rather* than that other people's views start to count. But that requires acceptance of the provisional nature of knowledge, truly scientific open-mindedness to new possibilities, however unforeseen, and that the rules of the existing paradigm are not pre-emptive of evidence that does not conform to those rules. To quote Polanyi again:

> A hostile audience may in fact deliberately refuse to entertain novel conceptions . . . because its members fear that once they have accepted this framework they will be lead to conclusions which they – rightly or wrongly – abhor. Proponents of a new system can convince their audience only by first winning their intellectual sympathy for a doctrine they have not yet grasped. *Those who listen sympathetically* will discover for themselves what they would otherwise never have understood. (My italics)

When it comes to the acceptance of a new paradigm, the saying "I'll believe it when I see it" is perhaps better rendered, "I'll see it when I believe it".[3]

A difficulty lies in the fact that the process of transition to a new paradigm may not be primarily intellectual. This is why it is very much a matter of changing hearts and minds at a level that is also intuitive. The popularity of an emergent paradigm may exceed its power to explain the phenomenon. I have already quoted Kuhn's warning that "the man who embraces a new paradigm at an early stage must often do so in defiance of the evidence". A decision of that kind can only be based on 'faith'.

Barker dubs people who are leaders in this process of transition 'Paradigm pioneers', and says, "The essence of the pioneering decision is: Those who (adopt a new paradigm) early do it not as an act of the head but as an act of the heart. They make a commitment to the tacit knowledge that Polanyi speaks of, to personal knowledge. They are following a heuristic process; a thought process for solving problems that cannot be cannot be handled by logic and probability theory alone . . . that we tend to use if not in the place of logic, at least as a short cut or empirical rule."[7]

This is not simply a matter of opinion or preference, and it does not bypass rational analysis. In Polanyi's terms, it is not license to speculate. It demands discipline, and rigorous discrimination of error, and discernment of its fruitfulness. This distinction is crucial.

In his essay, 'Demarcation of the absurd',[8] in which amongst other things he wittily castigates homeopathy for its "dilutions of grandeur", Petr Skrabanek quotes from *The comforts of unreason: A study of the motives behind irrational thought,* in which the author offers absolutely unexceptionable advice for any researcher: 'We must search our mind beforehand to find out what we would like to be true, and having got that clear, constantly discount our natural tendency in that direction'.[9]

But perhaps that quotation needs to be stated in the converse, too. David Reilly, a doctor responsible for producing some of the most convincing research evidence for the activity of those homeopathic high dilutions that Skrabenek derided, asked him how many positive randomised double blind controlled trials he would need to conduct in order to convince him. To which Skrabenek replied that he would never be convinced.[10] If we are to be innocent of intellectual double standards, we must *also* say, "We must search our mind scrupulously beforehand to find out what we would *not* like to be true, and having got that clear, constantly discount our natural tendency in that direction". *All* of us engaged in any pursuit of truth must be constantly aware of our susceptibility to the influence of what we want or do not want to be true.

The pros and cons of science

The achievements of science are literally awe-inspiring. They inspire awe at the beauty, the complexity, the diversity, the intricacy, the interdependence, and the fitness for purpose of all that exists and that is within the range of our consciousness. And at the intelligibility of it all that makes it accessible to our consciousness – from the grand scale of the universe to the smallest scale of elementary particles and genes. They have revealed a material reality that for many is completely satisfying and sufficient. These discoveries also inspire a different kind of awe at the astonishing technological achievements that they have made possible. The benefits have been immense. It is not surprising that modern science, the science of medicine to which it has given birth, and the model of medical practice built upon it have so captured the hearts and minds of people in the developed Western world, and are increasingly capturing the hearts and minds of people in the developing world. Why should we want to change anything?

Why should we be looking for any further evolution in our understanding of reality?

The answer must be that the reality revealed by modern science is *not* completely satisfying and sufficient. The dis-ease within medicine, and amongst patients, who despite their strong allegiance to the present model are constantly at the same time looking elsewhere for health and healing, reveals a restlessness (to paraphrase the earlier quotation from Keith Ward) to understand something more of the nature of things, of how things really are in their characters and relationships; a more satisfying and sufficient truth that we discern something of, even if it always lies beyond us in its fullness.[11] This is an understanding that ultimately all health care professionals, and all patients desire in order to achieve as faithful a response as possible to the unique problems that they present to us; the uniquely individual problems that Iona Heath described as the joy and the challenge of general practitioner care. Elsewhere she has written that, "The great gift of what we do is that every day, if we allow ourselves not only to listen but to hear, we are brought face to face with what we do not know, with the limits of the understanding and power of biomedical science".[12]

Perhaps the word that best sums up this need is 'meaning'. The thrust of the argument for paying more attention to 'stories of sickness', for health care professionals to enter into the experience of the patient, allowing the patient to express that experience, and participating together in the process of making sense of it, is to give validity, meaning and value to it. That in turn gives the patient a greater sense of control over their predicament. And these things are all powerful contributors to the 'contextual' healing effects of the therapeutic encounter;[13] the additional and indispensable effects that accompany the specific action of *any* treatment. David Moerman argues persuasively that there is meaning associated, explicitly or implicitly, consciously or unconsciously, with any treatment, active or inactive (placebo).[14] And that this accounts in part for the spontaneous self-regulatory component of the healing response.

The tension, and apparent contradiction within medicine between what EF Schumacher calls "science for manipulation" and "science for understanding"[15] is the philosophical, moral and ethical undercurrent that generates the momentum for change. It is an undercurrent that has flowed throughout the history of scientific medicine, as we have seen, and it has, so to speak, two main axes. One is what Lyng describes as the "polar dynamic that has featured so prominently in the evolution of medical knowledge . . . the movement between the reductionist and holistic poles in medical thinking".[1] The other axis is the 'polar dynamic' between the desire to control and the desire to enable; to control disease and enable healing.

But these different dynamics are not mutually exclusive. They are only apparently contradictory if we make them so. Bacteriostatic antibiotics render organisms more susceptible to the body's own defence mechanisms. The outcome of surgery depends absolutely upon the body's capacity for natural healing. No treatment will enable 'recovery' from Down's syndrome, but it may enable modification of functional symptoms that accompany it and improve quality of life. Complementary therapies are used in palliative care because, one way or another, they enable better tolerance of the symptoms and distress of terminal illness, or of the side effects of treatment. The holistic perspective above all is never inappropriate to health care in any context, even in the most immediate response to acute illness or trauma where it has at first a lower priority to the necessary control of the problem. Indeed, however much scientific medicine's emphasis on disease may at times invalidate the individual experience, the holistic perspective is rarely completely absent in even the most focused biomedical encounter, because it remains a core element of most heath care professionals' vocation.

Despite this, the fact remains that the entrenched position of the strict scientific paradigm, and the reductionist mechanistic tendencies of the biomedical model that result from it, do frequently pre-empt the underlying commitment to a holistic perspective and the essential and acknowledged contribution of self-regulating and self-healing processes. And they do oppose the proper scientific enquiry into the means by which these influences on health, illness and healing might be better understood and more fully exploited in patient care. The huge disparity between the investment in studying these parameters of health and in biomedical research is a consequence of this. This pre-emptive power is the reason why we need to take seriously the analysis of plausibility constructs, paradigms and models, of truth, proof, evidence, knowledge and reality that I have offered, if our science is to be moderated by wisdom, and our *scientia* properly harnessed to *caritas*.

Border disputes, or reconciliation and 'traffic in truth'?

As I point out when discussing the meaning of 'scientific medicine' in Chapter 3, this polarisation does not only arise from the restrictive and exclusive nature of the scientific paradigm and its medical model, and their rigid application; the alleged 'fundamentalism' of the randomised double blind controlled trial that I referred to earlier, for example. There is a very large middle ground occupied by clinicians working within the conventional model who have integrated unconventional methods into their practice, predominantly general practitioners. It is shared by practitioners of unorthodox therapies working with conventional healthcare professionals in multi-disciplinary teams. But there are also unorthodox practitioners who reject the biomedical model as vigorously as its strictest proponents would reject theirs, and so exacerbate the problem, as does any inevitably irreconcilable argument between fundamentalists.

Some practitioners and some forms of complementary and alternative medicine exacerbate the hostility of even the more liberal adherents of the biomedical model, including those who themselves have adopted some aspect of the alternative model that those practices represent. These are practitioners, whose beliefs and attitudes do reflect only what they want to be true, who act out those beliefs and attitudes in patient care uncritically; without proper understanding of the patient's condition, and without due regard to the appropriateness, wisdom, justification or limitations of their approach.

The polarisation of attitudes that is found among some proponents of the conventional medical model and some proponents of other models, particularly those from complementary and alternative practice, is in some instances reminiscent of the polarisation of attitudes between some fundamentalist proponents of religion and some scientists. Even when the differences are not so extreme and there is mutual respect between the protagonists in that particular debate, the two domains of thought can remain border territories where there is little prospect of trade or travel across the border, which properly understood should be a free-trade area for the exchange of intellectual goods. "Borders are where wars begin, and the border between (the different paradigms) has sometimes been seen by dwellers on both sides as a battleground. There is indeed a land on the other side, but its fate is to be conquered."[16] This is, unfortunately, too often the state of affairs across the border between different models of medicine. And unfortunately, as in any conflict, there is bound to be, in that hideous euphemism, 'collateral damage'. In a conflict between two medical ideologies the victims of that damage will be patients.

Paradigms and models can indeed be very dangerous, as the abuses of both communism and religion testify. And even a model that is in itself benign may be dangerous when it generates indirect risk. The indirect risk generated by the model on the catwalk is the anorexia of the young woman who is unduly influenced by the prescription for feminine beauty that is presented to her, pre-empting her choice of a more appropriate body image. The indirect risk of a therapeutic prescription, conventional or otherwise, arises when it pre-empts the choice of any other, possibly more appropriate or indeed necessary therapeutic approach.

When systematic attempts were first made to reconcile the difference between complementary and alternative practitioners and orthodox medicine, the word 'rapprochement' was used. It means 're-establishment or recommencement of harmonious relations, especially between States' (*Concise Oxford Dictionary*). In this context, the 'states' are the territories on either side of the paradigm border. Such a rapprochement is certainly essential if paradigm paralysis on either hand is to yield to the more creative endeavour of those in the middle ground. Fitzpatrick has argued that, "Just as reason cannot be integrated with irrationality, so orthodox medicine cannot be integrated with alternative medicine".[17] And he quotes Bruce Charlton, writing in the *Journal of the Royal Society of Medicine* in 1992, "Fringe therapies are a sort of cultural fossil, preserving a pre-scientific and pre-clinical mode of reasoning about medicine".

This represents the sort of blindness leading to suicide of the McNamara fallacy (Chapter 10). Kuhn suggested that different paradigms might prove to be 'incommensurable', not capable of being accommodated within the same frame of reference,[2] but I see no reason why this should be the case in medicine. What we really need, perhaps, to effect constructive change is not paradigm revolutionaries, but those paradigm pioneers Joel Barker refers to, who extend the frontiers without abandoning the fruitful territory behind. But to those settlers in the territory already occupied who only feel secure within their stockade, perhaps all pioneers look like revolutionaries.

In a paper following up his original critique of the biomedical model, George Engel comments, "Protagonists of the biomedical model claim that its achievements more than justify the expectation that in time all major problems will succumb to further refinements in biomedical research. Critics argue that such dependence on 'Science' is in effect at the expense of the humanity of the patient. This is a fruitless controversy . . .".[18] It is indeed completely unnecessary and inappropriate and thoroughly counter-productive. Engel continues, "The crippling flaw of the model is that it does not include the patient and his attributes as a person, a human being".

And yet it is surely not beyond the wit of medical man, and particularly perhaps of medical woman – who is now so numerous, important and influential a part of the medical workforce, to achieve a 'meaningful' synthesis. This is what patients desire and deserve, and it is what a more truthful understanding of the human condition requires.

That this is possible is evident (I use the word deliberately) in the writings of Howard Brody and Allen Barbour (hospital physicians) and of

Grant Gillett (surgeon) that I quote earlier;[19,20,21] and in the work of numerous other hospital doctors, general practitioners and practitioners of complementary and alternative therapies for whom the biomedical model is by no means anathema. We do consist of 'parts'. And those parts in themselves represent coherent wholes. At every level of complexity each whole is more than the sum of its parts, more than the sum of the separate wholes of which it is composed. And indeed, more than the sum of the influences in the social and cultural milieu we inhabit.

Poetry and science

In his essay, 'The meaning of a poem,' George Orwell writes, "I have tried to analyse this poem as well as I can in a short period, but nothing I have said can explain, or explain away, the pleasure I take in it. That is finally inexplicable, and it is just because it is inexplicable that detailed criticism is worthwhile. Men of science can study the life-process of a flower, or they can split it up into its component elements, but any scientist will tell you that a flower does not become less wonderful, it becomes more wonderful if you know all about it".[22] A similar point is made by Eric Cassell, writing about the importance of aesthetic appreciation in clinical decision making, and quoting Bernard Bosanquet: "It is not uncommon to take a work of art as an example of the compulsion by which the nature of a whole controls its parts, simply because that control, which is the essence of individuality, lends itself to analysis in a work that is pervaded by an especially harmonious unity".[23]

Cassell also describes the surprising ability of a professor of fine arts to distinguish at a glance between diseased and normal tissues on microscope slides by virtue of his artistic sensibilities; which recalls the tendency of mathematicians to judge the validity of an equation by its 'beauty'.

We need our botanists and our poets, art critics and artists, our reductionists and our holists, our mechanics, mathematicians and philosophers. We need elements of each, in different proportions of course, inside each one of us, for the sake of our own humanity and well-being (whole-being). And we need these attributes to coexist both symbiotically and synergistically (having an effect greater than their individual effects) not only within each of us but as attributes of our collective humanity, for its collective well-being and the proper appreciation of and respect for the world in which we live.

Medicine must change and evolve in this way. This is necessary if it is to fulfil its healing vocation. And because medicine is entangled with so much of human nature, the message of the model that it offers to society will influence the humanity and healthfulness of society as a whole. I believe medicine is changing and will change in this way, and in fact has always held these dynamics in creative tension as it has explored its particular view of reality. But it is time for the resistance to change that is particularly prevalent amongst strict proponents of the biomedical model to yield more imaginatively, more insightfully, and more graciously, to the pull of the undercurrents that indicate a turning of the tide.

BOX 11.1 *Resistance to change*

- Paradigm paralysis.
- Scientificism.
- The McNamara fallacy.
- Vested interests.
- Institutional inertia.
- Border disputes, tribalism.
- The culture of technology.
- The 'central dogma'.

Resistance to change (see Box 11.1)

The problem with paradigms lies in the paralysis and tunnel vision that afflicts adherents who become entrenched, in the military sense, on their side of the border between their own and another paradigm. This may be either a deliberately aggressive or defensive position in the face of a challenge that they see as offensive and unacceptable. It may be a conscious or unconscious defence against a threat to the sort of vested interests that Joel Barker describes. Or it may be that their commitment to one particular paradigm does not mean that they are opposed to what lies on the other side of the border, but that they simply cannot see over the parapet. To repeat the quotation from Kuhn, "When the anomalies – that signal a new paradigm arise they may be invisible to the majority of normal science adherents".[2] Just as the practice of medicine can generate both direct and indirect risk of harm, paradigms can generate both direct and indirect resistance to change. In practical terms it is often the models that the paradigms give rise to, and which determine the behaviours of the protagonists, in this case the practice of medicine, that inhibit the possibility of change.

The influence of technology and pharmaceuticals

> Physicians learn how to **cure** but little about how to **care**. One reason why doctors **overtreat** and **overstudy** and do not always talk with, or listen to, their patients is that they are too busy looking at organs and laboratory findings. Technology is overused because doctors expect to find an answer to every problem if they only look hard enough with the right instruments. (Howard Spiro[24])

One force tending to oppose change in medicine is the pharmaceutical and technology industries, that provide the tools of the biomedical trade. That is meant literally, not pejoratively. The ability to control and manipulate body function and disease processes that is biomedicine's strength, and for which we can be very grateful, depends upon the tools, which pharmaceutical companies, innovators in biological and medical technology, and manufacturers of medical equipment provide. We need them and they do a good job. But there are problems, which are generally well recognised. Any manufacturer has a two-way relationship with its consumer. It must meet the needs of the market, but it must also stimulate that need in order to be profitable.

In medicine, the research and development community must also pursue increasingly sophisticated and costly solutions to the more intractable medical problems, to an extent that becomes increasingly unaffordable while encouraging the expectation that the solutions can be found and should be afforded. Heated and agonised debates about affordability and rationing have become commonplace in the U.K., reflecting huge dilemmas for policy makers (the National Institute for Clinical Excellence), the purse-holders (Primary Care and Hospital Trusts), and carers, particularly frontline clinicians; not to mention great unhappiness for patients. It is an awkward situation. Doctors and patients want the tools because they are the only weapons on which they can rely to tackle disease. The availability of the tools, including diagnostic tools, encourages us to use them and want more and better versions of them. Their use focuses attention on what they can be used for and diverts attention from the wider and more complex question of why they are needed in the first place, which may have more to do with psychosocial or environmental factors than any inherent biological fault. In his critique of the medical model,

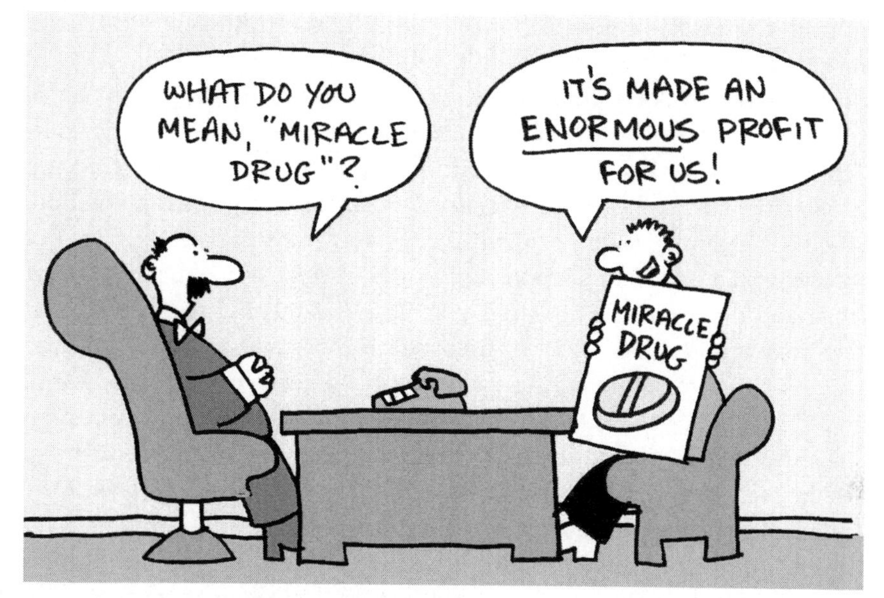

Figure 11.1 *Pharmaceuticals need to stimulate need.*

Engel remarks that, "The biomedical model . . . encourages bypassing the patient's verbal story by placing greater reliance on technical procedures and laboratory measurements".[25] This is as true today as it was 30 years ago. He refers to the suggestion of another critic of the model that, "while reductionism (which technology allows us to practise with greater precision) is a powerful tool for understanding, it also creates profound misunderstanding when unwisely applied. (It) is particularly harmful when it neglects the impact of non-biological circumstances upon biological processes". This is a helpful comment because it emphasises that it is not the tools in themselves that are the problem, but their unwise application.

The trouble is that the tools are a very seductive alternative to the more taxing and time-consuming investigation of non-biological circumstances. Technology breeds expectations and attitudes that reinforce the need for technology. Lyng refers to these tools as 'medical instrumentation', and points out that the need for both theory and medical instrumentation creates an intimate link between medicine and the basic biological sciences.[1] Through the use of theory and technological principles, basic scientists produce medical instrumentation that, in his somewhat high-flown language, become incorporated into "the subjective body of the clinician as a new transcendental structure or a new form of tacit 'knowledge' resulting in new powers of observation and direct interpretation". He suggests that in contrast to what is commonly believed, basic science does not serve an explanatory role for the clinician; rather, it creates the space for possible medical events.

In other words, basic science and the technology that it facilitates enable clinicians to do something about the disease that confronts them, encouraging what Lyng calls 'the interventionist thrust' of modern medicine and an appetite for and tacit dependence on the necessary instrumentation; science for manipulation, in Schumacher's words, at the expense of science for understanding.[14] In *Medical Hubris,* David Horrobin argues that what Illich and other critics of science were attacking was not true science but technology, and the control of patients in the course of controlling disease processes that technology exerts, with its consequent potential for harm, and nowadays, we would add, ethical dilemmas. More true science, he suggests, not less, would redress the balance. The true science he refers to would seek a better understanding of the proper balance between the extraordinary potency and superb effectiveness of bodily control mechanisms (self-regulation) and the need for technological intervention. There is too little of this science for understanding in medicine, and "unequivocally too much technology".[26]

This tacit dependence upon technology produces another indirect resistance to change. "(Likewise) companies manufacturing mammography equipment or tests for prostate specific antigen (for identifying cancer) can grow rich on the medicalisation of risk."[27]

And so do drugs encourage the need for drugs. Consequently, clinicians and the Health Service generally become entangled in the ethical and economic complexities of their relationship with the pharmaceutical companies who inevitably, and to an extent necessarily have a powerful vested interest in the continued pre-eminence of the biomedical model. Global pharmaceutical companies have a clear interest in medicalising life's problems, and there is now 'an ill for every pill'.[26]

The motivation, perhaps the compulsion, financial, scientific and political, for investment in pharmaceutical and technological research is so strong, that there is little appetite and virtually no inducement for research that might allow us to explore and exploit the low-tech and unprofitable components of medical practice. Although the sheer unaffordability of increasingly sophisticated and specialised drugs and techniques to control disease may eventually compel a change of direction, there is no serious commitment yet to meet the challenge to explore the potential to enable self-regulation and self-healing that we know to be inherent in all good medical practice. The challenge to establish, for example, "How the doctor himself, as a therapeutic agent, (can) be refined and polished to make of him a more potent agent".[23]

The 'Too much medicine?' editorial in the *British Medical Journal* that I am quoting,[26] also identifies, somewhat cynically perhaps in some instances, forces that tend to encourage greater medicalisation: Patients and their professional advocacy groups can gain moral and financial benefit from having their condition defined as a disease. Doctors, particularly some specialists, may welcome the boost to status, influence and income that comes when new territory is defined as medical. Although it is evident that single gene defects alone rarely if ever cause a specific disease, advances in genetics open up the possibility of defining almost all of us as sick, by diagnosing the 'deficient' genes that predispose us to disease. The implication being that we must invent drugs or technologies do enable us to do something about it.

Institutional inertia

> As members of a profession not always known for its humility, we need to remember and understand the blind alleys that medicine has gone down, the unnecessary suffering it has caused, the important innovations that have been ignored or suppressed, and the ancient professional rivalries that have led to our current divisions. (Fiona Godlee[28])

A sense of adventure and a spirit of exploration are obviously part of the human psyche, but paradoxically a certain resistance to change seems to be embedded in human nature too. Most of us can be pretty conservative in that sense, in our taste in food, clothes, music, people – and ideas. Though some of us thrive on variety, experiment, innovation and difference, there is often reluctance to move out of the comfort zone of the tried, tested and familiar. But science, by definition, is a process of exploration, discovery and innovation. The goal of science is the *Unended Quest*, as Karl Popper called his autobiography;[29] the unended exploration of reality, the unended quest for truth.

To return to Schumacher's distinction, science for manipulation is useful, indeed indispensable; but it has to proceed from and be subject to science for understanding.[14] There may be a limit to the kind of question that science can be expected to answer, but there must be no limit to the questions science is willing to ask with the tools available to it. And no limit to its willingness to expand its tool kit in order to be able to ask them. The development and increasing use of qualitative research methods, using a more descriptive and narrative approach to it subjects to overcome the limitations of the quantitative approach based on what can be counted and measured, is an example of this willingness. Medical science has even more reason to be open to new possibilities, because of its commitment to alleviating suffering and disability.

And yet – science and medicine both exhibit surprising examples of unwillingness to surrender cherished ideas, or to accept innovation. An example from contemporary science is presented by Oxford mathematician John C. Lennox in a fascinating discussion of the complexity of intracellular mechanisms and the processing of genetic material.[30] He describes with beautiful clarity the subtle permutations by which genetic material (DNA) is processed and transmitted in the production of the proteins that are the building blocks of our vast diversity of human characteristics (and indeed the even vaster diversity of the characteristic of all living things). He shows how these processes depend on mechanisms within the cell that act upon the DNA, and do not derive from the properties of DNA itself. He demonstrates that the proposition that the genome (our individual genetic code or template) accounts completely for an organisms inherited characteristics cannot be true. This proposition has long been regarded as the 'central dogma' of molecular biology; so called by Francis Crick the DNA pioneer. Lennox quotes from *Unravelling the DNA Myth* by Barry Commoner, Senior Scientist and Director of the Critical Genetics Project at the Centre for the Biology of Natural Systems at Queens College, City University of New York. He asks, with him why, in the light of the more recent knowledge he describes, this central dogma has continued to stand. In the context of what has been said about paradigms. Commoner's answer to this question, which John Lennox quotes, is interesting. He says: "To some degree the theory has been protected from criticism by a device more common to religion than science: dissent, or merely the discovery of a discordant fact, is a punishable offence, a heresy that might easily lead to professional ostracism. Much of this bias can be attributed to institutional inertia a failure of rigour, but there are other more insidious reasons why molecular geneticists might be satisfied with the status quo; the central dogma has given them such a satisfying seductively simplistic explanation of heredity that it seemed sacrilegious to entertain doubts. The central dogma was simply too good not to be true."

In *Bad Medicine – Doctors doing harm since Hippocrates*,[31] historian David Wootton gives an account of how little medicine achieved with its specific treatments until scientific method took hold: "If we define medicine as the ability to cure diseases, then there was very little medicine before 1865." Prior to this he gives three reasons for the status that medicine had achieved, and for the difficulty in recognising that medicine, as a technology, did not work:

- Doctors were trying to achieve outcomes that the body's natural healing processes were also working to achieve.
- The placebo effect meant that an ineffectual intervention could often result in a cure.
- In order to test a therapy (by comparing outcomes) you need a concept of a disease as . . . a typical condition of many patients.

In other words, it was other aspects of the therapeutic encounter that earned medicine what respect it deserved. That is no surprise. But more surprising to many of us I suspect is the catalogue of resistance within the medical profession to well-founded and often life-saving innovations that he presents. He suggests that the profession is culpable for the death and suffering that could have been avoided if those innovations had been adopted more promptly and willingly. His book is controversial for its use of hindsight, which some critics regard as unwarranted. And yet he makes a very strong case.

His examples include:

- The use of fruit and vegetables (particularly lemon juice) to prevent scurvy on long sea journeys; practised by seafarers since the beginning of the 17th century, but only adopted as standard practice at the end of the 18th.
- The frank hostility to the use of Nitrous Oxide as an anaesthetic, eventually adopted by doctors in Europe (1846) long after its anaesthetic properties were first recognised (1795) and subsequently adopted by American dentists.
- The reluctance to accept the evidence that puerperal fever was a contagious disease spread between women after childbirth by contact with the doctors and midwives attending them; first reported in 1795 but fiercely contested for more than 60 years.
- The resistance that persisted until 1866 to John Snow's demonstration, in 1849, of the water-born transmission of Cholera in London; a proposal depending on a germ theory of disease that flew in the face of the dominant miasmatic (bad air) theory.
- The reluctance to abandon blood-letting (bleeding) as a treatment until well into the twentieth century, because "the discovery of the circulation of the blood (1628), of Oxygen (1775), of the role of haemoglobin (1862) made no difference; the discoveries were adapted to the therapy rather than vice versa". (The *Lancet*, ironically, is one of our leading medical journals).

- And the delay between Fleming's discovery of Penicillin (1929) and the systematic investigation of its potential by Florey and Chain that demonstrated its clinical value (1939).

In fact, Wootton reports Joseph Lister's observation of the bactericidal properties of *Penicillium glaucum* in 1872, and its successful clinical use by Lister to treat an infected wound in 1884. And he says that "the true puzzle about penicillin is why it was not brought into medical use fifty years earlier". Possible, and perhaps excusable reasons for the two episodes of delay in exploiting the benefits of penicillin are Lister's preoccupation with antiseptic surgery, and Florey's preoccupation with the production of vaccines.

Wootton suggests that the real question is not 'What discoveries made it possible for medicine to develop as it did?', But 'What psychological, cultural or institutional factors represented an obstacle to medicine developing as it might have?' The reasons he suggests for these examples of apparent medical obtuseness are not flattering to the profession. Commoner's 'institutional inertia' would be a polite way of putting it. Wootton puts it like this: "Any history of medicine which focuses on what works immediately brings to the fore these uncomfortable questions about delay, resistance, hostility, and (if we use the word metaphorically) malpractice." His explanation of the failure in medicine to make imaginative or intelligent use of the microscope during some 150 years following the pioneering work of van Leeuvenhoek and others in the mid-17th century is indeed uncomfortable. Partly, he alleges, the microscope had gone out of fashion because there was no money in it, but also it was dismissed as a tool for serious research because "the medical profession had set it face against (it) and other followed where they led".

Wootton develops his answer to the question, 'Why was progress so slow?':

> Part of the explanation lies in the way in which people identify with their own skills, particularly when they have gone to great trouble and expense to acquire them. Just as surgeons wanted to go on being surgeons, and so were blind to the possibilities of anaesthetics, so doctors wanted to go on being doctors, and so were reluctant to sheath their lancets. . . . Conventional therapy (of the day) had enormous stability because both patients and doctors were educated to trust it. . . . There were psychological and cultural factors working against innovation.

Similarly, a recent commentary in the *British Medical Journal* suggests: "Various reasons for the slow pace of improvement have been identified, such as resistance to change among health professionals, organisational structures that block improvement, and dysfunctional financial incentives."[32]

It is particularly important to recognise the mutually reinforcing effects of attitudes within medicine and within society as a whole that are implied in that last paragraph. And indeed, to recognise the influence of social attitudes on change even when medicine leads the way. It was more than fifty years before political action ensured that the proven role of smoking as a principal cause of lung cancer imposed changes in our social behaviour. The role and function of medicine are very much socially as well as scientifically determined.

Wootton draws on Thomas Kuhn's theory of paradigms to identify the process of evolution in medicine in terms of laboratory science, of what is taught and written in text books, and of the structure of authority that holds communities together. He concludes that 'the primary obstacle to progress was not practical (Leeuwenhoek's microscope worked well), nor theoretical (the germ theory of putrefaction was not difficult to formulate), but psychological and cultural. It lay in doctors' sense of themselves, their awareness of their own traditions, their habit of conferring authority upon established canon and established therapies'.

The point is that alongside the momentum for progress in science and medicine, and all that has been achieved, there is an inherent tendency to cling on to 'central dogmas' of one kind or another. This is why paradigms are constructive *and* restrictive, motivating *and* paralysing; why models are necessary *and* dangerous. Whatever our occupation, whatever our world of ideas, we need to remember this so that our world view, paradigm or model helps us to work creatively but does not limit our horizons.

The example of complementary medicine

There is one contentions area of contemporary medicine that particularly challenges us to get this balance right. In Chapter 2, I mention complementary and alternative medicine (CAM) as one element in the 'evolutionary struggle', and in Chapter 3 as one of the existing symptoms of change in the model. CAM is a nebulous, ill-defined field which it is not the purpose of this book to document or examine; except in as much as it reflects or illustrates either arguments about the limitations of the biomedical model, or possible design principles for remodelling. The key issues concern the naturalness or otherwise of its various treatments; the extent to which it is or is not truly holistic; and the extent to which the subtle effects of its specific treatments and/or the non-specific, contextual or placebo effects of the therapeutic encounter and its routines, enable self-regulation and self-healing by comparison with conventional methods.

These matters will be touched upon more fully in Part 4. The relevance of the subject at this point is the attitude of medical science towards CAM; an attitude that risks throwing out the baby with the bathwater.

- In its broad generality CAM stands accused of being engulfed by post-modernism, anti-science, and regressive thinking;[33] a charge that certainly needs to be answered, even if it is presented in a provocative and tendentious style.[34] And there are manifestations of CAM that are certainly worrying.
- Of greatest concern is what is known as indirect risk. This is the risk of harm arising, not from what *is* done in the course of the treatment, but from what is *not* done because of the treatment; when the choice of treatment excludes other possibilities that may be more appropriate or even life saving for the particular patient.
- Less worrying are the relatively rare direct risks; harm caused directly by the specific treatment technique or medication.
- Another concern is the consequences for vulnerable people who make considerable and sometimes long-term emotional and financial investment in treatment of doubtful benefit; albeit they may also gain considerable encouragement and well-being from the relationship.
- There is also concern about the commercial exploitation of the CAM culture; the sale of products or aids to health over the counter or through the media. Not so much a problem when these are more of a lifestyle choice than a perceived medical necessity, but definitely a problem when they are mistaken for the latter.
- Finally, the profusion of CAM options can be thoroughly confusing for people who seriously want to do more to enhance their well-being and to take more control of their health, (one of the important reasons for the popularity of CAM), but just don't know what to do for the best.

For all these reasons CAM needs to be subjected to careful scrutiny, alongside the central issue of whether its methods yield real health gain for patients; and if so which, and how much gain do they yield. The problem is that in some fields of CAM that have been the subject of research, patients quite obviously benefit, while conventional research methods suggest that the specific treatments do not affect specific diseases. Patients get better but apparently the treatments do not 'work' in the accepted biomedical sense of the word. They are apparently 'effective', but they lack specific 'efficacy'. Their benefits are attributed to the incidental effects of the process, and therefore, it is implied, are not to be taken seriously. They do not fit the medical model. Patients get better, quite often when conventional treatment has not helped. But why? And how can this success be replicated in main stream medicine? Medical science it seems, does not want to know. Institutional inertia perhaps?

Complementary medicine provides a good example of the tension between a momentum for change and resistance to change. There is no doubt that its huge popularity represents a cultural phenomenon, a shift towards a new plausibility construct. In part it reflects a reaction to the materialist, reductionist, highly technological spirit of the age. In part it reflects patients' desire for more personal control and responsibility in healthcare. In part it has to do with a growing awareness of ecological issues, the intimacy of our relationship with our environment and the plants and animals that inhabit it with us. It has to do with a growing appreciation of subtle and complex dynamics of human nature and human well-being. Many of its methods are very old – acupuncture has been practised for thousands of years, homeopathy for 200 years. But their popularity now is sometimes represented as a symptom of the post-modern age, where 'anything goes' and there are no certainties or absolutes. I have no sympathy with the suggestion that the popularity of CAM is simply a manifestation of a post-modern culture. I believe it is largely because people seek in complementary medicine some or all of the qualities of therapeutic relationship, and indeed often the effectiveness, that they find lacking in orthodox medicine. Even though those qualities are no more the prerogative of CAM than of any other form of medicine. Our need of them is neither ancient, nor modern, nor post-modern, it is just essentially human.

In terms of medical science, complementary medicine represents a shift towards a new paradigm. Some commentators dismiss the language of paradigm. Andrew Vickers who has worked in complementary medicine research for many years is one.[35] He says that we should stop talking about paradigms in this context. He is right only in so far as the language of paradigms is used sloppily and inappropriately to "lend verisimilitude to an otherwise bald and unconvincing narrative", to quote Pooh Bah from W.S. Gilbert's *Mikado*. Properly used, in the sense I have presented it in the Introduction and in the previous chapter, 'paradigm' is the correct and appropriate term for a pattern of thought – the principles, the rules even – that determine the way we go about our business; whether in business and commerce (in Joel Barker's terms[3]) or in science and medicine.

There *is* a reductionist analytical scientific paradigm that complementary medicine, in its more coherent manifestations, says is inadequate to our understanding of the human condition and human well-being. The paradigm *does* give rise to the biomedical model that complementary medicine says is inadequate for the complexity of human healthcare. The reductionist paradigm insists on a model that depends on methods of controlling disorder, with wonderful results and huge benefits. Complementary medicine represents a more emphatically holistic paradigm that insists on a model that depends on methods of restoring order, and it claims positive results and great benefits for it. As this book repeatedly affirms, the two paradigms are not mutually exclusive and do already coexist. But complementary medicine, for all its confusing unregulated diversity and frequent lack of rigour, says we have got the balance wrong.

When patients benefit from complementary medicine in a manner that defies the conventional rules of medical efficacy, we have to ask 'Why? What is going on?' There are researchers who are asking these questions and trying to develop the scientific tools to answer them.[36,37,38] Others focus their efforts on what is not going on. They concentrate on using the tools of 'destructive analysis', predominantly the controlled clinical trial, to identify treatments that conform to the narrow definition of medical efficacy, and to dismiss those whose apparent or alleged benefits derive from other elements of the therapeutic package. A broad and accessible outline of this approach can be found in a book called *Trick or Treatment? Alternative medicine on trial*, one of whose authors is Emeritus Professor of Complementary Medicine at Exeter University.[39] It is an approach that is valuable and necessary to filter off some of the murky water in the plunge bath of CAM. But there is a healthy baby swimming about in there too, which has a lot to tell us if we are prepared to give it speech.[40]

This diversion into complementary medicine is a useful example of the tensions and difficulties that beset an attempt to evaluate truth, proof and evidence in patient care. And as an example of the unfortunate cross-border conflict between paradigms and models, when appreciation of their true complementarity and a more willing 'traffic in truth' should prevail. It should not distract us from the broader issue of the more general and long-standing dis-ease within medicine that is occasioned by the constraints of the biomedical model. Nor from the desire to augment its undoubted and immense benefits with a more subtle and more supple understanding of the dynamics of health and illness, and of medicine's role in managing them.

Barry Commoner and John Lennox wonder why the central dogma of DNA's role has stood for so long when there is good reason to question it, and attribute this to reasons more common to religion than science. The biomedical model has stood for far longer as the 'central dogma', we might say, of healthcare; and perhaps for rather similar reasons.

References

1 Lyng S. *Holistic Health and Biomedical Medicine.* New York: State University of New York Press; 1990.

2 Kuhn T. *The structure of scientific revolutions.* Chicago: University of Chicago Press; 1996.

3 Barker J. *Paradigms: The business of discovering the future.* New York: Harper Collins; 1992.

4 Harris C. Seeing sunflowers. *J R Coll Gen Pract.* 1989; 39:313–319.

5 Polanyi M. *Personal Knowledge.* London: Routledge; 2002.

6 Fuller S. *Kuhn vs. Popper. The struggle for the soul of science.* Cambridge: Icon; 2006.

7 Souter K. Heuristics and bias in homeopathy. *Homeopathy* 2006; 95:237–244.

8 Skrabanek P. Demarcation of the absurd. *Lancet* 1986; 1;960–961.

9 Crawshay Wiliams R. *The Comforts of Unreason: A study of the motives behind unrational thought.* London: Kegan Paul Trench Trubner & Co. Ltd; 1947.

10 Reilly D. Personal communication.

11 Ward K. *In defence of the soul.* Oxford: Oneworld; 1998.

12 Heath I. Uncertain clarity: contradiction meaning and hope. *Br J Gen Pract.* 1999; 49:651–657.

13 Miller FK. The power of context: reconceptualising the placebo. *J R Soc Med.* 2008; 101:222–225.

14 Moerman D. *Meaning medicine and the 'placebo effect'.* Cambridge: Cambridge University Press; 2002.

15 Schumacher E. *A Guide for the Perplexed.* London: Sphere Books (Abacus); 1978.

16 Polkinghorne J. *Traffic in Truth: Exchanges between Science and Theology.* Norwich: Canterbury Press; 2000.

17 Fitzpatrick M. Reclaiming Compassion. In: Ernst E. *Healing Hype or Harm? A Critical Analysis of Complementary or Alternative Medicine.* Exeter: Societas; 2008.

18 Engel G. The clinical application of the biosocial model. *Am J Psychiat.* 1980; 137(5):535–544.

19 Brody H. *Stories of Sickness.* New Haven: Yale University Press; 1987.

20 Barbour A. *Caring for patients: a critique of the medical model.* Stanford: Stanford University Press; 1995.

21 Gillett G. (2004). Clinical medicine and the quest for certainty. *Soc Sci Med.* 2004; 58:727–738.

22 Orwell G. The Meaning of a Poem. In: Orwell G. Orwell S. Angus I. *The Collected Essays Journalism and Letters of George Orwell My Country Right or Left 1940–1943 Volume 2.* Harmondworth: Penguin; 1970.

23 Cassell E. *The Nature of Suffering and the Goals of Medicine.* New York: Oxford University Press; 2004.

24 Spiro H. *The Power of Hope.* New Haven & London: Yale University Press; 1998.

25 Engel G. The need for a new medical model. *Science* 1977; 96(4286);129–136.

26 Horrobin D. *Medical Hubris – A reply to Ivan Illich.* Edinburgh: Churchill Livingstone; 1978.

27 Moynihan R, Smith R. Too much medicine? *Br Med J.* 2002; 324:859–860.

28 Godlee F. History will be the judge. *Br Med J.* 2010; 340:c2447.

29 Popper K. *Unended Quest.* London: Routledge; 1992.

30 Lennox J. *God's Undertaker: has science buried God?* Oxford: Lion Hudson; 2007.

31 Wootton D. *Bad Medicine: Doctors Doing Harm Since Hippocrates.* New York: Oxford University Press; 2007.

32 Grol G, Berwick D, Wensing M. On the trail of quality and safety in health care. *Br Med J.* 2008; 336:74–76.

33 Ernst E. Complementary/alternative medicine: engulfed in post-modernism anti-science and regressive thinking. *Br J Gen Pract.* 2009; 59(561):298–301.

34 Swayne J. Commentary. Complementary/alternative medicine: engulfed by post-modernism anti-science and regressive thinking. *Br J Gen Pract.* 2009; 59(561):301.

35 Vickers A. Research paradigms in mainstream and complementary medicine. In: Ernst E. *Complementary medicine: an objective appraisal.* London: Butterworth Heinemann; 1996.

36 Walach H, Falkenberg T, Fønnebø V *et al.* Circular instead of hierarchical: methodological principles for the evaluation of complex interventions. *BMC Med Res Methodol.* 2006; 6:29.

37 Fønnebø V, Grimsgaard S, Walach H *et al.* (2007). Researching complementary and alternative treatment – the gatekeepers are not at home. *BMC Med Res Methodol* 2007; 7:7

38 Verhoef MJ, Lewith G, Ritenbaugh C *et al.* Complementary and alternative medicine whole systems research: Beyond identification of inadequacies of the RCT. *Complement Ther Med.* 2005; 13:20.

39 Singh S. Ernst E. *Trick or treatment? Alternative medicine on trial.* London: Bantam Press; 2008.

40 Swayne J. Book review: Trick or Treatment? *Br J Gen Pract.* 2008; 58 (555): 738–739.

part 4

THE DIRECTION OF CURE

12

DESIGN PRINCIPLES

Summary

- Any attempt to consider how the way we do medicine might be, should be different, must be personal rather than theoretical.
- What would 'different' look like for me as a patient and/or, for my patients, if we were really to get it right? Why would I want it to be like that?
- A new design for the medical model must accommodate:
  - a clear understanding of what medicine is for;
  - a more complete understanding of what we mean by 'whole person care';
  - a greater appreciation of the importance of 'the story of illness' and the significance of symptoms;
  - a more profound understanding of the concept of healing;
  - a realisation of the importance of 'meaning' in the experience of illness;
  - a proper understanding of the therapeutic importance of self-regulation and self-healing in health care, and how to promote them;
  - a clearer awareness of the distinctive nature of health and well-being;
  - a proper appreciation of, and commitment to the principles of holistic, integrated and integrative health care.
- Many of the principles of a remodelling process are at least implicit in the preceding chapters. In this chapter some of them are discussed in more detail.
- It is a challenge to think critically, honestly and imaginatively about the way we do medicine, and how we might do it better.
- It is a challenge to explore these 'design principles' actively; to think 'outside the box'.
- A challenge to consider possibilities for change that would really make a difference.

Whole person care

The focus, the subject of healthcare is a person – you and me. Medicine has a responsibility for groups of people, families, communities, but its primary responsibility is the *person* in need of care, who may at the same time be a member of such a group. Every component that we put in place in our model of health care, every design feature, will depend on how we regard the person in our care; even when we are caring for groups or communities. So we have to know who this person is – the person who is the genetics, the biochemistry, the disease, the illness; the person who embodies their culture, environment, and relationships; who has their own story of aspirations and disappointments, achievements and failures; each one of us a unique and complex human being. Medicine cannot perceive, let alone respond to all of this in any one person. But it must be aware that

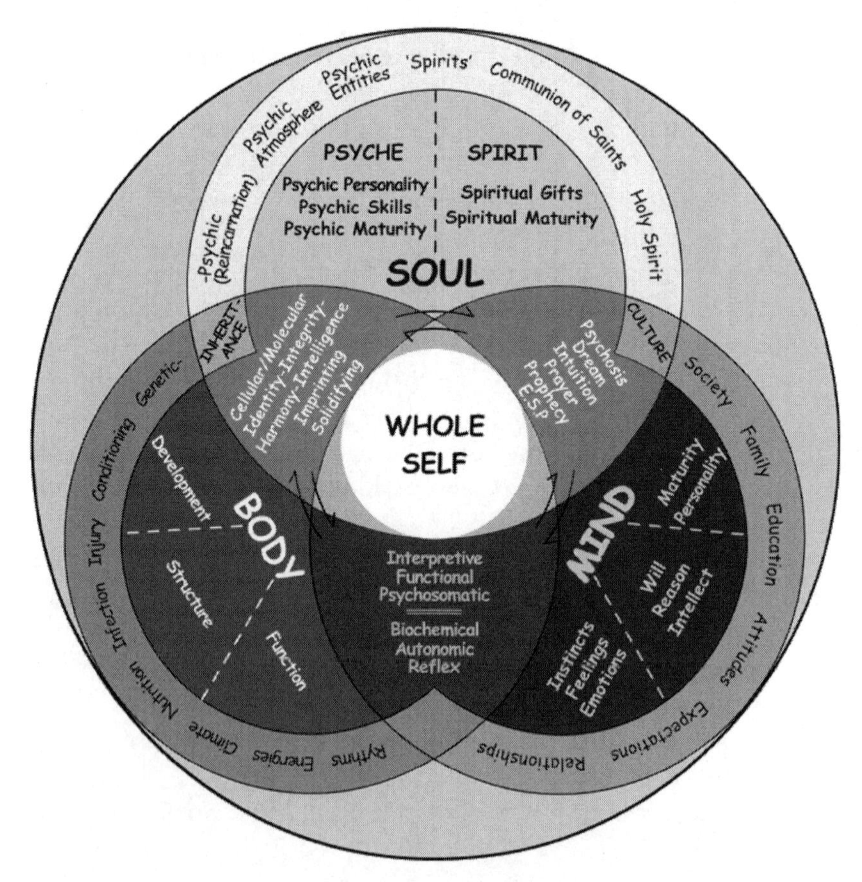

Figure 12.1 The structure of 'wholeness', showing body, mind and soul, their interaction within the individual, and between the individual and the circumstances of his or her life.

these are the things that make each of us 'tick,' and be perceptive of the part they may play in promoting or prejudicing our health and well-being.

So this chapter begins with a design that I call 'the structure of wholeness' (Figure 12.1). It represents a person, you and I, as possessing the three traditional attributes of body, mind and soul. It shows the dynamic interaction of these in the ellipses created by the overlapping circles. On the perimeter it shows the relationships that influence and sometimes control who we are, and through which we are part of a greater whole, a bigger picture. You might wish to change some of the details in the design, which does not pretend to be comprehensive. You may not believe that we are spiritual beings or have souls, for example. But I hope you will agree that it broadly represents what goes to make you who you are.

The whole truth and the whole story

> To achieve its enduring goals medicine must clarify what knowledge is represented by knowing who a person is, and mediate any conflict between the two kinds of knowledge, which we call the *scientific* and the *personal*. (Eric Cassell[1])

Whole person medicine is not just a romantic notion. It is probably what all doctors aspire to, but often find difficult because of the constraints of the biomedical model, and the targets and guidelines that are its political manifestation. In a survey of over 2000 Scottish GPs 87% felt that a holistic (whole person) approach was essential to providing good health care, but only 21% felt that primary care (general practice based care) was delivering high quality holistic care, and only 7% felt that the organisation of primary care was conducive to it.[2]

Reconciling the scientific and the personal is the holistic goal we strive for if we wish not only to control disease processes, but also to enable and empower the self-regulating and self-healing properties that we know our bodies and our minds to possess. To achieve this we have first to comprehend each person as a unique and integrated whole, body, mind and soul, expressed as dynamic, interpenetrating, interactive and interdependent elements of our being. And then to recognise each person's intimate connection with the physical, cultural, social, psychological and spiritual milieu of our lives.[3]

Few of us will have knowledge of all of this even in ourselves, let alone in any other person. But in any significant relationship, particularly a therapeutic relationship, we must be open and attentive to as much of it as is revealed to us. Such breadth of understanding of another person is a huge challenge, stretching our personal and professional resources to the limit. In medicine the narrow biomedical focus we are primarily trained and equipped for gets in the way. But if we lose sight of the *person* who is ill, and the *personal* ingredients of their illness, the problem in its totality will remain unresolved and we are likely to build up a bow wave of unresolved illness ahead of us: at least a burden of continuing high consultation rates and minor morbidity, at worst of real suffering.

This wholeness is the inherent truth of everyone's life. If medicine is not to be divorced from healing, then whole-making is part of its responsibility. There is an instinct for wholeness which is at work in everyone, whatever their condition, and however apparently lacking in self-awareness, or the ability to express themselves, or to determine the course of their lives. Medicine must be aware of this, and responsive to it.

And we can do so in the first instance by allowing and encouraging the person to tell (or have told for them by someone who knows and cares) the whole story – the story of sickness, the illness narrative; a story that will greatly exceed the scope of the formal medical history, and that will demand our whole attention.

The Physician or nurse cannot 'heal', that is make whole again, without feeling and knowing the nuances of a particular patient's predicament.[4] In its fullness, that capacity requires compassion, but it begins with a willingness to hear the whole story and to be open to the whole truth of the *person* who is the patient.

The 'meaning' of symptoms

I don't mean to imply the lesser importance of the body within the story. On the contrary, I strongly affirm the value and importance of the flesh and blood creatures that we are and for whom we care. I believe that practitioners must remain closely in touch (literally, if possible) with the wonder of our patient's body. However sick, damaged or distorted, it is the unique vehicle of a unique individual of unique value. Our patients' bodies should be an object of 'worth-ship', and our dealings with them a reflection of our sense of that worth.[3]

And of course, it is with the body, how it feels and how it behaves, that most medical consultations begin; unless they have a primarily psychological focus. But it is the tendency, following the biomedical approach, for the doctor to be most interested in those parts of the story that fit the model. As we have already seen any information that does not fit the model is likely to be ignored, or politely disregarded. But that is a terrible mistake. To disregard a patient's description of symptoms because the practitioner does not know what to do with it is wasteful and demeaning. It is demeaning in two senses – it puts the patient down, diminishes the value of their experience and them as a person, and it denies the possibility that the experience has any significance that is not strictly anatomical, physiological or pathological in the accepted biomedical sense. This is wasteful, because it also denies the possibility of really understanding the problem, and of formulating a truly appropriate response.

I still remember a talk by an experienced GP on my general practice vocational training course about the importance of understanding the metaphorical significance of the language of symptoms. 'Pain in the neck' was one example. The language of symptoms may be rich with metaphor, or cultural resonance, or personal idiosyncrasy; as well as unfamiliar but actual physiological significance. Truly understanding what the precise sensation associated with a presenting symptom in a particular patient means can disclose what is sometimes called 'the centre of the case'. Though of course we are not talking about a 'case' but a person whose core problem, whether there is accompanying pathology or not, is expressed in the character of that particular sensation. It could be the key to the whole story.

The body is very much part of the whole story, and proper attention to what it tells us is a way into the whole truth of the matter, and, moreover, an essential and effective part of the healing relationship. It is also, of course, essential to the accurate biomedical analysis of the problem, which our interest in the story is not meant to preclude. The irony is that increasingly, nowadays, investigation has displaced thorough enquiry into the clinical history, and thorough examination. Thus further 'de-humanising' the therapeutic encounter when the story is not properly heard, nor is the body properly 'worth-shiped'. We might rewrite the quotation from Kafka[5] to read, 'To order an investigation is easy. To come to an understanding with people is hard.'

The goals of medicine

> The patient, using the knowledge and advice of the doctor, must decide what goals (not what treatment) meet his or her best interests or purposes – no-one else can know that. (Eric Cassell[1])

> What is required is a deep-seated reflection which recognises and faces up to the false assumptions of the past, and is prepared to rethink questions about the nature of medicine and the goals of health care. (David Greaves[6])

Clearly we cannot decide what medicine should *do* and how it should do it unless and until we can decide what medicine is *for*. What are the goals of medicine? A very broad definition of my own that accommodates a variety of therapeutic approaches is that, 'Medicine is the *disciplined* use of any human attributes in the *service* of *healing*.' The words in italics are essential to the definition – discipline, service and healing. Foremost of these is healing.

Healing

> A healing decision or action focuses on restoring the patient to at least the state he enjoyed before he became ill, or to a state of higher satisfaction and health than has been achieved previously, if at all possible. 'Healing' is used here in its broadest sense. Even when it is not possible to cure or contain the disease, healing can occur if the patient is assisted to cope with her illness, is cared for as a continuing member of the human community, and is helped to confront dying and death when they are inevitable. (Pellegrino and Thomasma[4])

The most important characteristic of healing is that *it is creative, and not just remedial*. This will become clearer as I go on, but first, some general principles that govern the healing process as I understand it. These are: that it is *fundamentally similar at whatever level of our being it operates*; that *healing cannot be achieved without some degree of suffering*; and that it involves us in *changing attitudes and new responsibilities*.

General principles of healing

The proposition that *the healing process is fundamentally similar at whatever level of our being it operates*, is based on the observation that all healing involves, in some fashion, the following elements: understanding the problem, providing the conditions conducive to healing, mobilising resources to effect the healing process, new growth, and reconciliation. Wound healing provides a simple example. It requires that our body 'understands' what has happened; that it recognises and responds to the effects of trauma. It requires conditions that are conducive to healing – that the edges of the wound are brought together, that the wound is kept clean, and so on. It requires that the physiological resources of immunity to infection and tissue repair are effectively mobilised. There will be new tissue growth, which may even be stronger than the original tissue. And if the damage is sufficient, it will require 'reconciliation', some adjustment to compensate for any loss of function. These examples can readily be extended to the healing of psychological and spiritual wounds.

The second proposition is that *healing involves some degree of suffering*.

Suffering is not only the consequence of illness and trauma, but inherent in the healing process. This truth is represented in one of the most basic healing processes in the body, the inflammatory reaction; whose cardinal signs are redness, heat, swelling and pain. This is not an enjoyable experience, but we cannot do without it, and we are increasingly aware of the disadvantages of suppressing its discomforts with anti-inflammatory drugs. Pain, another normal physiological and emotional reaction, is a stimulus to change; to escape our predicament, or to seek healing. Understanding the source of the pain, responding to it and working through it is part of the healing process.

The third proposition is that healing always involves *reconciliation and change*.

At a physical level this may involve a change in relationship of one part of the body to another – one taking additional 'responsibility', so to speak, for another whose function is impaired. And of course it is likely to affect, and to require us to adjust the way we regard our body, our appearance, our physical abilities.

BOX 12.1 *The principles of healing*

- Embraces body, mind and soul.
- Similar on every level.
- Involves suffering.
- Changes attitudes.
- Brings new responsibilities.

More broadly, any illness, injury or disability affects our relationships with others, and with ourselves – as a person as well as a body; whether temporarily or longer term; through the limitations it imposes; because of its implications for our activities and prospects – lifestyle, occupation and so on. Illness affects other people's responsibilities towards us, and ours towards them. The responsibility of others towards us, including the community's responsibility to its sick and disabled, is for compassion and care. The responsibility of the sick person, subject to any absolute limitations, is to get well, because only when we are as well and as fully ourselves as possible can we fulfil our potential to contribute to the well-being of others. True healing will almost inevitably require some reappraisal of our own life, but it can never be a self-centred process

These essential characteristics of healing, summarised in Box 12.1, can be applied to all kinds of disorder that affect our physical or mental health, our relationships or our quality of life.

Paradox in illness and healing

There are aspects of illness and healing that appear paradoxical (Box 12.2). One such is the role of *Illness as the agent of healing*. This idea is simply exemplified in the development of immunity: a child's exposure to infection is necessary to the development of a mature immune system. In another instance of child development, bones need to bear weight and take strain, even in the pursuit of potentially risky activities, in order to form the correct lines of force. In other words, we need challenge, and the discomfort that challenge may produce in order to be fit and well, to develop as a well-integrated whole.

Mental and emotional illness, colloquially called a nervous breakdown, is often an essential prelude to the development of new psychological insights and strengths, and the healing of old wounds; the breaking down a necessary condition of rebuilding and new growth.

The idea that illness is the agent of healing is also reflected in the proposition that symptoms are the expression of the organism's *response* to disorder, its coping mechanism, rather than of its failure to cope.

BOX 12.2 *The paradox of healing*

- Illness as the agent of healing.
- Suffering from a 'wellness'.
- Healing need not involve cure.
- Cure does not guarantee healing.

Another paradox is that, *rather than suffering from an illness, we are often suffering from a 'wellness'*. The pain caused by a physical injury is the response of a healthy nervous system to trauma. The pain of rejection, abuse, the denial of love and of self-worth, is the healthy response of our wounded humanity. We suffer because we are denied some quality of life that is fundamental to the fulfilment of our unique potential as a person, and that we know, perhaps subliminally, that we need; just as hunger is the response of a healthy body to lack of food. The eventual consequences of suffering may be psychological illness. But the *experience* of suffering affirms our unique personhood; just as an immune reaction to a foreign substance or to an implanted organ that is 'not self' affirms our unique physiological identity.

A third paradox is that *healing does not necessarily involve cure, and cure does not necessarily involve healing*. Indeed, the pursuit of cure may allow destructive influences that produced the disorder to persist. And within the constraints of an incurable illness an individual may achieve the personal and spiritual growth, the integration and reconciliation that amount to healing in the fullest sense. This is why a large dose of humanity, fed by sufficient exposure to the humanities during medical education, is absolutely essential to the work of any physician or practitioner. Properly integrated with the sciences, as Brendan Sweeney says, "This cross-fertilisation can produced a different sort of doctor: one who is richer and deeper as an individual (and) has the ability to relate to and communicate with people whose lives cannot be transformed (by medical science) but can be enhanced by support and the palliation of suffering".[7]

The goal of healing

What is the goal of these healing processes? It is suggested by my earlier assertion that healing is not just remedial, but creative. But is the ordinary physiological healing of a commonplace and uncomplicated injury really a creative process? Yes, it is. There is always something to be learned from the circumstances of the injury; about the clumsiness, carelessness, mischance or risk that induced it. As a person we learn from the experience, we hope. As a body we may develop better coordination or sensory skills, or some other adaptive physiological process. All the characteristics of healing that I have described will be in some small measure a creative experience. Depending on how we use them, and what we make of them, they can help us to become a better integrated person, in ourselves and in our relationship with others. They can help to make us whole.

The goal of healing is wholeness.

> Healing: To restore wholeness or, if this is not possible, to assist in striking some new balance between what the body imposes and the self aspires to. (Edmund Pellegrino[8])

The spiritual dimension

It will be obvious from my concept of the structure of wholeness that for me a complete understanding of the concept of healing must include an understanding of the spiritual dimension of human nature. This understanding underpins my whole approach to medicine and health care. It is not necessary to share it to understand and endorse the broad principles of healing presented here, but to ignore it is to neglect a dimension of people's lives that is fundamental to their well-being, whether they regard themselves as 'religious' or not. In fact, religion is often a barrier to the recogniton of this common denominator of human nature.

During many years dealing with chronic and complex health problems, it became apparent that whatever the presenting problem and its physical and psychological components, there was often an element of the story that had something to do with the person's spiritual life (Box 12.3). The spiritual experience revealed in the story of sickness might relate to the aspirations of the human spirit,[9] without holding any explicitly religious or theological associations for the patient. It might be to do with some lack of meaning or value that has to do with more than worldly needs, or with some sense of unfulfilled potential in life, but that is not seen as having anything directly to do with God. On the other hand it may very well have to do with experience of religion, often, sadly, bad experience (for example, what I call 'doctrine abuse), or with some unsatisfied sense of God-consciousness. And the feeling of lack of value, meaning or fulfilment may arise from that deeper instinct that I call vocation, and which I find to be inseparable, at least in some small degree, from that sense of God-consciousness. I came to recognise the striving for integrity and wholeness on this level as an inherent instinct comparable to the body's instinct for self-regulation and repair in the face of physical damage and disease. I realised, too, that these mechanisms and this instinct have the common characteristics that I have described here, at whatever level of our being they operate.

BOX 12.3 *Spiritual malaise*

- Lack of value and meaning.
- Unfulfilled potential/vocation.
- Sense of wrong, badness, failure.
- 'Doctrine abuse.'
- Unsatisfied God-consciousness.
- Hunger for integrity, wholeness.

Soul matters – as General Practitioner Mabel Aghadiuno claims in the title of her book on the spiritual dimension of healthcare.[10] This is a most important book that compellingly affirms the reality and importance of this dimension of health and healing, and should be compulsory reading for all healthcare professionals. Please read it. But for my purpose I will quote from it the (rather surprising) OFSTED prescription for the spiritual development of the child:

> (The spiritual dimension is the) non-material element of human being which animates and sustains us and, depending on our point of view, either ends or continues in some form whew we die. The spiritual dimension is concerned with identity, self-worth, personal insight, meaning and purpose. It is about a person's spirit. Some people would call this 'personality' or 'character'. Others would call it a person's 'soul'. (Ofsted[11])

Soul

The soul is one dimension of ourselves that we seldom discuss. I do not believe that medicine and the healing professions will ever be able to do full justice to people's need for healing and healthcare unless and until they recognise and understand the soul as the core of our being; and understand that illness can involve, and even arise in the soul.

The soul has been described as 'the information bearing essence' that expresses our unique identity as a person.[12] In Figure 12.1, I represented this essence as comprising, in my understanding, psyche and spirit. But a difficulty arises from the various uses of the words psyche and psychic. The Greek word *psyche* has entered the English language and acquired a life of its own. Not only does it have to accommodate the concepts of psyche in modern psychology, but also the phenomena that are commonly described as psychic.

The psychic dimension of our nature has been called 'the intermediate dimension';[13] intermediate between mind and spirit. It embraces the unconscious elements of our personality, and the collective unconscious described by Carl Jung. It includes those attributes that are described as extrasensory or paranormal. It is a common mistake to melodramatise the psychic dimension; to associate it automatically, for example, with the occult. It is worth remembering that electricity was once regarded as occult before its true nature was understood. We live in an environment of electromagnetism, radiation and gravity – natural phenomena, energies, that infuse our everyday lives. Psychic energy is another. We inhabit a complex network of relationships – electromagnetic, gravitational, ecological, emotional and psychic. We all possess some psychic sensitivity and some psychic attributes, to a greater or lesser degree. It is, for example, what makes some people charismatic. The psychic dimension is a normal aspect of human nature and of the world we inhabit. Its moral and spiritual value, as with all human attributes, such as intellect and sexuality, depend upon the use we make of them.

Psychic nature is not bound by time or space. It helps to form and is formed by our personality. We are all susceptible, to a greater or lesser degree, to psychic influences, which can affect our body functions and our personality. It is by the exercise of their psychic gifts, working initially through the psychic nature of the patient, that some therapists, variously but often inappropriately called faith healers or spiritual healers, operate.

It is on this level of psychic rapport, in addition to our emotional empathy and our psychological insight, that any of us may develop a healing relationship with another person; whether within a professional health care relationship or in everyday life.

Our psychic nature can be represented as the matrix of the soul; the element in which our spiritual identity is formed and develops, through the imprint and working out of our life experience, and by the presence in the core of our being of the Spirit, the divine essence – by its action within us, and our response to that action.

It is through the intermediate dimension of the psyche that prayer is effective in promoting healing, by the agency of the Spirit, usually in the absence of any overt psychic gifts in those who pray.

In short, I would say that the structure of our personal wholeness is the interactive, interpenetrating and interdependent relationship of body, mind and soul, infused by the spirit of God, in whom we live and move and have our being, and in whom we have unique value in relation to one another and to the 'bigger picture' of creation as a whole.

Of course, it will not often be the case that in our healing relationships we need to address the state of the other person's soul. And just as we may lack certain clinical or psychological skills, we may not be equipped to do so anyway. But an awareness of our limitations does not preclude an awareness of the possibility of such a need in the other, nor a willingness to be open to it, to be accepting of it, and seek the discernment that is needed that we perhaps cannot provide.

To ignore or neglect this dimension of a patient's life may be to deny something essential to the meaning of that life and to the prospect of greater wholeness and well-being.

Meaning

> Encounter with meaning is central to the human experience. (John Polkinghorne[12])

> Meaning is inescapable: that is to say, illness always has meaning. . . . To understand how it obtains meaning is to understand something fundamental about illness, about care and perhaps about life generally. . . . The experience and meanings of illness are at the centre of clinical practice (Arthur Kleinman[14])

> The meaning that patient attaches to illness and suffering, especially in chronic or fatal illness, is critical for the healing process; and that meaning is accessible through the patient's illness story. (James Markum[15])

All illness, all suffering, is part of the narrative of a unique life. All pain is part of a story. All pain has a story behind it. Unless we can comprehend the 'story of sickness', and engage with it compassionately and creatively; unless we can help patients to find some meaning in it, I doubt the capacity of scientific medicine to achieve much at all that we could properly call healing. But 'meaning', is an imprecise word; it has many ingredients.

BOX 12.4 *The ingredients of meaning*

- Identity, personality, integrity, intactness.
- Relationships.
- Roles – family, community, work.
- Hopes, dreams, aspirations, purpose.
- Shame, guilt, regret.
- Conflicts – conscious/unconscious.
- Self-esteem, value.
- Loneliness, belonging.

(*After Cassell*[1])

The five core ingredients of 'meaning' are underlined in Box 12.4:

- Identity – Who am I?
- Integrity, or integratedness – Is my life authentic, real?, What makes me who I am?
- Purpose – Why am I here?
- Value – What is my life worth?
- Belonging – Am I truly loved? Where am I really 'at home'?

These questions are the essential framework of our lives. The answers are the scaffolding that supports us or the fault lines that undermine us. The overlap with Box 12.3 is obvious.

If we see medicine as a healing vocation it must comprehend and make real the meaning of our own and of our patient's life. And the uncomfortable truth is that this understanding must start with the understanding of ourselves. This 'meaning' is critical for the healing process in ourselves and in others. And it is revealed and can be explored and made whole through our stories.

> There is a human need to make sense of everyday events. To create a framework of meaning and causality. The framework doesn't have to be scientifically valid (much less 'true'), but it does need to work for us, as a day-to-day explanatory model. (David Misselbrook[16])

Throughout the 100 years or so since scientific medicine became established, partly despite and partly because of its great achievements, this kind of perspective has become subordinate to the biomedical model; the subordination of the person to the disease. "By reducing the body to a collection of parts, the patient as a person vanishes before the physician's gaze. That is literally *de-meaning,* and it does happen."[15] This tension between holistic instinct and biomedical process is a poignant paradox in medicine, as we have seen. It is present in doctors' expectations of themselves, and in patients' expectations of their doctors. And it demands of us a difficult intellectual and perceptual juggling act, as Iona Heath explains in the following quotation that I used earlier. "While using the generalisations of biomedical science (we have) a constant duty to refocus on the individual, – their experience and the meaning they attach to (it). . . . We cannot see (both) simultaneously – we have to choose one way of seeing or the other. To maximise our understanding, (and)not become stranded and impotent at one pole of the dualism, we must learn to oscillate our gaze."[17]

In 'Reflections on the Doctor–Patient Relationship', Moira Stewart reconciles these two main roles, within a framework of understanding, meaning and truth; summarised in Box 12.5.[18] And she includes that other indispensable ingredient of a healing relationship – trust; fittingly emphasised in the earlier quotation from the *Oxford Handbook of Clinical Medicine.*[19]

BOX 12.5 *Meaning, truth and trust in medicine*

Two main roles

- To sort out and understand the process of health to illness and disease.
- To make meaning of the process.

which require

- The doctor's trust in the inherent truth of the patient's experience.
- The patient's trust that the doctor will remain steadfast in helping to make sense of things.

(*Moira Stewart*[18])

The service of healing

If healing is medicine's proper vocation, as I believe it is, one way of representing the goals that serve that vocation is by the precepts suggested in Chapter 7; restated in Box 12.6.

BOX 12.6 *Medicine's four responsibilities for healing*

- To support the natural capacity of the body to regulate and heal itself,
  - by encouraging a healthy life-style;
  - by enabling those self-healing and self-regulating processes;
  - by helping to avoid or remedy situations that are detrimental to those processes;
- To teach people to understand and manage distress and disorder that is within their personal competence for self-care or for the care of one another.
- To intervene, but only as far as and for as long as is necessary, in ways that relieve suffering and control disorder when those natural resources are impaired and until they are sufficiently recovered, or where that personal competence is too limited to cope.
- To respect the unique value of each individual, and to act in such a way as to enhance their quality of life, regardless of the prospect of 'cure'.

The more succinct list in Box 12.7 assumes the goals in Box 12.6. They may seem obvious and uncontroversial, but their implications for 'remodelling' are not necessarily so straightforward.

BOX 12.7 *The goals of medicine*

- The relief or mitigation of suffering of mind or body.
- The relief or mitigation of disability.
- The treatment of individual illness, sickness or disease.
- The well-being and quality of life of individuals or communities, compromised by illness, sickness or disease.
- The control of causes of illness, sickness or disease, where causes are amenable to medical knowledge, insight or skill.
- The acquisition of appropriate knowledge, insight and skill.

These goals will be served first and foremost by personal care: the care of individual patients, and the insights gained by their care; secondly by the care of communities; thirdly through insights that make possible social or political solutions to health care problems; and finally, by research that enhances medicine's ability to do these things. All these parameters of health care are reflected in Figure 12.1, the picture of the person whose care is the overarching goal of medicine.

Suffering

Although the first goal of medicine is the relief of suffering, that statement needs some qualification. The goal is the relief of suffering *caused by damage or disorder* of mind or body. It is not the relief of *all* suffering, because much suffering is not the result of any such disorder. Suffering may be caused by many varieties of distress, adversity or abuse that are not the direct responsibility of medicine, though disorders of mind or body that are the responsibility of medicine may result from these. Medicine has a responsibility to treat the disorder and a responsibility of advocacy for the victims; for identifying but not for removing the cause.

Fiction provides two famous examples of doctors' failed advocacy in attempting to remove the cause of suffering. In Ibsen's play *An enemy of the people*, Dr Stockman's advocacy to remedy the contamination of the water supply that is causing illness amongst the tourists using of the town baths not only fails because of the townspeople's determination not to lose the income from the baths, but leads to his denunciation as a lunatic and the eponymous 'enemy'. The general practitioner in AJ Cronin's novel *The Citadel* finds a drastic solution to his failed advocacy by blowing up the town's leaking sewer in the cause of better public health.[20]

One form of suffering of this kind, that may come to be the responsibility of medicine is what I have called suffering from a 'well-ness'. This is suffering caused by the normal and healthy response to some kind of adversity or insult, some destructive experience. Physical pain is a normal response to physical trauma, and mental and emotional pain to emotional trauma. The eventual consequences may well be some serious disorder of mind or body, but the original distress is a healthy response to some insult to our human nature. Physical and emotional malnourishment, for example, hunger and lack of love, cause suffering that may result in illness, but the distress they cause is the normal response to the denial of an essential human need.

Medicine may have a responsibility to treat the consequences, and in the process to understand the factors causing or predisposing to the problem. This understanding should be part of the diagnostic process, and is often an essential part of the healing process because it confers meaning on the suffering and its consequences. It also affirms the essential humanity of the sufferer that has been damaged by the destructive experience, the value of those attributes of human nature that make us vulnerable to adversity or abuse. It may offer the possibility of gaining some control of the situation; another important aid to well-being and healing.

The problem is that much illness that presents to doctors is a symptom of that primary suffering, and not of any actual disorder. As we have seen, if the story is not heard the opportunity for appropriate resolution of the problem is lost. Further medicalisation may result, leading farther away from the real solution.

So medicine's most obvious goal, the relief of suffering proves to be ambiguous. Where to draw the line? Is a line to be drawn at all? Is the general practitioner, for example, always to be the mediator of all suffering that is construed or experienced as an illness? If so, his or her biomedical acumen needs to be augmented with a high degree of emotional intelligence and discernment. Or the healthcare team, or the healthcare system, must be flexible and versatile enough to accommodate and share the diversity of need that presents to it; and to direct the patient towards the appropriate solution, or the appropriate provider of a solution.

Precarious living

> **Precarious**: Held during the pleasure of another; question-begging, taken for granted; dependent on chance, uncertain; perilous. From Latin – *precarius*: obtained by entreaty (*prex, prec-* prayer). (*Concise Oxford Dictionary*)

I have a book called *Precarious Living; the path to life.*[21] It is an excellent title – discomforting, challenging, exciting. It reminds us that life is precarious – dangerous, unpredictable, dependent on circumstances and other people. But it says that unless we accept the precariousness of life, if we try to escape it or insure ourselves completely against it, we will not be fully alive. Nor will life be the adventure, the process of discovery – of our world and more importantly of ourselves – that it should be.

This precariousness is built into the picture of 'wholeness' in Figure 12.1. It is built into the way we are made: our genetics, our constitution, the circumstances of our birth, our life situation and relationships – our nature and our nurture. All that is represented in the circles and at the interface between them, and all that is represented in perimeter around them, is precarious. But at the same time the picture has built into it the means of our survival of that precariousness, and of our growth and flourishing as a person despite it. And not only despite it, but also *through* it. It represents the challenges and opportunities that make possible a full life, and the resources available to us for making the most of them: the path to life. Those resources include the biological processes by which life survives, processes of self-regeneration, healing and repair. They include the resources of mind and spirit. And they include the resources that exist in our relationship with other people and our environment.

For every person the balance between the precariousness of life and the resources to meet it will be unique. For some the precariousness is great and the resources are scarce. For some it is the other way round. Some with apparently scarce resources transcend the precariousness of life. Others with apparently ample resources are overwhelmed by it.

For everyone there is some degree of personal freedom. It may seem perverse to say that of people whose mental or physical disability is so severe that any possibility of freedom of choice or action is denied them. But no one's life is without the possibility of meaning and dignity. No one's life, is worthless, or not deserving of 'worth-ship'. They may lack the resources for this within themselves, when it is the responsibility of the caring community to affirm it. But there is always, nevertheless, some freedom within that person, however deeply imprisoned by their disability, to respond to care that affirms their dignity and value, even if it is only at that level of their being that I have described as the soul. Our response to that instinct for wholeness described earlier, which is at work in everyone whatever their condition, can evoke this free response in any person in our care. But most of us are not so afflicted and have considerable freedom, and the responsibility that goes with it, to make what we can of life. This means living with its precariousness, the 'learning curve', that is our path to life.

Medicine has to live with the precariousness of life. Often it has to pick up the pieces. Often it has to contain the inevitable suffering of life's inherent perils. It has to accept the unpredictability and uncertainty of life. It has to understand and work with the balance of precariousness and resourcefulness, of freedom and responsibility in individual lives.

Certainly medicine has its responsibility for advocacy. It has a responsibility to teach and explain (part of the meaning of being a doctor), to warn, to admonish even. Where it can help to mitigate the precariousness or increase the resourcefulness for individuals or communities it must do so. It can and should have a salutary (health-making) influence, its role in 'salutogenesis', but it cannot sanitise life.

Above all, the fact that medicine is so deeply implicated in the precariousness of life, that its first task is to confront the precariousness of individual lives, and that the life of every healthcare professional is just as precarious as the life of each person they care for, requires and is the ground for compassion.

Natural medicine and natural healing

One of the popular epithets applied to complementary and alternative medicine (CAM) is 'natural medicine'. This is by no means always appropriate. The highly sophisticated methods of acupuncture treatment and of homeopathic pharmacy, for example, are not at all natural. At least in the sense that a therapy is the application of readily and naturally available remedies in response to the particular need. The use of herbs and touch and tender loving care might by contrast be called natural. What is more important, and actually 'natural' in these and other therapeutic approaches, very definitely including conventional medicine, is not the method of treatment but the response in the patient; the natural *healing* that is evoked. In the case of CAM, of course, the therapeutic benefit is often dismissed by conventional medical scientists because it is attributed exclusively to this natural healing effect; whereas in conventional practice this effect is marginalised or disregarded in relation to the effect of the medical intervention itself.

Chapter 7 discusses some of the general principles of healing in relation to medicine. Many of these depend upon evoking and mobilising the natural self-regulating and self-healing mechanisms and resources that are a recurring motif in this book. A key design principle for the new model will be to re-evaluate these and give them a higher priority in our whole approach to health care.

Placebo

First we need to sort out a confusion of language. The term 'placebo' has come to be used to describe any effect of treatment that cannot be attributed directly to the specific effect, sometimes caused the 'characteristic effect' of the treatment method – the drug, the surgical procedure, the acupuncture needle, the manipulation, etc.[22,23] But this is a mistake that limits our understanding of what is going on 'off the ball', as a footballer might say. Used correctly a 'placebo' is a sham treatment, an inert (inactive) replica of a drug for example. It is given so that, literally, 'I please' the patient, and encourage a positive response – when a specific and active treatment is not available, or not appropriate, or when the practitioner is uncertain what to do, or when he or she feels compelled to do *something* when no active intervention might be an appropriate, possibly better choice.

So the primary meaning and use of 'placebo' is as an alternative to a specific and active treatment for the patient's problem. When I was a child in the 1940s, on visits to my father's GP surgery, I would sometimes be given a pleasant white tablet from a jar in the dispensary as a treat. These were placebos, occasionally and deliberately dispensed to encourage a positive response in the patient for one of the reasons given in the last paragraph; and given to reinforce the healing power of the prescription already dispensed in the course of the consultation, namely 'the drug doctor' as it has been called. In those days, of course, the repertoire of investigation and specific treatments was much more limited than it is today.

Nowadays, actual placebos of this kind are rarely if ever dispensed, except in the course of placebo controlled trials of drugs or procedures, when they are used to distinguish between the specific, characteristic effects of those drugs or procedures and their 'non-specific', or 'incidental' effects. This is necessary because it is very well known that the *experience* of *any* medical intervention, including the consultation, the process of diagnosis, investigations (X-rays, blood tests, etc), and surgery, can have a positive (or indeed negative) effect on the patient's well-being, symptoms or body functions, regardless of the actual and intended effect of the treatment. This needs to be 'discounted' against the overall effect of the specific treatment so that its actual effect (efficacy) can be determined, and its superiority to placebo assessed. The fact that this kind of experimental method creates an artificial and partial understanding of the therapeutic process has already been discussed elsewhere (Chapter 6). But it is an explicit example of the true meaning of placebo as a deliberate and sham alternative, often a very effective one, to a specific medical intervention.

The deliberate giving of sham treatments in actual therapeutic situations may be very rare nowadays. But the giving of *active* treatments for the very same reasons as I listed for giving true placebos in days gone by still goes on. Many prescriptions are given to please patients who expect, even demand, that something be done. The giving of inappropriate antibiotics for self-limiting infections is by now a familiar example because exhortations to doctors not to do it have appeared in the newspapers and not just in medical journals. Prescriptions are given to make life easier for doctors when an explanation, or education, or a fuller enquiry into the nature of the problem, would be more appropriate; but time, perhaps, does not permit it.

Treatments such as these, given when there is no clear and necessary indication for the drug or procedure's specific action, so that it is actually irrelevant to the clinical situation are by no means inert. But they fulfil the same purpose as a true placebo.

To summarise the discussion to this point:

- Self-regulation and self-healing are inherent biological properties of all organisms, and inherent properties of the human body, mind and spirit.
- Many experiences can stimulate and support their effectiveness in ordinary everyday life.
- Experiences that have a medical context provide particular and powerful stimulus and support to these processes.
- This effect is independent of the characteristic, intended and active effect of a particular medical intervention.
- The effect may be stimulated by an inactive or sham treatment, or by an active treatment not specifically indicated for the problem.
- The effect accompanies to some degree every medical encounter and every specific intervention.
- The effect is a response of the patient to the whole experience of the encounter and the intervention.

According to this account the use of a true placebo is actually a *specific* therapeutic act intended to effect a positive response by means of an inert or sham treatment. This is a very clearly defined use of the term. And the 'specific' nature of a true placebo effect is confirmed by the knowledge that substances that are technically inert nevertheless trigger the release of naturally occurring, physiologically active chemicals in the brain. Confusion arises when *any* spontaneous improvement in the condition of the patient that is independent, or perceived to be independent of the specific action of a medical intervention is described as a placebo effect. In fact, this improvement may have nothing at all to do with the therapeutic process. It may be due to the natural course of the disease, fluctuations in the symptoms, regression to the mean (a statistical fact that if a variable is extreme on its first measurement it will tend to be closer to the average on its second measurement, and if it is extreme on a second measurement, it will tend to have been closer to the average on the first measurement), bias in the reporting of symptoms by patients, or some other concurrent treatment.[24] But allowing for these possibilities, one way of overcoming the confusion caused by the use of 'placebo' to describe all the incidental effects of a therapeutic process rather than just the sham treatment, has been to describe them as the 'non-specific' effects.

Non-specific effects

But this really only adds to the confusion. Because we have to ask, "When is non-specific, specific?", and vice versa. Here we meet a paradox, or at least a conceptual difficulty. When we deliberately use a non-specific factor of the therapeutic encounter, does it not become specific? The process of paraphrase – restating what the patient has said in our own words, either to be sure we have understood, or to encourage her or him to reflect on what was said – is likely to promote new and helpful insights. For some practitioners it will not be a 'technique' but an instinctive and unconscious response to the patient's narrative; it will be part of their non-specific repertoire. For a psychotherapist it will be a specific technique. The distinction between the specific and non-specific elements of a therapeutic encounter will often be a matter of context and usage, as Charlotte Paterson and Paul Dieppe explain in their review of characteristic and incidental effects in complex interventions.[22] For a complex therapy, such as physiotherapy or complementary medicine, the history taking process (the narrative), the diagnostic process particular to that therapy, discussion of the therapeutic theory, exploration of personal circumstances and lifestyle issues, patient education, the listening and the talking, may be inseparable from the specific treatment and its characteristic effects. The diagnostic process and the specific treatment may emerge from the process as a whole, and each part of the package may be contingent on another. The process of case taking in some disciplines that require particularly detailed enquiry and attentiveness may be a specific technique whose purpose is an intellectual analysis of the case history in order to identify the indications on which to base a treatment strategy. But it is also therapeutic in its own right.

An active drug (specific agent) will always have an added placebo component (non-specific effect). One clinician's non-specific approach is another's specific technique. This dual effect of various aspects of the interaction between practitioner and patient is common to all medical disciplines. The specific–non-specific dualism is in many instances as artificial and unhelpful as the mind–body dualism that still permeates much of medicine. This fact of life does not excuse us from studying and seeking to define and manage the different elements of the specific/non-specific or mind/body continuum appropriately. But we must remember that they are at best ambiguous, and at worst misleading distinctions, to prevent us getting the analysis of those different elements out of perspective.

What it boils down to is that the outcome of any medical endeavour depends (in varying degrees) on a combination of the direct effect (the *efficacy*) of whatever technique the practitioner employs and of the

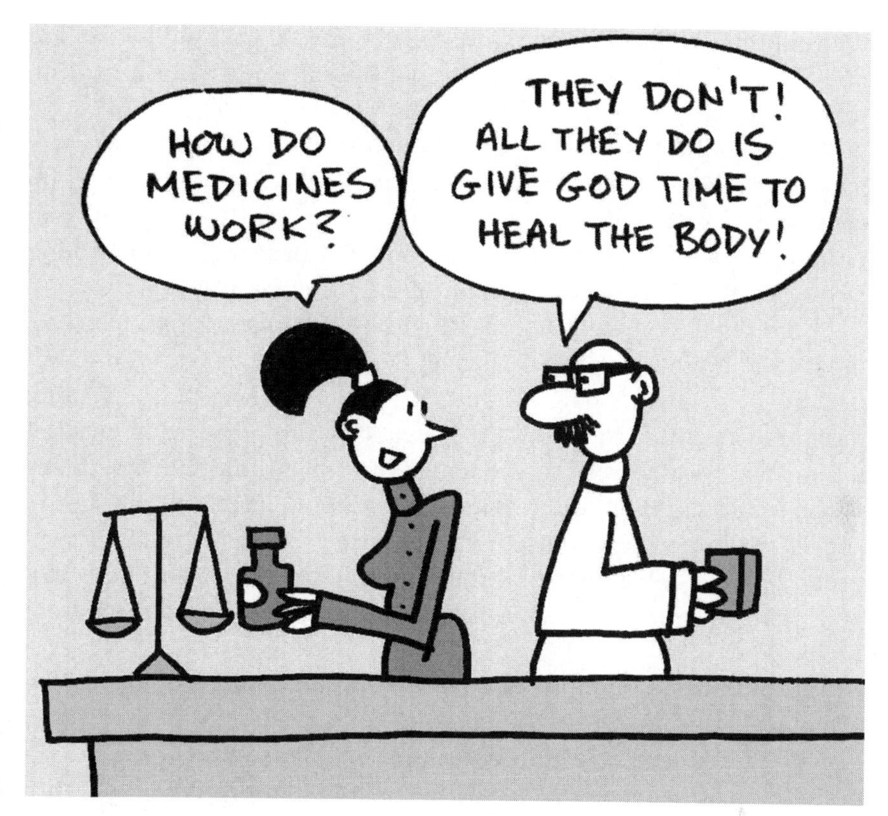

Figure 12.2 *Pharmacology's big secret.*

therapeutic experience as a whole. It is a package deal. All therapeutics is what is sometimes known as a 'black box', whose component parts are difficult to define; their separate contributions to the outcome (the overall *effectiveness* of the treatment) difficult to distinguish.

It is important to investigate the efficacy of a specific technique in order that we may be sure of its active role (to 'prove' it); in order that we may understand it; and in order that we may improve it. It is equally important that we acknowledge and investigate the role of the therapeutic experience as a whole, so that we may understand that; and so that we may use it well and maximise its contribution to the therapeutic process – to the outcome, or effectiveness of the treatment.

Context and Meaning

Two concepts have been introduced recently into the discussion of healing processes associated with medical procedures that I have labelled 'natural'. They help to describe, clarify, and to an extent explain them, overcoming the confusion of 'placebo' and 'non-specific' effects. They are *context* and *meaning*. Together they describe the essential elements of the whole therapeutic experience.

The significance of context has already been discussed briefly. Its more important role is its contribution to the overall effectiveness of the therapeutic process. And its most important determinant is the quality of relationship between the practitioner and the patient; in which other factors like the physical environment of the encounter play a part.

In the conclusion to their paper *The Power of Context: reconceptualising the placebo effect*, Franklin Miller and Ted Kaptchuk write: "Contextual healing is precisely what has been off the radar screen of scientific medicine, which has focused on therapeutic benefit produced by medical technology. Fixation on the specific efficacy of treatment interventions obscures the fact that the technological tools of medicine are always applied in some context, which itself may contribute significantly to therapeutic benefit. . . . We should see the context of the clinical encounter as a potential enhancer and in some cases the primary vehicle of therapeutic benefit."[25]

The importance of 'meaning' in the therapeutic encounter or healing relationship, has been discussed already. The attitude of the practitioner, and the rapport and dialogue between practitioner and patient, are obviously key contributors to the patient's sense of meaning in the experience of illness. Diagnosis is part of this dialogue, and as Howard Brody argued, 'diagnosis is treatment'.[26] In this paper he is primarily writing about the role of diagnosis in assisting what he describes as the 'placebo effect'. He gives a brief account of characteristics of the placebo effect, including what I have called the 'pure' placebo effect. But he goes on to say, "To understand the placebo effect . . . it is crucial to avoid a narrow focus on the sugar pill or other inert medication, and to look instead at the physician–patient relationship – there is a placebo-effect component to virtually every physician–patient encounter".

So he moves from describing the pure placebo effect (the direct effect of the inert or sham treatment) to describing the contextual healing effect of the relationship. And he goes on to explain how important this process is to conferring meaning on the patient's experience of illness; and how important that is to the healing process. He describes the therapeutic value of the diagnostic process and the caring encounter together as the 'meaning model'. In this paper thirty years ago he anticipated the two concepts or mechanisms, *context* and *meaning* that are now proposed as the key components of the therapeutic process for promoting natural healing – self-regulation and self-healing.

'Meaning' as a vehicle for healing is explored thoroughly in *Meaning, Medicine and the 'placebo effect'* by Daniel Moerman.[27] There is a huge literature on the various manifestations of 'placebo', but this book provides a thorough and challenging review of the subject. In it, he explores how various 'placebo' phenomena achieve their effect through their meaning for the patient. These include, for example, the different placebo effects of different coloured tablets in different cultures because of the meaning associated with that colour in that culture.

For the purposes of this book, in addition to other specific references that crop up, for general reading I recommend that book by Moerman, and one other, *Understanding the placebo effect in complementary medicine: theory, practice and research*, edited by David Peters,[28] as providing a sufficient overview of the subject of 'placebo' from different perspectives. Factors determining the working of the placebo effect are summarised in Box 12.8.

BOX 12.8 *Some determinants of the 'placebo' response*

- Colour of the drug.
- Number of doses given (more doses, bigger effect).
- Power of the brand name (well-known name, bigger effect).
- Cost (more expensive drug, bigger effect).
- Method of delivery (injections/acupuncture bigger effect than pills).
- Frequency of the treatment (more often, bigger effect).
- Expectation (patient expects good result).
- Knowing the drug is being given (as opposed to not seeing it happen).
- Conditioning (it has happened before, so it is likely to happen again).
- Newness of the treatment (the newer the better).
- Expectation and behaviour of the clinician.
- Compliance/commitment of the patient to treatment.
- Setting of treatment (pleasant environment, bigger effect).

Not all 'natural' healing requires the reinforcement of placebo, context or meaning. Some conditions and some patients would get better anyway without recourse to medicine of any kind. But although we know this is so, the extent to which it is so is impossible to measure, because even a 'no treatment' group in a research study will have been affected by both the

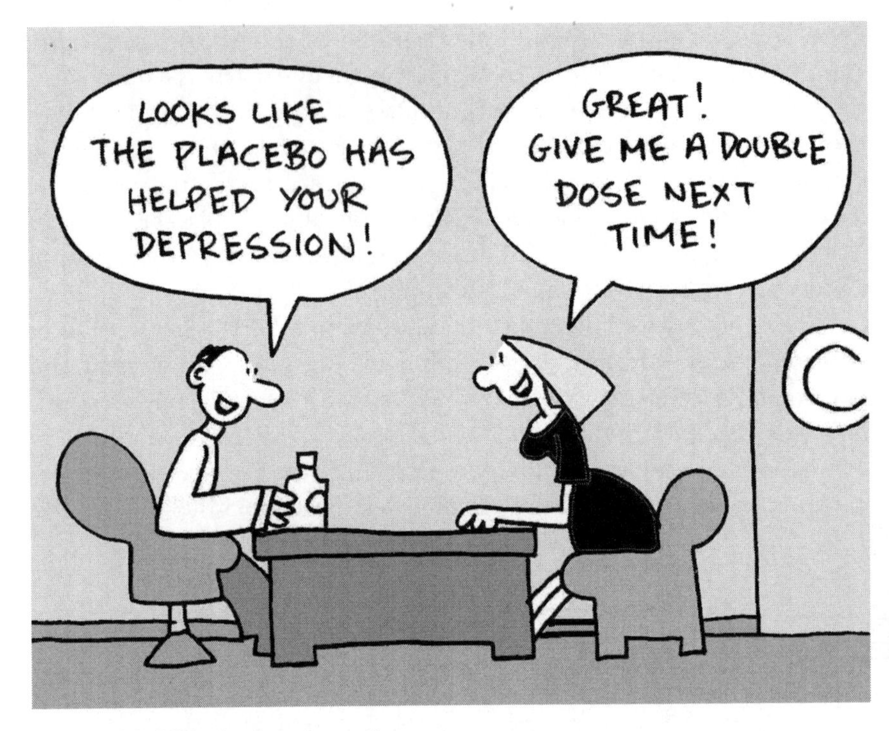

Figure 12.3 With placebos, size matters.

context and the meaning in the process of recruitment into the study. And those patients who simply do not present their problems to a healthcare professional and just 'let nature take its course', will by definition never be identified at the time of the illness. A retrospective, qualitative study of such 'non-patients' after nature has been allowed to take its course would presumably be possible, and would certainly be very interesting. But as far as I know has never been attempted. And in our pervasively health conscious culture, such people must be very few anyway.

Suffice it to say that there is general agreement within clinical practice and medical science, (a) that spontaneous healing processes can be stimulated by factors incidental to *any* specific treatment technique, and (b) that the effectiveness of *all* specific treatment techniques is derived in part from a 'placebo' component. In other words, for example, the *effectiveness* of a drug of proven pharmacological *efficacy* is part pharmacological and part 'placebo'. A recent review of biological, clinical and ethical issues related to 'placebo' effects states in its summary. "Recent research shows that placebo effects are genuine psychobiological events attributable to the overall therapeutic context, and that these effects can be robust in both laboratory and clinical settings. There is also evidence that placebo effects can exist in clinical practice, even if no placebo is given. Further research will allow advances in the ethical use of placebo mechanisms that are inherent in routine clinical care, and encourage the use of treatments that stimulate placebo effects."[24]

An irony

Returning to the opening paragraph of this section, you may now notice an irony. The benefits of some CAM therapies are dismissed because they are attributed exclusively to factors other than the direct action of the treatments themselves; factors that in fact, as we have seen, are fundamental to the overall effectiveness of all therapeutic procedures.

Rheumatologists Paul Dieppe and Michael Doherty have investigated the role of context and meaning in the response to treatment of patients with osteoarthritis.[23] Studying 193 clinical trials, they found a significant placebo effect accompanying all forms of treatment; and an effect size in the placebo response that in some instances exceeded the effect size of the active treatment. It is a useful paper because it provides a succinct summary of the various determinants of placebo responses, including those shown in Box 12.8, many of which are dealt with at greater length in Moerman's book.

They review factors that enhance or inhibit 'contextual healing', with particular reference to the quality of the practitioner–patient relationship – focused and unhurried attention, comfortable environment, listening, thorough examination, good explanation, addressing any concerns, pointing the way forward; and say that "it is obvious . . . that practitioners should capitalise on the impact of context effects to enhance the benefits to their patients, as a professional responsibility." And they conclude, "Practitioners of complementary and alternative medicine (CAM) often do this very well, and seem ahead of us more traditional physicians. . . . We often label practitioners of CAM as charlatans and explain their treatment success as 'just placebo effect', apparently oblivious of the large effect size of such 'non-treatment' benefits. But if we did learn from the research literature, from practitioners of CAM, and from simple observation, and optimise these meaning responses in our clinical practice, the benefits of such 'contextual healing' to the population of people with osteoarthritis would be huge."

The editorial introducing the themed edition of the *British Medical Journal*, *'Ceci n'est pas un placebo'*, said much the same thing: "Is it possible that the alternative medical community has tended historically to understand something important about the experience of illness and the ritual of doctor–patient interactions that the rest of medicine might do well to hear?'[29]

The article to which the editorial related reported a study involving patients with irritable bowel syndrome in which no 'specific', active treatment was given. One group had no practitioner contact at all, but were on a waiting list for treatment. The second received a placebo treatment, sham acupuncture, with minimal interaction with the practitioner involving no attention given to the patient or conversation other than to explain the scientific nature of the study. The third received the sham acupuncture during an interactive practitioner–patient relationship 'augmented' by warmth, attention and confidence. The proportion of patients in each group reporting 'adequate' relief of symptoms was 28%, 44% and 62%, respectively; and for those reporting 'moderate to substantial' relief it was 3%, 20% and 37%. The authors point out that the proportion of patients in the 'augmented' group reporting adequate relief is comparable with the responder rate in clinical trials of drugs used in the treatment of irritable bowel syndrome. They conclude, these results indicate that such factors as warmth, empathy, duration of time, and the communication of positive expectation might indeed significantly affect clinical outcome.[30]

This study is a good example of the fact that, for all that has been said about their limitations, and the limited value of the *efficacy* they demonstrate, randomised controlled trials have an important role in investigating and elucidating the 'incidental' effects that contribute so much to the *effectiveness* of treatment. But, of course, in the context of this trial, the 'augmented' style of consultation was the 'specific' intervention.

Health, well-being and quality of life

The question of what is meant by 'health' and how it relates to 'well-being' is subtle enough and complex enough to occupy many chapters, if not many books. Here is a simple account of the two concepts; sufficient I hope to guide us in the remodelling process.

Health is not a commodity

Health, well-being and quality of life are not standardised 'commodities'. They are highly individual. There are sociological and medical instruments for measuring them, questionnaires of one sort or another, and these may give a measure of change, in response to medical care for example. But both the absolute measurement and the degree of change will depend on individual characteristics other than the need for social or medical help or its effectiveness. They will depend as much on the person as the predicament. Our perception of ourselves or of our world, our expectations and aspirations, our culture, religion, and personality, our circumstances, and other factors besides no doubt, make all the difference. They will variously affect our evaluation of our health, our sense of well-being, our quality of life (what we are able to do with our lives), and our quality of *living* (what we can get out of life, regardless of our actual limitations or opportunities).

This is really just another way of saying that a proper understanding of a person's health, well-being and quality of life requires knowledge of the *person*, and of the narrative of their illness. And it also requires an understanding of the way that medicine can affect, and unfortunately sometimes distort rather than enhance that narrative.

Health is a process

Health is often regarded as a state – the condition I am in at a particular time. But it is better regarded as a process. Health is dynamic. It involves constant readjustment and self-regulation of the functions of body and mind to maintain their harmony and integrity in respect of our innate constitution (the way we are made genetically, are born and nurtured), and with regard to the subsequent circumstances and events of our lives. These are the ingredients of the three circles in Figure 12.1, the dynamics of the overlapping areas between them, and the relationship between these and the context of our lives outlined on the perimeter. Our health is a biographical process, not just a biological state. Health care must take account of what we have been, what we are and what we may become.

Health is also dynamic in that it concerns the process of living and the progress of our lives. It has to do with the maintenance and development of our 'capabilities',[31] our potential to make the most of our lives, which will be enhanced or threatened by those constitutional and contextual factors. Medicine may have no control over the circumstance of people's lives, but gaining insight into their healthful or harmful effects, promoting the one and warning against the other, will be one of its goals. More obviously it has a responsibility to overcome or mitigate their adverse effects, as well as seeking to remedy or mitigate whatever constitutional defects impair our capabilities.

Health is not necessarily the same as well-being

Screening programmes, as we have seen, are designed to detect disorder in people who are feeling well. Some are designed to predict future disorder where there is none present. The so-called 'worried well' may be the victims of screening programmes ('partial patients') or health scares or old wives tales. They may also include the fit and healthy man who strains a chest muscle in the course of some physical activity. Failing to attribute the subsequent pain to its actual cause may provoke the fear of heart attack, and induce for the first time a disconcerting awareness of his mortality. Depending on his personality, the experience might permanently change his perception of his body, and his interpretation of the inevitable and usually benign variations of function and sensation that we all experience from time to time. Two people with large ears, or small breasts, or similar birth marks, may regard them quite differently – normal and unexceptional to one, a disfigurement to another. Both are equally healthy, but in each case one is unwell.

Well-being may not depend upon good health

> In the months that followed I learnt that illness is multifaceted and complex; that it is a process, not a static entity; and that it is possible to go on living well and experiencing wellbeing even within the context of a terrible and incurable illness. This surprised me, as I had always thought of health as the sine qua non of happiness. And yet, all of a sudden, I found myself changing, responding to constraints, learning to make sense of my life in the light of my illness. The work of realigning my life, its values, and the meaning I gave its different elements surprised me. (Havi Carel[32])

Serious and terminal disease may co-exist with a surprising degree of well-being. Personality, spirituality, relationships, life history and personal circumstances will variously affect tolerance of symptoms, ability to cope and the capacity for positive experience. Quality of life may be impaired in terms of what the patient can do, but quality of *living* may transcend those limitations.

Well-being as distinct from health and the treatment of disease receives little attention in mainstream medical education. But it is of central importance in assessing the needs of the patient and the outcome of treatment in complementary medicine, it is central to the holistic approach to health care (see 'The holistic perspective', below), and it is even the subject of government sponsored research undertaken by the Centre for Well-being unit of the New Economics Foundation (www.neweconomics.org/projects/five-ways-well-being).[33]

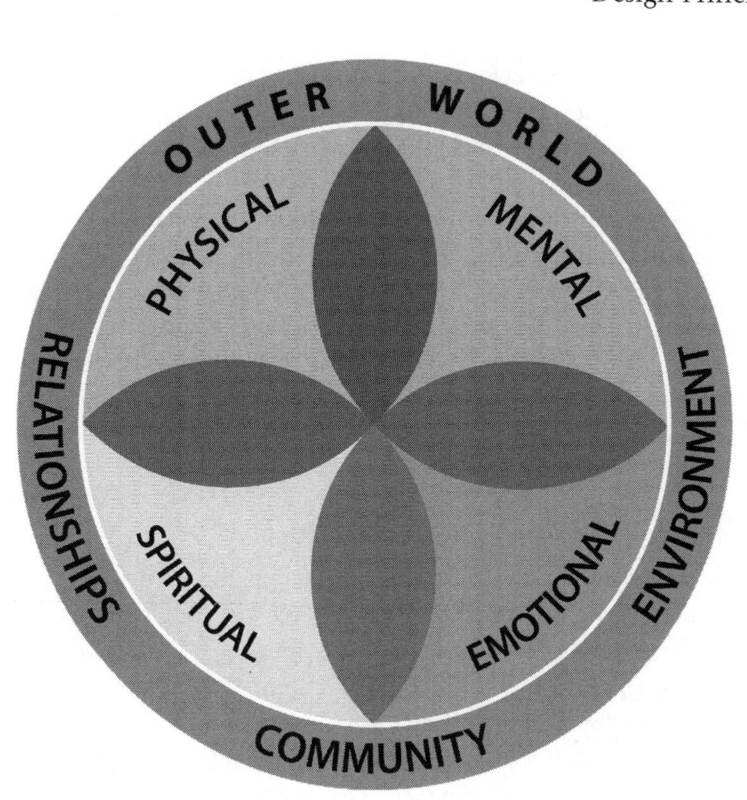

Figure 12.4 *Well being.*
(Reproduced with the permission of Jan Alcoe and the Editor, *Journal of Holistic Healthcare*)

But the concept of well-being is vague, not clearly defined. By contrast with 'health', which is generally regarded as having objective criteria to do with bodily and mental structure and function and the absence of disease states, 'well-being' is subjective and has many dimensions including our physical, emotional, spiritual, social and environmental condition and circumstances. A helpful distinction is made in a paper on wellbeing by Craig Brown and Jan Alcoe.[34] It includes a diagram representing the dimensions of wellbeing (Figure 12.4), similar to my structure of wholeness diagram (Figure 12.1), but much simpler. They state, "If we are physically unwell, we can still redress the balance by enhancing our wellbeing on the emotional, mental and spiritual levels. Wellbeing is essentially about how we relate inwards to ourselves and come to understand ourselves through the four dimensions (physical, mental, emotional and spiritual). There are further aspects of wellbeing, which is how we relate outwards – to others, our community and our environment".

They quote a patient whose experience makes their point: "I recently joined a choir and it's made me feel like I'm part of something again [*spiritual*]. The singing seems to have reduced the pain I experience from my arthritis [physical] and all the laughing we do has given me a lift [*emotional*]. I'm even beginning to get my head around reading music [*mental*]".

But another contributor to the same journal's themed edition on well-being warns about the risk of creating a well-being industry. "No one could have missed the explosion of wellbeing commodities and magazines for sale. Academic departments of psychology are rushing to develop competing measure of wellbeing (with pages of statistical analysis)."[35] Well-being must not become just another health care commodity, and a vehicle for more 'targets'.

Health and culture

There is considerable literature in anthropology on one or another aspect of health and culture. *Culture, Health and Illness* by the late Cecil Helman is a good introduction.[36] For the immediate purpose it is probably sufficient to recall that perceptions and interpretations of health and illness are indeed affected by cultural differences – geographical, ethnic, national, religious and social. If we invite them those differences will be revealed in patients' illness narratives. And if they are neglected, or worse still violated by being forced into an alien interpretive framework, the illness is likely to be compounded.

The relationship between medicine and society was discussed in Chapter 4, and the subject of culture and society recurs as a theme in Chapter 17.

Health and healing

The remarks about health and well-being highlight the confusion in our thinking about health. Is perfect health (should such a state exist) equivalent to complete well-being (should such a state exist)? Is health a measure of the functioning state of our bodies and minds, regardless of our perception of well-being? Is well-being primarily a mental state regardless of our physical condition? Or is a fair degree of satisfaction with our bodily condition and the working of our mental faculties necessary to feel well?

There is no satisfactory answer to that sort of question. Health (again) is not a commodity that can be measured. It is a subtle and personal thing. It is a "balance, a state of equilibrium, not only within a person's body and psyche, but also in that person's relationships with the other people around them, (and) with the natural environment". That is a quotation from another book by Cecil Helman,[37] but it is very close to the description of wellbeing in the earlier passage. Here, Helman is commending the traditional healers that the World Health Organisation saw as possible allies of the medical system, and who Helman says really are as holistic as the WHO says they are; because their's is – "A view of illness that takes it outside the body, its diseased organs and the purely physical, and then places it in its wider personal social and cosmic context. Whatever else is going on in their lives, for peoples and healers in these communities, health is harmony – and illness not just the malfunction of a particular organ".

These concepts of balance, equilibrium and harmony are helpful in several ways. They help us to understand what is meant by 'holistic', a concept we will shortly dissect more fully; they help to define 'health'; and they bring health, well-being and healing to a point of convergence. We have considered health as a process; a biological and biographical process, and a precarious one. It is in fact a continuous balancing act. Homeostasis is the process by which our bodies tend towards a healthy balance in response to changes in our internal and external *milieu*. Balancing on one leg on a windy day is not a fixed postural state, but a process of continual adjustment of physiological function in response to external influence. It is a dynamic process. And health is a dynamic process, a process of continual adjustment, striving to keep our whole being in balance.

Healing promotes balance, equilibrium and harmony of the whole person in the holistic sense that Helman describes. But where health can be seen as a process *maintaining* those attributes, healing is *creative*. It is directed towards progressively greater balance, equilibrium, harmony and wholeness, as discussed above and in Chapter 7. Health is a process that incorporates well-being, whole-being. Healing is a process of whole-*making*.

The holistic perspective

The term 'holistic' is more seriously abused by some complementary and alternative therapists than the word 'natural'. I have a leaflet in front of me advertising 'holistic massage'. We might as well speak of holistic plumbing. Your plumber might indeed have a holistic attitude to your central heating system; taking account of your personal metabolic needs and susceptibility to cold, your personality (thrifty or extravagant), the vagaries of climate change and your carbon footprint, the international market in copper, and so on and so forth. But his plumbing technique, his fixing of your pipes, could in no sense be called holistic.

What the advertisement presumably means is that the masseuse may but will not necessarily, take as broad a view of your needs as I have described

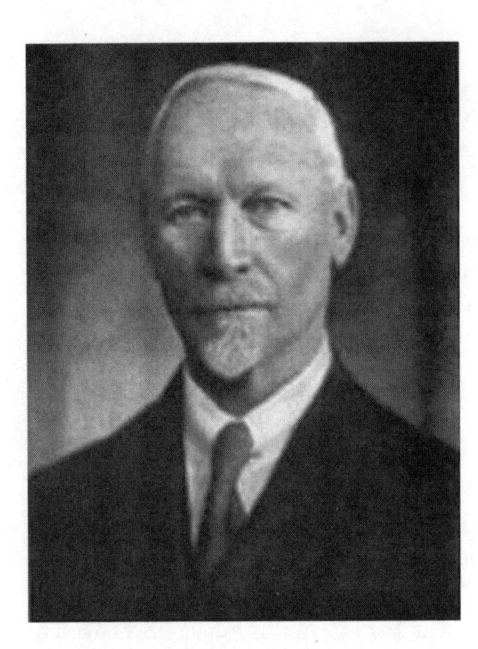

Figure 12.5 *Jan Christian Smuts (1879–1950)*

for your plumber, and may counsel you accordingly. But then, so will (or should) your GP, or your orthopaedic surgeon. And he will not describe his work as holistic hip replacement. Complementary medicine, so often described as 'holistic', is not *necessarily* any more so than conventional medicine; certainly not by definition any more so.

Holism is an attitude, a perspective; the perspective depicted in Figure 12.1. It is a statement of the relationship between parts of a system that makes the whole of the system greater than the sum of those parts. And it is a statement of the interdependence of the parts in determining the well-being of the whole.

The holistic 'perspective', this sense of the relationship of things as parts of a greater whole, must have been in the consciousness of humankind since pre-history. But the term 'holism' is less than 100 years old. It was coined by Jan Smuts the South African statesman (Figure 12.5), in 1925, and adopted by the *Encyclopaedia Britannica* two years later. A brief and helpful account of the holistic instinct that lead Smuts to write *Holism and Evolution*, the book that introduced the concept, can be found in *Holism and Complementary Medicine* by Vincent di Stefano.[38]

> A philosophical system directed towards an understanding of whole systems, rather than particular events or phenomena. (He) sought to counter the mechanistic and deterministic view of life that had increasingly dominated the emerging scientific world by reaffirming the co-centrality of the mind and life in creation. For Smuts, the study of matter alone did not provide an adequate understanding

of the world. Through his exploration of 'wholes', Smuts offered a broader and more comprehensive perspective on the nature of reality than that provided by reductionist science.

Reductionism and holism are complementary

Di Stefano ends his account of Smuts' work by making a point that needs emphasising today, and in the context of this book. "The philosophy of holism can therefore be seen to be *complementary* to that of reductionism, which holds that phenomena can be understood by an analysis of their individual components. Holism offers a systemic view of reality that emphasises (both) autonomy *and* interdependence, and accepts that matter, life and mind are implicate and integral to the phenomenal world." (My italics)

Holistic medicine is sometimes represented as the antithesis of bio-medicine in the sense of being in direct opposition to it. It is not. Holism is the antithesis of reductionism only in the sense of being in strong contrast to it. They are complementary, and necessarily complementary, views of reality. And as far as medicine is concerned, I want my doctor to have a holistic perspective *and* a repertoire of the biomedical knowledge and skills necessarily informed by reductionist analytical science. All science, and medicine in particular, must possess that versatility if it is to have a true hold on reality; if they are to perceive and elucidate the 'whole truth' – of a particular field of scientific enquiry or of the predicament of the particular patient. Without this balanced perspective, healthcare professionals will be able neither to make sense of the problem, nor to bring meaning to the patient's experience.

Figure 12.1 at the beginning of the chapter is explicit in its representation of this balance. Our detailed knowledge of its component parts and their interaction is essential to our ability, when necessary, to control and manage those parts and processes. And that can only be achieved by reductionist methods. But the true value and ultimate success of our ability to do that depends on our appreciation of the relationship of those parts with the whole, and with the wider holistic landscape depicted in the perimeter of the diagram.

Integrated care

The word 'integrated' can be applied to healthcare in a number of ways, some of which are too vague, or misrepresent the 'actuality'. According to the *Concise Oxford Dictionary*, the verb 'integrate' has to do with the completion (of an imperfect thing) by the addition of parts; or, the combining of parts into a whole. In a social sense it means bringing or coming into equal membership. The adjective 'integrate' means made up of parts, whole complete. While 'integral' means of, or necessary to the completeness of a whole; whole, complete; or, forming a whole. These are helpful definitions because it seems to me that they describe what integrated health care should be about.

What is called integrated medicine or integrated care may not be like this at all. It is often a loose aggregation of different therapeutic methods, resources or services, perhaps within a geographical or administrative framework. They may not share any common model of disease processes, healing processes or whole person care. And they may not engage in any process of shared management that effectively integrates their different methods and perceptions within a coherent care plan for the individual patient. This is not integrated care. There is no sense of a service combining its parts into a whole. It is still a fragmented service, likely to have a fragmenting effect on the patient within it.

Alternatively, the process of integration may be sufficiently close, represent a sufficient level of interprofessional awareness, and be sufficiently mutually respectful and mutually supportive to achieve a highly effective level of shared care or appropriate interprofessional liaison. A service like this can properly be described as integrated. It conveys a sense of completeness and wholeness in itself. And rather than tending to the fragmentation of the patient by emphasising the separateness of the 'parts', it will emphasise their relatedness. It will be integrative.

Integrative care

A properly integrated service will be conscious of this integrative function and will deliberately seek to serve it. It will be integrative of the patient because, by its very nature, bringing together different perspectives of patient care it will encourage a holistic understanding of the patients' needs. Note that it is the bringing together of different *perspectives* that is necessary to achieve this. Not just the bringing together of different skill sets. And it will be integrative of the care professionals and care teams involved because of the need to explore and share different perspectives.

This will be particularly true when the integrative process involves the physical, psychological, social and spiritual dimension of care, as ideally it must. And as indeed it already sometimes does, particularly (but not exclusively) in some primary care settings, some mental health care settings, and in palliative care.

And where integrated care and the integrative process reach out into the community, embracing these perspectives and being seen to do so, it will be integrative of the wider community. Then its healthful influence, and its opportunities for effective advocacy, will be greater. And in this context it is worth recalling a kind of integration that I referred to in Chapter 4; the integrated provision of personal care, scientific knowledge, professional skill and advocacy that will be integrative because it relates the well-being of the individual to the well-being of society.

So here we come full circle. Real integration and its integrative effects will be informed by a holistic perspective, and will in turn serve the holistic principle. The implications for holistic and integrative clinical practice are discussed in Chapter 15.

Complementary medicine

This discussion of 'natural' medicine, holism and integrative medicine has inevitably raised the question of the place of complementary medicine in health care, which requires some clarification of what is meant by 'complementary' medicine, and how valid and distinctive a concept it actually is.

Complementary medicine, often simply called CAM, has metamorphosed, in name at least, from 'quackery' (still a proper designation in view of some conventional doctors and scientists), through 'fringe medicine' and 'alternative medicine', to 'complementary medicine'. Many of its proponents now prefer to regard it and promote it as 'integrated medicine' or 'integrative medicine', and this perceived ideal for the future role of CAM, or some CAM therapies, within a broad spectrum of healthcare is discussed later in Part 5. As it is, the justification for describing any CAM practice as 'integrated' or 'integrative' is as much subject to the provisos I have stated as any other healthcare practice.

The labelling, definition or classification of CAM presents a number of problems. These include – where to draw the line between CAM therapies and conventional therapies, the nebulous nature of CAM and the variety of practices that may or may not belong under the CAM umbrella. The use and appropriateness of the terms 'holistic' medicine and 'natural' medicine in the context of CAM have already been discussed.

Conventional complementary medicine

If the question whether and in what sense a therapeutic method can be described as 'natural' or 'holistic' does not serve to distinguish complementary from conventional practice, we also have to recognise that the existing repertoire of conventional therapeutic methods does not fall conveniently into one or other of these categories. It is sometimes suggested that the syllabus of a conventional Western medical school curriculum distinguishes conventional from CAM. But the General Medical Council now requires medical schools to include familiarity with some CAM therapies within the syllabus, and many medical schools offer special study modules in certain CAM therapies. For a long time, the professions allied to medicine, such as physiotherapy and occupational therapy, have been augmented by disciplines such as art therapy and music therapy. Nutritional medicine and dietary therapies are represented within and without conventional services. Referral from conventional doctors to CAM practitioners is now commonplace, chiefly from general practitioners but also hospital doctors, and referrals in the opposite direction are gradually increasing. General practices and some hospital departments (pain clinics, palliative care units) include CAM skills and/or practitioners in their teams.

The so-called 'big five' CAM therapies are acupuncture, herbal medicine, homeopathy, chiropractic and osteopathy. Reflexology and aromatherapy have been found of value in helping patients in palliative care, and both are now represented by National Occupational Standards, along with acupuncture, homeopathy and hypnotherapy. Acupuncture, herbal medicine, homeopathy, hypnosis and manipulative medicine have all for a long time, been represented by well-established groups or organisations within the conventional medical profession. Spiritual healing has possibly the best research profile of the whole range of CAM therapies. Osteopathy and chiropractic are now statutorily registered health care professions in the UK, and acupuncture and herbal medicine are in the process of acquiring formal registration. Doctors and other registered health care professionals are regulated by their own professional bodies, and to an extent by the organisations responsible for their particular discipline; the Faculty of Homeopathy, for example. This list reveals the vague, even non-existent boundary between what has been traditionally regarded as orthodox and conventional and what was previously regarded as unorthodox, alternative or complementary.

In fact, many conventional therapeutic methods and interventions are ancillary, adjunctive or complementary to one another. Think of surgery, chemotherapy and radiotherapy in the treatment of cancer – three very different therapeutic methods; let alone any of the CAM therapies that are integrated with them, sometimes to mitigate their adverse effects. It would hardly be stretching a point too far to say that *all* conventional therapeutic methods are complementary, in the sense that any of them may have a part to play in treating the developing health care needs of any one of us at various times in our lives, either separately or in combination.

There are some therapeutic practices that are found on the 'fringe' of CAM, crystal therapy for example, which even committed CAM practitioners might consider too way out to be included under the CAM umbrella. But others might not. Visitors to centres of New Age thought such as Glastonbury will see evidence of 'healing' practices that lie beyond the limit of what many CAM adherents would find comfortable. It is also, incidentally, the home of a general practice that has pioneered the active integration of a number of CAM practices with conventional healthcare.[39]

Defining CAM

The dividing line between CAM and conventional medicine is erratic and unclear, in practical terms at least. The clearest distinction is in terms of the mechanisms involved. There are those that can be described, explained, understood, and therefore justified in terms of our current knowledge of physics, chemistry, anatomy, physiology, cellular and molecular biology and genetics, and which are readily acceptable as orthodox and conventional. And there are those which cannot be so described, and which as a result, generally speaking are not readily accepted. But although medical science may only acknowledge mechanisms that it finds plausible, and whose efficacy can be proved in the idealised context of formal randomised controlled trials, patients, and indeed increasing numbers of doctors, are more pragmatic, and choose therapies that they find to be effective in the real world. These issues of proof and evidence were explored in Part 3.

So, mechanism of action can be used as a legitimate demarcation between conventional and CAM. In Petr Skrabanek's paper 'The demarcation of the absurd', he decries non-science (as he sees it) such as homeopathy. He suggested that homeopaths suffer from 'dilutions of grandeur'.[40] Some doctors and scientists still do regard much if not all of CAM as absurd, which is to say the least discourteous towards the many patients who find it effective.

The book is not directly concerned with examining the specific complementary therapies that one way or another are making a contribution to the total spectrum of UK healthcare, but with acknowledging that they do make this contribution, that there is a great deal to be learned from them, and that they have an indispensable role in developing the holistic and integrative principles that must be central to the remodelling of medicine.

References

1 Cassell E. *The Nature of Suffering and the Goals of Medicine*. New York: Oxford University Press; 2004.
2 Hasegawa H, Reilly D, Mercer SW, Bikker AP. Holism in primary care: the views of Scotland's general practitioners. *Primary Health Care Research and development* 2005; 6:320–328.
3 Swayne J. Homeopathy Wholeness and Healing. *Homeopathy* 2005; 94:37–43.
4 Pellegrino E, Thomasma D. *The Virtues in Medical Practice*. Oxford: Oxford University Press; 1993.
5 Kafka F. *A Country Doctor in In the Penal Settlement*. London: Secker and Warburg; 1949.
6 Greaves D. *Mystery in Western Medicine*. Aldershot: Avebury; 1996.
7 Sweeney B. The place of the humanities in the education of doctor. *Br J Gen Pract*. 1999; 48:998–1002.
8 Pellegrino E. The healing relationship: the architectonics of clinical medicine. In: Shelp E. *The Clinical Encounter: the moral fabric of the patient–physician relationship*. Dordrecht: Reidel Publishing; 1983.
9 Fitzpatrick M. *The tyranny of health*. Abingdon: Routledge; 2001.
10 Aghadiuno M. *Soul matters: the spiritual dimension of healthcare*. Oxford: Radcliffe Publishing; 2010.
11 OFSTED. *Promoting and evaluating pupils' spiritual moral social and cultural development*; 16th March 2004. Available online at http://tinyurl.com/6h66s46.
12 Polkinghorne J. *Theology in the Context of Science*. London: SPCK; 2008.
13 Israel M. *The Intermediate Dimension*. London: The Churches Fellowship for Psychical and Spiritual Studies; 1970.
14 Kleinman A. *The Illness Narratives: suffering healing and the human condition*. New York: Basic Books; 1988.
15 Marcum J. Biomechanical and phenomenological models of the body the meaning of illness and quality of care. *Medicine Health Care and Phlosophy* 2004; 7:311–320.
16 Misselbrook D. *Listening to Patients*. Newbury: Petroc Press; 2001.
17 Heath I. *The Mystery of General Practice*. London: Nuffield Provincial Hospitals Trust; 1995.
18 Stewart M. Reflections on the doctor–patient relationship. *Br J Gen Pract*. 2005; 55(519):793–801.
19 Longmore M, Wilkinson I, Turmezei T, Cheung CK. *Oxford Handbook of Clinical Medicine*. Oxford: Oxford University Press; 2007.
20 Cronin A. *The Citadel*. London: New English Library; 1983.

21 Israel M. *Precarious living: the path to life*. London: Hodder and Stoughton; 1976.
22 Paterson C, Dieppe P. Characteristic and incidental(placebo) effects in complex interventions such as acupuncture. *Br Med J*. 2005; 330:1202–1205.
23 Doherty M, Dieppe P. The "placebo" response in osteoarthritis and its implications for clinical practice. *OsCar*. 2009; 17:1255–1262.
24 Finnias D, Kaptchuk TJ, Miller F, Benedetti F. Biological clinical and ethical advances of placebo effects. *Lancet* 2010; 375:686–95.
25 Miller FG, Kaptchuk TJ. The power of context: reconceptualising the placebo effect. *J R Soc Med*. 2008; 101:22–225.
26 Brody H. Diagnosis is treatment. *J Fam Pract*. 1980; 10(3):445–449.
27 Moerman D. *Meaning medicine and the 'placebo effect'*. Cambridge: Cambridge University Press; 2002.
28 Peters D. *Understanding the placebo effect in complementary medicine: theory practice and research*. London: Churchill Livingstone; 2001.
29 Spiegel D, Harrington A. What is placebo worth? *Br Med J*. 2008; 336:967–968.
30 Kaptchuk TJ, Kelley JM, Conboy LA *et al*. Components of placebo effect: randomised controlled trial in patients with irritable bowel syndrome. *Br Med J*, 2008; 336:999–1000.
31 Lyng S. *Holistic Health and Biomedical Medicine*. New York: State University of New York Press; 1990.
32 Carel H, Johnson S, Gamble L. Living with lymphangioleiomyomatosis. *Br Med J*. 2010; 340:c848;148–149.
33 Michaelson J. Work at the Centre for Well-being. *Journal of Holistic Healthcare* 2010; 7(1)13–15.
34 Brown C, Alcoe J. The heart of wellbeing. *Journal of Holistic Healthcare* 2010; 7(1):24–28.
35 House W. The wellbeing industry. *Journal of Holistic Healthcare* 2010; 7(1);50.
36 Helman C. *Culture Health and Illness*. Fifth edition. London: Hodder Arnold; 2007.
37 Helman C. *The Suburban Shaman*. London: Hammersmith Press; 2006.
38 di Stefano V. *Holism and complementary medicine: Origins and Principles*. Sydney: Allen and Unwin; 2006.
39 Peters D, Chaitow L, Harris G, Morrison S. *Integrating Complementary Therapies in Primary Care*. Edinburgh: Churchill Livingstone; 2002.
40 Skrabanek P. Demarcation of the absurd. *Lancet* 1986; 1:960–961.

13

PRINCIPLES IN PRACTICE

Summary

- The approaches to patient care of other healthcare professions have a great deal to contribute to the evolution of a better model.
- This is chiefly because their approach accommodates biomedical knowledge and skills within a holistic perspective.

This chapter presents two examples. The first is from a specific discipline – occupational therapy. The second is from work that embraces the whole field of disability and rehabilitation.

1 The Occupational Therapy Model[i]

There is no single theoretical model of occupational therapy, but several different models of both theory and practice. The model/s that an occupational therapy (OT) practitioner is taught or uses may depend on their geographical location (the Australian and Canadian occupational therapy communities have each developed their own models), and the local syllabus. OTs work in widely differing clinical situations, and some models lend themselves better to some than to others, and therapists may choose a model to work with accordingly. Or an OT may use several different models to guide her clinical practice, including the biopsychosocial model and the cognitive behavioural approach as well as discipline-specific OT models. Two models are described here.

The Australian Occupational Performance Model

This model describes the task of occupational therapy in terms of the Internal (Figure 13.1) and External (Figure 13.2) context of the patient's experience:[1]

---

i I am indebted to Sara Jane Kelly for the information on which the following account is based. It represents her personal view, except where other sources are cited.

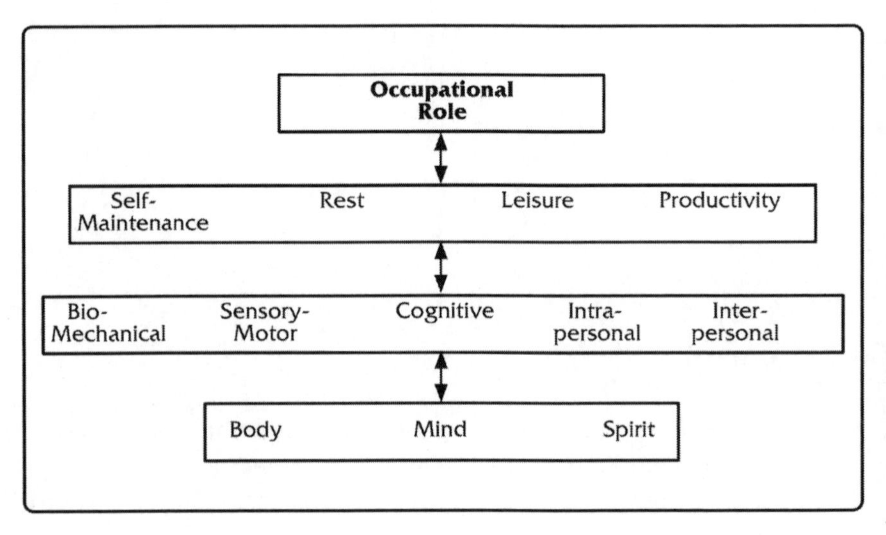

Figure 13.1 *The internal context.*

The diagrams speak for themselves of the tasks, the practitioner–patient relationship, and the inter-professional collaboration required for effective treatment and care; and graphically represent the holistic perspective of the occupational therapy profession.

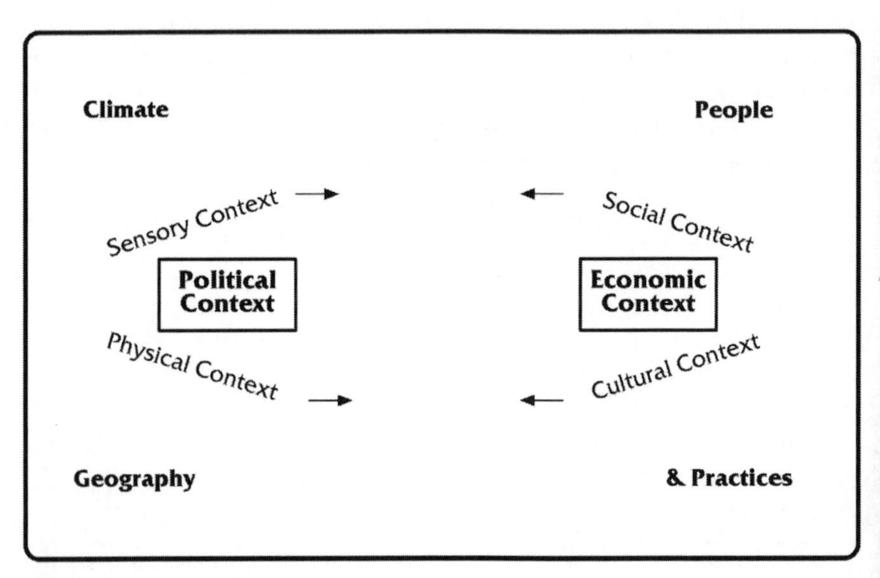

Figure 13.2 *External Context.*

The Model of Human Occupation:

The Model of Human Occupation (MOHO), first published in 1980, grew out of the work of Gary Kielhofner in the United States and hence is associated with his name. He has continued to be involved in its development, which is now the work of many people and has become one of the leading theories in occupational therapy practice worldwide. These notes are taken from the MOHO website (http://www.moho.uic.edu/intro.html).

The introduction gives a sense of the diversity of models used in OT. A National Board for Certification in Occupational Therapy (NBCOT) study of U.S. entry level practitioners asked respondents to indicate their top three frames of reference. The Model of Human Occupation was identified by 11 per cent of practitioners. According to the NBCOT report, it was the occupation-based model most frequently used by practitioners and its use is comparable to that of other major occupational therapy models – e.g., the biomechanical (17%), the neurodevelopmental (14%), the sensory integration (13%) models.

What does MOHO theory address?

MOHO seeks to explain how occupation is motivated, patterned, and performed. By offering explanations of such diverse phenomena, MOHO offers a broad and integrative view of human occupation. Within MOHO, humans are perceived as being made up of three interrelated components: volition, habituation, and performance capacity.

- Volition refers to the motivation for occupation.
- Habituation refers to the process by which occupation is organised into patterns or routines.
- Performance capacity refers to the physical and mental abilities that underlie effective occupational performance.

MOHO also emphasises that to understand human occupation, we must understand the physical and social environments in which it takes place, and the effects of that context on the occupational problem.

Theoretical refinement has taken place over the years to achieve a clearer and more accurate explanation of how these four factors (volition, habituation, performance and environment) interact to influence what people do in their *everyday*, occupational lives; and to explain why problems can arise in the face of chronic illness and impairments, and when environmental factors interfere with occupation.

For whom and where is MOHO applied in practice?

MOHO is intended for use with any person experiencing problems in their occupational life and is designed to be applicable across the life span. For example, MOHO has been applied with such diverse groups as adults with chronic pain, children with attention deficit hyperactivity disorder, persons with traumatic brain injury, older persons with dementia, persons living with AIDS, and adolescents with mental illness. It has also been applied in situations dealing with children and adults who are homeless, with battle-fatigued soldiers, and with victims of war and social injustice.

MOHO is also used in a variety of therapeutic contexts. For example, in hospitals, outpatient clinics, residential facilities, nursing homes, rehabilitation programs, work programs, prisons and correctional settings, and community based organisations.

Descriptions of MOHO from other sources

Emily K Schultz gives the following overview of MOHO:[2]

- The Model of Human Occupation (MOHO) is a practice model designed to provide theory along with practical tools and strategies for occupational therapy and related rehabilitation practice.
- MOHO concepts focus on how people are motivated toward their occupations (i.e., work, play, and self-care), how they learn and sustain occupational patterns in life, and how they engage in physical, cognitive, and social action.
- MOHO also focuses on the importance of the environment on occupation. MOHO emphasises that through therapy persons are helped to engage in doing things that maintain, restore, reorganise, or develop their capacities, motives, and lifestyles.

Cole and Tufano describe the focus of MOHO as:

- A systemic, holistic approach for persons of varying needs and populations across the lifespan.
- Stresses the importance of the mind/body connection in its depiction of how motivation (internal) and performance of occupations (external) are interconnected.
- Human occupation described as the 'doing' of work, play, or activities of daily living within a temporal, physical, and sociocultural context.
- The interactive nature of the relationship between the person and his environment and how this contributes to people's source of motivation, patterns of behaviour, and performance.[3]

Conclusion

What unites the two models described here, and others like them, is that they are 'holistic', addressing an individual's occupational performance in terms of the physical body, cognitive processes and social context. Some also include spiritual aspects.

The implications of this for occupational therapy training is that students receive *equal* tutoring in psychology and psychiatry as they do in biology and medicine. This may be quite unique in health care and usually means that when an OT approaches a patient for the first time, she or he is considering their function in activities of daily living on many different levels.

Therapy outcome measures for rehabilitation professionals[4]

This is the title of a manual for speech and language therapists, occupational therapists, physiotherapists, rehabilitation nurses, and hearing therapists. It is not hard to imagine the huge population of patients, and the great diversity of problems cared for and treated by this vital group of healthcare professions; nor to understand why I said in my apology in the Preface 'Without the energy and influence of those other professions and services, it is the medical profession that would be lost.' Doctors, and a multitude of patients, would indeed be lost without them.

I can claim no more than that I am aware of this work, and have dipped into it on the internet. But even such scant acquaintance reveals the indispensible contribution that these professions have to make to the evolution that this book seeks to encourage. It moves first from a traditional perspective of Disease-Impairment-Disability-Handicap to enlarge this spectrum by including Well-being. It then develops these into four other categories for assessing the outcome of care and therapy – Impairment, Activity, Participation, and Well-being. Each of these has three parameters to be assessed:

- Impairment – Abnormality, Structure/Function, Body/Mind.
- Activity – Restriction, Abilities, Person.
- Participation – Disadvantage, Circumstances, Society.
- Well-being – Upset, Feelings, Satisfaction.

To my eye, these groups of words reflect the various permutations and dynamics of Disease/Diagnosis+Context/Meaning/Value+Sickness/Suffering+Healing/Wholeness that are the goal of medicine, and of the 'remodelling' project. The manual is inevitably an academic work, but it encompasses the human predicament within an outwardly formal account of what whole person medicine and a healing vocation actually mean.

This vision is illustrated in the early pages by a few case studies. For example, Mr C:

Impairment	Mr C is a 40 year-old man with cerebral palsy, quadriplegic (paralysed in all four limbs), and dysarthric (impaired speech).
Disability/activity	He is wheelchair-bound, but totally independent, with an adapted wheelchair and living in adapted accommodation. He can communicate in all situations with a communication aid, adapted for the telephone.
Handicap/participation	He works as a solicitor, is an active member of the disability movement, has a full social life, and his views are sought and valued by a number of people.
Well-being/distress	He experiences occasional frustration resulting from restrictions in access and negative attitudes occasionally encountered.
Summary	This gentleman, who has a severe level of impairment, has been able to overcome his difficulties so that, while restricted, he is independent and not socially disadvantaged in any particular way.

Principles in practice

This short chapter makes the point that there are already models of treatment and care within medicine that represent many of the principles that this book sets out to affirm. They are practised by professionals that used to be called 'ancillary' and are still thought of as 'allied' to medicine. Their example and their role are in fact central to the ethos and goals of medicine. This glimpse into their work has important relevance to the themes of holistic and integrative practice (Chapter 15), interprofessional awareness (Chapter 16), and interprofessional education and collaboration (Chapter 19).

References

1 Occupational Performance Model (Australia). Available online at http://tinyurl.com/6e3y3we
2 From: Cole M. *Applied theories in occupational therapy: a practical approach instructors manual*. Based on: Cole M. *Applied theories in occupational therapy: a practical approach*. Thorofare, NJ: Slack Incorporated; 2008. Available online at http://is.gd/eZfpgr (requires PowerPoint reader)
3 From: Cole M. *Applied theories in occupational therapy: a practical approach instructors manual*. Based on: Cole M. *Applied theories in occupational therapy: a practical approach*. Thorofare, NJ: Slack Incorporated; 2008. Available online at http://www.efacultylounge.com.
4 Enderby P, John A, Petheram B. *Therapy Outcome Measures for Rehabilitation Professionals*. Chichester: Wiley; 2006.

14

EXPERIMENTAL MODEL

Summary

- The experience of conventionally trained doctors using the homeopathic method provides an experimental model with which to explore contrasting paradigms in science and medicine and the 'design principles' discussed in previous chapters.
- It exemplifies some of the characteristics of a Kuhnian 'scientific revolution'.
- The homeopathic method emphasises the neglected science (and art) of 'pathography', and has a contribution to make to epidemiology.
- The important question is 'why' do patients often do better under the homeopathic method than under conventional treatment? What is going on in 'the black box'?
- This would seem to justify huge investment in its investigation.
- But the homeopathic method is also susceptible to some of the undesirable traits of the biomedical model.

An experimental work in progress

The previous chapter draws attention to branches of mainstream medicine whose practice is modelled on a very broad understanding of the what is required to enable people to live with, and as far as possible overcome the effects of disease and disability. Biomedical science informs their work, but for most of them it is the patient's whole experience that determines how they construe the problem and seek to resolve it. Earlier chapters show that there are many doctors and other mainstream healthcare professionals whose *attitude* to patient care is not dominated by the biomedical model, even though their day-to-day *practice* may be constrained by it. But there is one group of clinicians whose practice illustrates several of the themes discussed in previous chapters particularly well. These are conventional doctors and other statutorily regulated healthcare professionals who use the homeopathic method.[1] They include dentists, nurses, pharmacists, podiatrists, and a few representatives of the professions referred to in the previous chapter. They are operating what is in effect a working model through which to explore several aspects of the evolution of medicine and the remodelling process. It achieves excellent clinical results, however much controversy surrounds the question of how they are achieved. In fact, it is that question that makes their method, and their model so interesting and worth exploring; so important in fact.

The characteristics of the method and its clinical effects are set out below and grouped according to the relevant theme in other chapters. Some of these are peculiar to the method, but many are characteristic of all good medical practice. They represent just one of several models amongst complementary therapies which may also be integrated with mainstream medicine in the same way that homeopathy is used by this group of doctors. But they offer a particularly close comparison that makes the method helpful as an 'experimental model'.

Paradigms and models

- Conventionally trained users of the homeopathic method have adopted a new paradigm without abandoning the paradigm in which they were trained. They are *paradigm pioneers*.
- They practice to a different model integrated with the orthodox Western model.
- The motivation of clinicians and patients who use homeopathy as complement or as alternative to the acknowledged power of the biomedical approach, arises from 'anomalies' of the sort predicted to lead to paradigm shift.
- Resistance, sometimes amounting to hostility, to the implications for clinical practice and medical science of their new working method is characteristic of resistance to paradigm shift, of *paradigm paralysis*.

Truth, Proof and Evidence

- The scientific challenges homeopathy presents are at odds with a research agenda that is dominated by cellular and molecular biology and genetics, and by pharmaceutical and technicological considerations. Clinical outcomes challenge the prescribed criteria of evidence based medicine.
- Doctors using homeopathy integrate a variety of 'ways of knowing' (Chapter 10) together with research evidence in assessing and managing their patients. This eclectic 'mindlines' approach to decision making is

well recognised in general practice,[2] but looked askance by medical science.

- Formal evidence of efficacy from reductionist research methods gives inconsistent results.
- Clinicians using this method demonstrate a 'scientific passion' for their work; a new sense of discovery in their understanding of health and illness; a realisation that every patient does, in Conrad Harris's words,[3] present them with a research project.

Medicine and the individual

- The 'story of sickness', the narrative approach is fundamental to the method.
- The method focuses on the person as a whole. Even in acute and circumscribed conditions the reaction and state of the person and the context of the problem are considered as well as the pathology, and may be used diagnostically.

The illness

- The inevitably multifactorial nature of any illness, and its multifaceted presentation in the individual patient is taken into account.
- The patient's detailed experience of the illness is taken seriously.
- Predisposing factors and susceptibility, and psychological and social factors ('meta-organic' factors), are essential components of the diagnostic process.

The therapeutic process

- The therapeutic process consciously involves factors and dynamics over and above the prescription of a homeopathic medicine.
- It seeks to avoid the disadvantages of 'digital medicine' and clinical damage (Chapter 8, 'Being a patient').
- Homeopathic medicines in dilution have no known *pharmacological* property capable of controlling disease processes or manipulating body function.
- The homeopathic method has many contextual features conducive to a self-regulatory response.
- Empathy is an essential quality in the therapeutic process.
- But the 'ingredients' of the method mirror most clinical practice (Box 14.1).

BOX 14.1 *The ingredients of medicine*

Rx	The Mixture
1/3	Placebo
1/3	The Doctor The Manner The Mystique The Relationship The Consultation
1/3	The Therapy The Technique The Prescription
	SHAKE WELL BEFORE USING

The healing process

- Change in symptoms, body functions and personal characteristics in response to treatment are followed up in greater detail than in conventional practice.
- The observed dynamics of the healing process are more subtle and various than those described in conventional practice, including known contextual or placebo effects.
- The response to treatment (consultation + prescription) is attributable to self-regulating processes, whether the specific homeopathic medication provides some subtle stimulus or not.
- Clinical outcome is consistently shown to be better in many conditions, for whatever reason, than has been achieved in those patients by conventional treatment.[4]
- In many instances the healing process extends beyond the remedying of specific disorder in the individual patient to include changes in self-awareness, behaviour, life-style and relationships.

Medicine and society

- The popularity of homeopathy, along with other CAM therapies, defies scientific scepticism, and is part of a wider cultural phenomenon.

- The particular holistic perspective of this approach to the understanding of the causes of illness complements the conventional epidemiological and public health perspective.
- The method begs interesting questions concerning the 'medicalisation of life'.
- It promises allegedly greater cost-effectiveness relative to the spiralling costs of conventional treatment.

The context of care

- Because the homeopathic method has been supported by the NHS since its inception, its practice and its practitioners, its clinics, the patients who choose to seek its help and the doctors who wish to refer them for it, are caught up in the political, organisational, funding and rationing issues of the present day health service. These currently threaten to disenfranchise both patients and providers of homeopathic care in the NHS.
- The constraints of evidence based medicine upon all medical practice in the UK compromise its clinical status.

It is clear from this list that the work of these doctors, and other conventionally qualified and regulated healthcare professionals, additionally qualified to use homeopathy within defined limits of competence, provide a useful experimental population for the remodelling process and a potentially fruitful 'laboratory' for exploring it. They are practising a developed model of medicine according to a more flexible and expansive paradigm, involving, the meticulous observation of the evolution of illness and the dynamics of disease processes and healing processes, and achieving enhanced clinical and quality of life outcomes for the patients in their care.

A detailed exposition of all the points on the list would require a book of its own, but to select a few examples, what might we already learn from this experimental model?

Paradigm shift

Trevor Thompson, Consultant Senior Lecturer in General Practice in the Academic Unit of Primary Health Care at the University of Bristol, has written a PhD thesis exploring the experience of doctors who had adopted homeopathic practice:[5]

> We took the experience of a group of 20 medical doctors of diverse backgrounds, who had taken up the practice of homeopathy to various extents. We then related their subjective experience with homeopathy to the precise articulation of Kuhn's views of paradigmatic transition from *The Structure of Scientific Revolutions*.[6] Our purpose in doing this was to understand if the individuals' journeys of engagement with homeopathy could be convincingly demonstrated to have these Kuhnian features – treating each person's transition as a small revolution in itself. Our conclusion is that the experience of these doctors is in accordance with what is predicted on the basis of Kuhn's theories.

Remember that in Kuhn's terms we are concerned with a *scientific* revolution. Not one motivated primarily by moral sentiment or metaphysical speculation, (though these are present in some degree in all scientific thinking), but one "inaugurated by a growing sense . . . that an existing paradigm has ceased to function adequately in the exploration of an aspect of nature to which the paradigm itself had previously led the way." The motivation for these doctors to work in a new way had to be because the biomedical scientific paradigm and model in which they had trained and which had 'led the way' in their practice of medicine did not do the job for which they had trained sufficiently well. 'Anomalies' (situations in which the paradigm failed) had to have accumulated to such a degree as to cause a 'crisis' that precipitated change. The new way of thinking and working had to be based in a new paradigm that addressed the anomalies in a completely new way. The anomalies that made Ptolemy's model of a universe centred on the earth inadequate were resolved by Kepler's and Copernicus's model of a universe centred on the sun. For these doctors, the anomalies thrown up by the biomedical method had to be resolved by the homeopathic method if Kuhn's predictions were to be fulfilled in this case.

The biomedical paradigm has been a great success, but as Kuhn pointed out, great success is not the same thing as complete success. A paradigm may enable us to achieve insights that are true for one aspect of reality, but that are not universally true. Newton's insights remain true in one field of mechanics, but not in the field of quantum mechanics. The insights of the reductionist biomedical paradigm are true insights but cannot be completely true within a more holistic perspective. Thus for doctors to adopt the homeopathic method to resolve anomalies in their biomedical repertoire is not to deny the power of the biomedical model nor to abandon its usefulness, but to acknowledge its incompleteness for the task in hand.

Thompson's 'experimental' subjects demonstrated the characteristics prescribed by Kuhn as criteria of 'revolution' leading to the commitment to a new paradigm, while not denying the inherent value of the old. The critical anomalies included the potential for harm resulting from biomedical interventions, particularly adverse drug reactions; their ineffectiveness or limited effectiveness in many conditions; the failure of the model to accommodate many of their patients' symptoms; its failure to explain or offer a solution to many patients' illness; its focus on specific parts rather than to comprehend the totality of the problems that many patients present; its neglect of the narrative of the patient's illness.

The encounter with the homeopathic method came as a timely solution to these anomalies. It offered a way of construing and responding to patients' problems that overcame the shortcomings of the orthodox model. And it worked. How it worked was, and still is, something of a mystery, which is explored elsewhere in this chapter. The point being that their decision, as predicted by Kuhn, was taken in defiance of the evidence; their continuing commitment based on their informed empiricism; their empirical judgments informed by clinical skills learned within the orthodox paradigm. As Thompson says, "These transitions are not mediated by conventional empirical considerations, such as scientific data, but by local empirical events such as a patient getting better. . . . (For these doctors) their conversion to homeopathy is not based on theoretical considerations, but on how it solved for them the paradoxes of their previous (situation). So in terms of Kuhn's ideas, we have the anomalies, and we have a new (paradigm) for their explication".

Solving the anomaly that orthodox biomedical therapeutics often does harm by adopting a method in which direct risk, such as adverse drug reactions, is extremely rare is an obvious motivating factor in making the transition. Other anomalies, which relate to points in the above list of the useful experimental characteristics of the homeopathic method, need teasing out more fully. These include the problem of engaging with the narrative of the illness, and the problem of 'irrelevant' symptoms.

There are two provisos that need to be added to this analysis. It is not quite correct to say that these doctors adopted a 'new' paradigm. The basic principles of the homeopathic method were established some 200 years ago, and several of them were not original even then. They embraced the importance of detailed symptomatology (not unlike Sydenham's pioneering clinical method) that took account of changes in the ill person as a whole, knowledge of the patient as a person in addition to their symptomatology, and recognition of the ability of the body and mind to heal itself when conditions conducive to that process obtain. It is worth noting that conditions conducive to healing that were stressed in the early literature of homeopathy were primarily conditions related to issues of life style, diet and public health that are relevant today and that were well ahead of their time. The other specific condition conducive to self-healing was, of course, the subtle stimulus of the homeopathic medicine selected by the painstaking study of the patient.

So doctors encountering homeopathy for the first time are encountering a model of practice whose conceptual framework is not new-minted in the process of their discovery of it, as a new Kuhnian paradigm is meant to be, but comes to *them* as a new discovery; a conceptual framework that transforms their approach to patient care. This transformation is not just a new diagnostic approach and way of prescribing, it affects the way they perceive the patient and the illness and their role as a doctor.

In a small survey of the effects of the study of homeopathy on their working life, doctors reported that they had relearned the art of taking a patient's history, had learned to listen more and be less dismissive of what their patients had to say, had developed a new outlook on chronic disease, had become more aware of natural healing, had begun to see patients more as a whole and not as much at a cellular biochemical level; that they were more aware of patients as individuals and that it was the whole person that sought treatment, that it had rekindled interest in clinical medicine, and that practice was richer and more fascinating as a result.[7] Numbers reporting these reactions in this particular study were small, but these are typical of the reactions of generations of doctors encountering the homeopathic method. They are, of course attitudes we would hope to find as commonplace amongst all doctors; and the attitudes expressed may well have been those with which these doctors originally came into medicine. The clinical method and perspective that they encountered in homeopathy may not have been strictly 'new'. The experience of medicine that it engendered for them may have been at least implicit in their original vocation to medicine. But the encounter resulted in a transition from a biomedical paradigm within which they had learned a model of medicine defined by it, to an inescapably different way of construing the challenge of illness and the possibilities of health care.

The second proviso is that it can be argued that adopting the homeopathic method as a working model does not represent a paradigm shift because it does not subsume or displace a previous paradigm in the way that Kuhn predicts, and that the Copernican 'revolution' in astronomy exemplifies. Certain limitations of the biomedical model may be highlighted by this experimental model, but it remains valid and useful. By contrast with Ptolemy's astronomy which was obviously no longer true once Copernicus's observations were shown to be correct, the reductionist paradigm on which the biomedical model is based remains true within its own terms.

This investigation of doctors' encounter with a changing paradigm and a changing model when they encounter the homeopathic method and these two provisos, are helpful in considering how a new model should be designed. The fact that a patient's cellular biochemistry is awry, and may need correction by the application of biomedical technology, is not rendered invalid by recognising that the problem is related to his job situation (or lack of one), his marriage, or his guilt, shame or anger about some other situation in his life. Nor by the fact that some other subtle or non-specific therapeutic process, or some psychosocial change in his life, could help the body to readjust. While the destructive situation persists as a maintaining cause of illness the subtle influence may not be effective, and the biomedical intervention may be life-saving. As I have emphasised, the remodelling process is not a competition between models, it is a balancing act and a process of reconciliation.

Kuhn says that the new and the old paradigms cannot be commensurable (measurable by the same standard), and often that will be the case, as with the astronomy of Ptolemy and Copernicus. But the challenge of relating different paradigms is not perhaps that they should be commensurable, rather that they might be commensurate – that is, coextensive, covering the same ground; landscape seen from the ground and from the air, but the same landscape. Newtonian physics remains valid within its own terms, relativity and quantum mechanics notwithstanding. Physicists seek a unifying theory for all three, which is an exciting prospect if elusive. But each is useful on its own terms. It is just not helpful to try to solve one kind of problem by applying a different frame of reference. The challenge is to apply the appropriate frame of reference at the appropriate time. The homeopathic method recognises that the maintaining causes of malarial infestation, displaced fractures, and lack of Vitamin D cannot be remedied solely by seeking to enhance self-healing, though it may have something to contribute to the recovery process when the main cause is remedied.

The homeopathic method provides us with an experimental model from which we can learn, not a panacea. Like all models it has its dangers, which we will return to later in the chapter.

Medicine and the individual

An intriguing aspect of the homeopathic method is its ability to accommodate a great diversity of information about the patient, objective and subjective, within the pattern that is reflected in the treatment strategy. In a contribution to *Narrative Based Medicine*, Marshall Marinker quotes a monograph by Michel Foucault which refers to a Chinese classification of animals into a number of bizarre categories that have no apparent relationship to one another whatsoever. They include: belonging to the Emperor, embalmed, tame, fabulous, frenzied, and drawn with a very fine camelhair brush. Marinker goes on to compare this list with the list of the sign and symptoms presented by a patient, Hilda Thomson. These include her build and appearance, the physical features of her arthritic joints, the serology, her resentment at her husband's disability, her anger at the government's treatment of small shopkeepers, and an array of medication of no benefit prescribed by other doctors in their unsuccessful attempts to help her. This is typical of the complex narrative that many patients present in general practice and that must be comprehended if the problem is to be resolved satisfactorily.[8]

A doctor applying the homeopathic method to this 'case' would not only hear and take seriously its disparate features and attend to its biomedical and pharmaceutical elements, but would seek to assemble its historical, situational, constitutional, emotional and physical components into a recognisable pattern that would be reflected in the materia medica of a similar homeopathic (like to the suffering) prescription. A favourable outcome could be attributable to the coherent meaning conferred by this process on the patient's experience of illness during the consultation, or to the prescription, or both; the point being the narrative approach essential to the outcome rather than the attribution of effectiveness to the process or the prescription.

Whatever the therapeutic method, positive expectation giving hope will enhance it. Avoidance of unrealistic expectation and false hope is an ethical priority. But this experimental model suggests that the threshold of expectation and hope is sometimes set too low.

Informed empiricism and pathography

Before considering possible objections to the homeopathic model, some other issues raised by the list of experimental characteristics: Firstly the 'informed empiricism' that in turn informs the doctor's experience of the method. A survey of the characteristics of 184 doctors using the homeopathic method published in 1987 revealed that the average interval between qualification and beginning their study of homeopathy was 12 years.[9] The predominant use of homeopathy was in general practice (64%). The average number of consultations each year in general practice at that time was approximately 7,000. So if, say, nine of those years were in full time general practice for most of those GPs, each would have brought the accumulated experience of 63,000 patient encounters, along with their conventional medical education and training, to their study of homeopathy.

This is a pretty sound basis on which to build the fundamentally similar if more open and detailed disciplines of case taking and clinical observation that the homeopathic method encourages. It is reasonable to suppose that the patterns of pathogenesis (the development of disease), the pathography (the description/picture of the disease), and of change in response to treatment that they came to recognise, would be as accurate and reliable as the data from their previous wholly conventional clinical method. The key difference is their openness to and willingness to accept the data that did not fit the old model, or that revealed unfamiliar possibilities in treatment outcomes.

In his foreword to a book on homeopathic method, Conrad Harris, Professor Emeritus of General Practice in Leeds University medical school, writes, "I came across the old term 'pathography' – describing what's wrong with a patient – in the writings of Oliver Sacks, and I saw that it was a neglected phase of research, tailor-made for general practitioners. Since then, trends in general practice have made it less likely that they will take up the challenge. It was a joy, therefore, to learn that pathography is not an optional extra for homeopathic practitioners, but an essential part of their methods, and safe in their hands. I hope they will make their findings known outside their own literature, as an important contribution in medicine".[1]

This is an important consideration. Because discussion of homeopathy is almost invariably confined to questions of plausibility and efficacy (how could such extremely dilute medicines possibly 'work'; and do they 'work' any better than placebo), and neglects the clinical phenomena that the method describes. These are a matter of clinical acumen, regardless of the nature of the therapeutic agent involved.

Specific, non-specific, contextual and meaning effects

There seems to be little argument that patients do benefit from treatment by the homeopathic method. A study of 6,500 patients seen over the course of six years in the NHS outpatient clinic at Bristol Homeopathic Hospital showed that some 70% of patients benefited (slightly better, better, or much better), particularly children under 16. Some 50% overall are reported better or much better, and some 60% of children. All patients were referred by their general practitioner. Many had been treated by conventional specialists before seeking homeopathic treatment. Many were able to reduce, and some to stop their conventional medication.[4] This study, corroborated by studies from other NHS homeopathic clinics, reports real results in really sick people. It was dismissed by sceptical critics, not because they disbelieved the reported good outcomes, but because they did not believe that the homeopathic prescription was responsible for them. A variety of other explanations were ascribed to the results, particularly the placebo effect. The results were held to be inconclusive because the study was not controlled. There was no comparison group of patients deliberately treated with a known placebo that would have allowed a real effect of the homeopathic medicine to be detected.

What *is* conclusive is that patients got better to a degree that exceeds conventional expectations. What is really interesting is the question 'Why?' What was going on? The research method certainly does not allow us to conclude that the prescription only was responsible for the effect. It may or may not have been. It may have been so in some patients but not in others. We certainly can be sure that contextual healing and the placebo effect contributed to the outcome. It always does. It will have done so to a greater or lesser degree in different patients, because we know that it affects different individuals differently, and affects the same individual differently on different occasions. But, even if due entirely to placebo, if the results are so much better than would be expected, why is that? And how can it be achieved in other clinical settings?

Evidence that homeopathic medicines have *specific* effects is inconsistent and controversial. But it does not conclusively exclude the possibility that they do. The investigation of that possibility must continue and must be rigorous, because if it is real the scientific paradigm really will have to shift. But regardless of that fascinating challenge, the other possibility, the power of its *non-specific* effects is just as fascinating and important.

The term 'enhanced placebo' has long been current amongst doctors who use homeopathy. This is in part because in the absence of any possible pharmacological effect or any known biophysical effect that can manipulate body function, any active property they do possess must operate by enabling the 'natural' self-regulating mechanisms discussed in Chapter 12 – just like placebo. The homeopathic method is a useful experimental model because it allows us to investigate ways of achieving this that may inform the remodelling process.

The homeopathic method exemplifies several factors that contribute to the contextual or placebo effect, again not necessarily more so than in other clinical methods, but perhaps more consistently and more deliberately:

- It is closely attentive to the patient's (or carer's) account of the illness. Even in an acute episode or circumscribed ailment (an injury, for example) it takes account of as much of the 'story' as it is practical to elicit. In a more chronic or complex illness, a very full narrative may be elicited. The old medical word 'anamnesis' is still sometimes used in homeopathy and its meaning – calling to mind, recollecting – is evocative of *the narrative approach* to medical case taking.
- Because it integrates physical details (sensation, appearance, localisation etc.), emotional details (taciturn, weepy, agitated, angry, etc.), general features (appetite, thirst, sweating, restlessness, etc.), and contingent factors (effect of movement, temperature, emotion, etc.) in the clinical description of the complaint, it has an intrinsically *'whole making'* effect. The patient may never have thought of themselves in this integrative way before.
- *Empathy* is an essential ingredient of the doctor–patient relationship. Not only as a compassionate response to the patient, but also to elicit sensitive information.[10,11,12]
- *Trust* in the relationship goes hand in hand with empathy. ('Where there is no trust there is little healing'. OHCM aphorism[13])
- *Hope* is likely to be a strong motive to recovery in people seeking an unconventional solution to their problem. Nevertheless, a recurring feature of doctors' experience of patients' response to the homeopathic approach is the relatively low level of expectation that patients bring to the consultation. Knowing that they are to receive a different form of treatment may encourage the *expectation* of improvement in the presenting complaint, but they often have little or no expectation of other improvement beyond that. The improvement in general well-being or other symptoms that may be part of the response to treatment, and which may precede any change in the presenting complaint, surprises them. This will then naturally encourage hope of further progress, which will reinforce the overall therapeutic effect. If the practitioner is explicit about the possible extent of the benefit of treatment at the outset, that therapeutic impetus of hope as against expectation and past experience may be at work from the start. But expectation is not a consistent ingredient of the process. Some patients are extremely sceptical, and may have been 'sent', by their spouse for example, against their better judgement. And expectation, hope and trust can decline, in patient and practitioner, when a series of prescriptions prove ineffective; until even in such inauspicious circumstances yet another change of prescription may well 'work'.
- It is commonly assumed that the *time* given to the patient during a consultation accounts for much of the benefit of the homeopathic

method. 'Time to allow healing' (OHCM aphorism[13]) is undoubtedly conducive to the placebo effect. But working with this model does not always involve time. General practitioners use it within the constraints of routine surgeries. In one survey of the use of homeopathy by doctors in the UK , the 49 GPs prescribed honmeopathic medicines in 25% of 5,620 consultations.[9] In the Bristol Homeopathic Hospital (NHS) outpatient survey, consultation times were similar to other specialist outpatient departments.[4] Time can indeed be an important non-specific therapeutic agent. But the quality of the *attention* paid to the patient and of the case taking process, which have their own therapeutic value, are not necessarily dependent on time.

- And finally, of course, there is the mysterious little pill or powder or bottle of drops; although these have none of the colourful characteristics that have been shown to enhance the placebo effects of some conventional drugs.[14]

The remodelling of medicine will need to take account of both the possibility of specific influences on the functions of body and mind more subtle than the mechanistic biomedical interventions we are familiar with, and the possibility of making more effective use of the non-specific effects of treatment. But then, of course, if we learn to make better use of non-specific effects deliberately, they will become specific effects. Which is a contradiction inherent in medicine anyway. The incidental psychotherapeutic quality of a good GP consultation, though focused on a specific intervention for a specific complaint, is part of its non-specific content. For a psychotherapist it is the specific intervention.

Evidence

It is 'evident' that the homeopathic method involves a complex therapeutic process of which the prescription of a specific medicine is only a part. This is true of many medical procedures, which is the justification for research methods that are designed to isolate the effect of the specific medicine or technology from everything else that affects the process in order to determine its specific efficacy. That is both a strength and weakness in evidence based medicine, as earlier chapters have argued. The limitations of this quantitative method of research is one reason for the increasing use of qualitative research, which allows for the generation of rich data and the exploration of 'real life behaviour'. . .[15] Qualitative research would take account of the role of informed empiricism, and the scope for clinical judgement whose demise is so much regretted by many GPs, in the decisions of doctors using the homeopathic method. It would also take account of the extent to which its popularity amongst the public is due to the fact that it has 'resonance', that it has meaning for them.

The description of pathogenesis, pathography and the response to treatment that emerges from the homeopathic method is also a rich and neglected terrain for epidemiological study; a point that is developed a little later in the chapter.

As an experimental model, homeopathic method presents a challenge and an opportunity for applying a diversity of research methods to provide a variety of evidence to inform our understanding of disease processes and healing processes and our ability to modify the one and enable the other.

The context of care

The homeopathic method has been practised within the NHS since its inception in 1948, and is as much subject to factors that determine the context of care as any other branch of medicine within the health service: resource allocation, patient access, patient choice, the 'postcode lottery' (some Primary Care Trusts will pay for it, some will not), waiting lists and follow-up intervals, 're-disorganisation', and so on. Problems arising from these are compounded by its controversial status and the small number of clinical and teaching centres. Its most numerous practitioners within the medical profession are general practitioners using it within or alongside routine practice, or who have specialised in its use as private practitioners.

Its experimental value in this regard is in the extent to which it exemplifies the difficulty of developing a model that accommodates the problem of resources, organisation and delivery, but more importantly the extent to which it models possible solutions to some of these. One of the claims of the homeopathic method is that it has something to offer in chronic conditions where conventional treatment depends on often costly maintenance treatment that does little to remedy the disorder and may carry a burden of adverse effects. Clinical outcome data from the Bristol survey quoted above support this claim.[4] Arguments about the specific *efficacy* of the homeopathic medicine are secondary here, because if the treatment package with its various components is *effective* in controlling the condition, improving well-being and quality of life, *and* reducing the social and economic burden of long term illness, to put it crudely – who cares how it does it?

The promise of such health, social and economic gains, would, you might have thought, justify huge investment in its investigation. But there is none. Here, paradigm paralysis really is a debilitating condition. The inhibiting influences discussed in Chapter 11, including the fact that there is not much money to be made by developing a methodology that reduces the demand for drugs and technology, seem to conspire to create a situation in which medical science is cutting off its nose to spite its face. It is unable to pick up the scent of a trail that might lead it in a direction it is not keen to go.

The epidemiological aspect of the homeopathic method that I have referred to also has something to contribute to the context of care in the study that it makes of psychosocial factors in the evolution of an illness. These may lie within a very small compass of personal experience, but they may also offer insights into broader issues of community and public health; into cultural and social trends and circumstances whose better understanding could encourage greater personal and social well-being. There is nothing especially new in the insights gained by this method, except in the realisation that they contribute to the pathogenesis of the illness more often and to a greater extent than is commonly realised. The model simply enhances this particular epidemiological insight.

Resistance

Whatever the qualifications of the homeopathic method as a 'new' paradigm in the terms of Thompson's analysis, it certainly evokes responses characteristic of the *resistance* to a new paradigm referred to in Chapter 12 in the work of Thomas Kuhn and Joel Barker, and described in relation to new knowledge by Michael Polanyi. Despite the existence of National Occupational Standards for Homeopathy,[16] the fact that its practice is unregulated except in the hands of healthcare professionals who are already statutorily regulated, does attract legitimate concern and criticism; a problem that is addressed here by confining this description of the homeopathic method as an experimental model to its use by conventionally trained and formally regulated clinicians. But considering that much of the criticism is levelled at doctors using the homeopathic approach and at NHS provision for it, the level and tone of hostility is extraordinary. Over the years 'absurdity' is one of the milder epithets employed by its more vocal detractors.[17] 'Blasphemous' is a more vigorous example,[18] and 'Witchcraft'[19] perhaps the most extreme – all the pronouncements of eminent clinicians and academics.

This is largely explained by the focus of the debate on the implausibility of the alleged activity of ultramolecular dilutions (no molecule of the source material remains) and the inconclusive nature of the evidence for efficacy in formal controlled trials. These are reasonable causes for scepticism. But failure to perceive even the remote possibility of a new horizon in medical science and to be at least curious and even perhaps excited about it, and unwillingness to acknowledge the seriously interesting characteristics of the experimental model that I describe here, do represent the resistance to change I discuss in Chapter 11. At its most vehement it represents a kind of scientific tunnel vision; Joel Barker's 'paradigm paralysis'.[20] This attitude is reminiscent of the original reaction of surgeons to the innovation of anaesthesia. Fifty years elapsed following the recognition of the anesthetic properties of Nitrous Oxide in 1795 before the eventual acceptance of anaesthesia by the surgical profession in London after its pioneering use in America, originally by dentists. In the study of the recurrent delays in adopting important innovations in the history of medicine, referred to in Chapter 11, David Wootton describes this example of this kind of paralysis: "it is clear from the inexplicable delay, the extraordinary hostility expressed towards its inventors, from the (pejorative) use of the phrase 'Yankee dodge', that there was something at stake, some obstacle to be overcome. That obstacle was the surgeons' own image of themselves – the emotional investment (they) had made in becoming a certain sort of person with a certain set of skills and the difficulty of abandoning that self image."[21] It is to be expected that any remodelling that accommodates the more challenging principles exemplified in this experimental model will meet similar resistance.

But it has to be said that contemporary proponents of the homeopathic method, in common perhaps with other complementary therapies, have done too little to articulate and explore systematically the clinical and scientific implications of the phenomena described in this analysis. There are understandable reasons for this: their numbers are few; the great majority are committed to direct patient care rather than the academic study of what they do; resources to investigate it are very limited; the methodology appropriate to its investigation is not well developed; dealing with criticism of the plausibility and efficacy of the method has been a major preoccupation; and survival as a clinical service in an inhospitable medical environment has been a priority. Nevertheless, if the homeopathic method is to serve and be of value as an experimental model as has been suggested here, its practitioners and proponents must find a way of making the case more fully, more clearly, and with greater scientific passion and cogency. Otherwise their predicament may justly be compared to Wootton's account of the failure of the mid-19th century Hungarian obstetrician Semmelweis to persuade colleagues of his revolutionary approach to the prevention of cross infection in maternity wards, "It is difficult not to sympathise with Semmelweis, who certainly knew how to reduce deaths from puerperal fever. But it is also important to acknowledge that his arguments deserved to be met with puzzlement and scepticism".

Objections to the model

The homeopathic method provides an experimental model with many potentially fruitful design features, but part of the experiment must be to identify limitations that we would not want to reproduce in the remodelling process; or to be aware of features that could be dangerous if handled carelessly. This particular therapeutic method replicates two potentially serious flaws that are inherent in the conventional model. These are the 'pill for every ill' scenario, and the 'medicalisation of life' scenario.

Because doctors using this method are aware of its potentially powerful non-specific effects, it has been suggested that to allow for this and to reduce the wrong attribution of change to the administration of the medicine, at the first consultation, in chronic conditions at least, no prescription should be given; at the second a deliberate placebo should be given (medicated and unmedicated doses are indistinguishable); and only at the third consultation, when any changes resulting from the first two have been carefully noted, should the specific prescription be given.[i]

But this is a counsel of perfection, similar to that proposed by David Horrobin in *Medical Hubris*, where he discusses the ambiguous effect of many conventional medical interventions and points out that only controlled trials of treatment against no treatment would help to resolve the matter.[22] The expectation of the patient and the inclination of the practitioner are to receive and to give a prescription, whether in conventional or homeopathic practice, and both are difficult to resist and may be similarly ill-advised in either case, reinforcing the expectation for the future and making it increasingly difficult to resist when some other therapeutic approach is actually more appropriate. This is a kind of indirect risk present in all medicine – the risk of encouraging inappropriate dependence on medical intervention.

Secondly, because of its respect for and attention to the detail of the story of the illness, the homeopathic method risks replicating the tendency that is recognised in conventional general practice in particular, for every

i In my own use of homeopathy I would often and explicitly decline to give a prescription at a consultation because of its contextual and meaning content, or its sometimes obviously psychotherapeutic content.

aspect of the human predicament to be construed medically. This is the indirect risk of any all-inclusive approach to the illness narrative. It has become a truism, for example, that in many instances general practice has assumed the role of the priest. The biomedical perspective avoids it by virtue of its reductionist focus. In that case the indirect risk is the opposite – neglect of the personal and psycho-social factors that may be essential to the proper diagnosis and resolution of the problem. This central dichotomy in medicine is nicely exemplified in this experimental model.

Thirdly, the homeopathic method (like other complementary methods) *can* be applied in quite a mechanistic fashion, with a directive style of consultation and a rigid diagnostic and treatment protocol, that is less truly holistic than, for example, a good GP consultation.

An opportunity too good to miss?

In the integrated and integrative use of the homeopathic method by conventionally trained and experienced doctors and other healthcare professionals, we have available to us an experimental model for the evolution of medicine of great value. The painful irony is that far from being welcomed as an exciting opportunity for scientific and clinical exploration it is being driven underground by a level of hostility amongst a small number extreme sceptics that is difficult to comprehend.

A detailed account of the breadth of clinical observations of disease processes, symptomatology and healing processes is given in Appendix 14.1.

References

1 Swayne J. *Homeopathic Method: Implications for Clinical Practice and Medical Science.* Edinburgh: Churchill Livingstone; 1998.
2 Gabbay G, le May A. Evidence based guidelines or collectively constructed "mind lines"? Ethnographic study of knowledge management in primary care. *Br Med J.* 2004; 329;1013–1017.
3 Harris C. Seeing sunflowers. *J R Coll Gen Pract.* 1989; 39:313–319.
4 Spence D, Thompson E, Barron S. Homeopathic treatment for chronic disease: A 6-year University-Hospital outpatient observational study. *J Altern Complement Med.* 2005; 11(5):793–798.
5 Thompson T. *Homeopathy: exploring the popularity paradox. A multi-method study of the players process and outcome of homeopathic care by UK medical doctors.* Thesis, (PhD) University of Bristol; 2005.

6 Kuhn T. *The structure of scientific revolutions*. Chicago: University of Chicago Press; 1996.
7 Reilly D, Taylor M. *Developing integrated medicine. Report of the RCCM Research Fellowship in Complementary Medicine: The University of Glasgow 1987–1990*. London: Research Council for Complementary Medicine; 1993.
8 Marinker M. Sirens stray dogs and the narrative of Hilda Thomson. In: Greenhalgh T, Hurwitz B. editors. *Narrative based medicine: dialogue and discourse in clinical practice*. London: BMJ Books; 1998.
9 Swayne J. Survey of the use of homoeopathic medicine in the UK health system. *J R Coll Gen Pract*. 1989; 39:503–506.
10 Mercer SW, Reynolds WJ. Empathy and quality of care. *Br J Gen Pract*. 2001; 52 (Supplement): S9–S12.
11 Mercer SW, Watt GC, Reilly D. (2001). Empathy is important for enablement. *Br Med J*. 2001; 322:865
12 Mercer SW, Reilly D, Watt GCM. The importance of empathy in the enablement of patients attending the Glasgow Homoeopathic Hospital. *Br J Gen Pract*. 2002; 52:901–905.
13 Longmore MW. *Oxford Handbook of Clinical Medicine*. Seventh edition. Oxford: Oxford University Press; 2007.
14 Moerman D. *Meaning medicine and the 'placebo effect'*. Cambridge: Cambridge University Press; 2002.
15 Kuyper A, Reeves S, Levinson W. *Qualitative Research: An introduction to reading and appraising qualitative research. Br Med J*. 2008; 337:404–407.
16 Skills for Health. *National Occupational Standards for Homeopathy* 2009; Skills for Health. Available online at www.skillsforhealth.org.uk.
17 Skrabanek P. Demarcation of the absurd. *Lancet* 1986; 1;960–961.
18 Miller J. In: After Dark. (television broadcast). London: Channel 4; September 3rd 1988.
19 Baum M. Quoted in: Homeopathy is worse than witchcraft'. *Daily Mail* 2007 May 1st.
20 Barker J. *Paradigms: The business of discovering the future*. New York: Harper Collins; 1992.
21 Wootton D. *Bad Medicine: Doctors Doing Harm Since Hippocrates*. New York: Oxford University Press; 2007.
22 Horrobin D. *Medical Hubris – A reply to Ivan Illich*. Edinburgh: Churchill Livingstone; 1978.

APPENDIX 14.1

Clinical Observations in 'The Homeopathic Method'[1]

Epidemiology

- *Patterns of disorder in the family history* of an individual that predispose to and may predict the pattern of illness they will themselves experience are recorded. The familial influence may be multifactorial, and will differ from the inherited traits for single specific disorders whose genetic mechanism is recognised.

  If these patterns are a reality this would be confirmed by epidemiological investigation of the association between family history and personal history.

  These patterns are identified with certain homeopathic medicines. If the specific action of the medicines associated with them is demonstrated, the recovery of patients from disorders whose history is consistent with the particular familial pattern would corroborate the epidemiological data.
- *The history of illness during the life of an individual* is perceived as the manifestation of a continuous process. All episodes of illness are related to this process over time. At any one time the clinical picture forms a coherent whole. Different syndromes that coexist in the one individual are related parts of this whole.

  These clinical pictures, which are effectively discrete epidemiological entities, are identified with specific homeopathic medicines. The identity of these clinical patterns and their consistent occurrence should be susceptible to epidemiological investigation.

  The response to treatment includes change in any or all of the co-existing syndromes that comprise the pattern.

  If their specific effect is confirmed, the response of the patient to their action confirms the reality of the clinical/epidemiological entity so described. If it is not, the fact that separate syndromes change concurrently or sequentially in response to the one stimulus still implies a relationship between them.
- *Constitutional characteristics* of healthy individuals or of patients in between episodes of illness are associated with a predisposition to certain symptoms and disorders.

  The existence of these constitutional types can be investigated epidemiologically.[2,3] The clinical states associated with them could be similarly investigated.

If the specific action of constitutional medicines is demonstrated, the clinical outcome could be used to corroborate the epidemiological data.

- All these propositions have implications for preventive medicine.

Pathogenesis

- Toxicology and experimental pathogenesis (observations of the effects of the experimental administration of homeopathic medicines or their source materials in healthy volunteers), as well as study of the natural history of diseases, show the wide variety of systemic disorder that can result from a single pathological cause. This variety is reflected in the observed clinical versatility of the homeopathic medicines derived from the pathogenic agents. These patterns of symptomatology, of coexisting or sequential disorder, are found in patients who have not been exposed to the pathogenic agent concerned. The patterns of coexistence or evolution imply relationships between pathological processes that we often do not understand at present, and may not even recognise.
- The existence of these patterns is a matter for epidemiological study, as discussed above. Their significance in terms of our understanding of disease processes is an even greater challenge. The descriptive task, the natural history or pathography, is the first step.
- Once proven, the response of these patterns of disorder to specific medicines will help to confirm their co-inherence. The experimental pathogenesis of the medicines may then help us to understand the disease processes themselves better.

Aetiology

The relevance of a wide variety of aetiological factors are taken into account in construing and treating an illness. No systematic study has been made of the association between specific aetiological factors and the types of morbidity attributed to them in homeopathy, as far as I know. This would be interesting. Once again the proven effect of specific medicines associated with specific aetiologies would reinforce the value of the study.

Total pathography

In many of its treatment strategies, homeopathy seeks a total pathography. It construes the problem comprehensively in terms of family history, personal history, constitution, pathogenesis and aetiology, as a whole. It does this to provide the grounds on which to base prescriptions. In the process it develops a view of the dynamics of illness. This in turn informs the process of case taking and analysis.

This broad schema of pathography is far from being satisfactorily worked out and defined. It contains too much diversity of interpretation, too much unsubstantiated 'doctrine', too much speculation. These are the manifest weaknesses of homeopathy, and they undermine its strengths. Nevertheless this integrative view of illness has its underlying consistency. Better intellectual discipline, better analysis will make it truly useful in informing contemporary perceptions of disease processes. As with many aspects of homeopathy it is a stimulus medicine needs.

Healing processes

The inflammatory reaction is one of the fundamental processes of physiological healing. Its components and phases have been painstakingly described, from cellular level to symptomatology. We know that changes in blood supply and white cell activity on one level, and redness, swelling, warmth and pain on another, are all part of it. These are the local tissue changes of the healing reaction.

In its observation of the response to treatment, homeopathy has mapped out a process as intricately orchestrated but on the level of the organism as a whole. The question whether this process or aspects of it are common to all pathways of self-healing is intriguing. But its manifestations have no counterpart in any conventional account of mechanisms of healing. (They may be reflected in the literature of other complementary therapies that I am not acquainted with.) They are highly distinctive and deserve to be known and investigated by others outside homeopathy. In summary they are:

- Aggravation: the primary phase of the biphasic response. A therapeutic aggravation of existing symptoms should lead to an improvement.
- Well-being: this often improves in the early stages of the response. Sometimes it precedes specific symptomatic change. It may improve during aggravation of other specific symptoms.
- Elimination: this includes discharges, sweating, diarrhoea or rash occurring in the early stages of a positive response.
- Improvement in multiple symptomatology from one medicine.
- Improvement in incidental or unconsidered symptoms.
- Improvement in constitutional traits.
- Return of old symptoms: transient return of symptoms that had resolved or become dormant at some time in the past.

- Resolution of symptoms in the reverse order to that of their appearance.
- Improvement in more important systems before less important (e.g. mind before joints).
- Improvement in more deep-seated organs before more superficial (e.g. lungs before skin).

These are all well documented in clinical records, but far more systematic recording and analysis are required to provide the basis for further investigation. We need to confirm, clarify and define the changes we observe. We need to examine the relationship of the patterns of healing changes to the disease processes from which they arise. Are particular patterns of family history or pathography associated with particular patterns of healing change? Are particular clinical states more likely than others to show strong primary reactions during treatment? Are particular histories more likely to lead to the return of old symptoms than others? Once proven, the specific efficacy of particular medicines producing particular changes in particular clinical circumstances will provide a tool for investigating these processes in addition to their therapeutic value.

We need also to examine the influence of previous conventional treatment upon the pattern of healing change. Are certain changes more common after long duration of conventional treatment? For example, are skin eruptions more likely to show aggravation after long suppression with steroid preparations? Do allergies respond poorly to homeopathy after previous conventional desensitisation?

The implications for clinical practice and medical science presented by the phenomenology of the homeopathic method, regardless of, and over and above the question of the activity of homeopathic medicines, represent a scientific challenge of considerable interest and importance.

References

1 Swayne J. *Homeopathic Method: Implications for Clinical Practice and Medical Science.* Edinburgh: Churchill Livingstone; 1998.

2 Ives, G. Validation of the homeopathic theory of type. *Midlands Homeopathy Research Group Research Newsletter* 1981; 5:23–26.

3 Ives G. Constitutional types and homeopathy. *Communications British Homeopathy Research Group* 1985; 13:11–17.

part 5

REGIME CHANGE

PROLOGUE

A minor revolution

If we are to remodel medicine, as we must, it will require a minor revolution, or at least a metamorphosis. Not a major revolution certainly, because all the elements, the parts of this new whole are already available. There will be a marked change of emphasis, but nothing needs to be completely discarded – except some attitudes to health and health care, and a few political initiatives perhaps. And nothing needs to be invented. But something of a revolution it will be, none the less. For most health professionals it should be the sort of revolution that consists of throwing off their chains. What is now a biomedical straight jacket will become a less restrictive and more comfortable garment; though still as useful, indeed more so. The organisation of health care will set health professionals free to use their knowledge and their skills, and particularly their 'virtues' (see later), in a greater flourishing of the therapeutic relationship in which they themselves will be a more effective agent. *Caritas* will operate effectively hand in hand with *scientia*, which will be its more humble partner. Patients will discover the satisfaction of understanding and accepting their responsibilities for their own well-being.

A scientific revolution will be required, but only by way of refocusing the scientific gaze and the scientific effort. There will be a shift of medical science's ontological gaze – its vision of the way things really are, to embrace new possibilities. There will be a change of emphasis in its epistemological repertoire – its ways of knowing about the way things really are, to accommodate and validate new insights. Although these may not be *new* possibilities and insights so much as possibilities and insights that are longstanding but neglected, or even hitherto despised – like contextual healing and the 'placebo' effect. Science will redirect its efforts to understand better how we may promote healing rather than control disease. We will have more 'science for understanding' rather than 'science for manipulation'.[1]

There will be a minor revolution in the delivery of health care to make it conducive to the treatment of the patient as a person with a story to be heard rather than a problem to be analysed. This will in turn permit the health gains and economies that will result from achieving the hard task of understanding people instead of resorting to the easy but expensive task of writing prescriptions, ordering investigations or planning technological interventions.

There will also need to be a change in medical morality; a surprising suggestion, perhaps, which was mooted in Chapter 9, and that will be addressed again later in the context of medicine's relationship with our culture and society (Chapter 16).

A change of emphasis

To repeat – a new model of medicine will not be composed of any completely new parts because all the necessary elements are already available, if only on the margins. It will comprise familiar elements in a new structure, a new order. So there will be elements of the new design that prompt the response, 'Yes, but that's already happening.' It may be happening, but is it bearing fruit? Is it effective? Is it happening in practice?

For example, the humanities are often included in the medical school curriculum now. Art and literature offer students insights into human behaviour and the human condition, reflecting experiences and truths that they will encounter in the lives of their patients and in the course of their relationship with them. That is very good. But in the surgery or clinic, or on the hospital ward, amidst the technical demands of the job, and the constraints of time and targets, will they have the inclination or opportunity to recall those insights and use them to enhance the quality of care, and possibly enrich the life of the person who is their patient? Even though the principle is built into the present model of medical *education*, the present model of medical *practice* makes this unlikely, or at best very difficult. And colleagues involved in medical education tell me that clinical leaders and role models in the training system often do not exemplify it. The new model will make it possible to apply its principles in practice. The ideals of the medical curriculum will be refined, and will be modelled by the teachers and trainers, and the delivery of care will expect and allow their application in the real world.

David Greaves identifies two contrasting approaches to the relationship between medicine and the humanities.[2] The first equates medical humanities with the medical arts as a set of subjects which can be set against as well as complement medical sciences; the second focuses on the humanities as relevant to the whole fabric of medicine. The first restricts the medical humanities to an engagement of medicine with the liberal arts without any unifying conception, other than the contrast made with science; providing a 'balance' to medical science, rather than having any direct influence on it. The second provides an innovative and unified approach which transcends the present structure of medicine as a divided discipline – with separate realms of art and science – and is to be preferred because it holds out the prospect of developing new ways of resolving current difficulties.

In David Greaves' vision the change of emphasis resulting from a wider conception of medical humanities requires not just an addition to the curriculum, but a permeation and change of orientation of the culture of medicine, which will transform not only clinical practice but also the theoretical basis and social structures of medicine and healthcare. The medical arts can be treated simply as an ornament to medicine, whereas the medical humanities must be an integral part of it. The medical arts are aimed at humanising practitioners, medical humanities is aimed at humanising medicine. In the lecture by Brendan Sweeney that I referred to in the discussion of knowledge and wisdom in Chapter 10, he goes even further than this, suggesting that a proper balance between science and humanities in the education of a doctor would not only be beneficial to the profession but to society as a whole.[3] This theme of medicine's responsibility towards the society and the culture of which it is part will recur later.

What will 'different' look like? And how do we get there?

So, what *will* 'different' look like? And how *do* we get there? It is tempting to answer the second question immediately with the old chestnut, "If that's where you're going, I wouldn't have started from here!" Previous chapters have suggested the necessary direction of change, and that there is momentum for change. But they have also revealed the formidable obstacles to change that exist because the status quo is so firmly established. Whatever the new model comprises, it will be hard to get there from where we are now; and any proposal for remodelling must include not only the design of the model, but also the process for achieving it. Both are equally challenging.

The first question, "What will 'different' look like?" was posed within a small group of doctors and other health care professionals, meeting over the past two years to explore the means by which the sort of remodelling described in this book, or more specifically a more holistic perspective in medicine might be promoted. 'Remodelling' is my word for it, but generally speaking the group's purpose is the same. We have challenged ourselves to translate vague ideas, about what 'holistic' means for example, into processes that actually enhance medical practice and the well-being of patients. The group includes some with a background in general practice, some in academic medicine, specialists in rheumatology, mental health, and palliative care, some with experience of complementary medicine, several with research experience. All of us are addressing the challenge not only of offering effective whole person care to our own patients, but also of representing that principle within our professional communities, and of being true to it in our personal lives. This is a considerable challenge, even for a group of people persuaded of the need for change, and committed to working it out in practice as well as in theory. How much more difficult to share and promote that vision within a medical culture that is by no means so persuaded and committed? We are under no illusion as to the difficulty of effecting change.

The difficulty was anticipated in the Introduction. 'To promote these ideals as primary goals of medical culture, education and practice, and healthcare policy, will require a very considerable effort of will and imagination. It will require a redeployment of resources and some restructuring of the process of care. It will also require some humility on the part of all who have a vested interest in maintaining the status quo, in the intellectual, clinical, political or commercial power that the structure of the existing model confers. Modern medicine is successful and powerful, and does confer power on those who plan, manage and practice it. The reordering of power, even quite slight, that remodelling will involve, might be difficult for some to accept.'

Nevertheless, the conviction that the change is imperative and that it is possible prevails.

The 'prescription' presented here is largely my own but owes a great deal to the wisdom and insights of the colleagues with whom I have explored this theme, and to the many others whose ideas and experience are reflected in the quotations and references throughout the book.

'The ravelled sleave of care'

For all that the National Health Service dominates the medical landscape of the UK and the biomedical paradigm dominates medical thinking and practice, that dominance is in fact not so secure. The fabric of healthcare is at the same time both ravelled (entangled, confused, complicated) and proceeding to unravel (to distinguish separate threads, or subdivisions). This apparently contradictory state of affairs has a number of causes. One is the recurring 'redisorganisation' of healthcare by policy makers. This will continue under the UK's 2010 coalition government, though there is some hope that a more coherent strategy may emerge. Another cause is the increasing specialisation of biomedicine as it becomes more technologically sophisticated. The third and most important cause is the attitude and behaviour of patients. 'We', the patients, are reshaping the medical landscape and dismantling the medical model. 'We' are also the medical practitioners who in our role as patients are by no means always as wedded to the model as we may be in our practice. I may be an eccentric example, but I suspect not altogether untypical of some medical colleagues. Over the past five to ten years I have been very grateful for skilled biomedical intervention but have also benefited from homeopathy, osteopathy and acupuncture, and over-the-counter first aid advice from pharmacists. I have also used the internet to add to my existing knowledge of my health problems. And I have probably been influenced to some degree, though I might be reluctant to admit it, by what I have read in the newspapers. I am sure I am not the only doctor who has adopted such an eclectic approach to their own health care, and I am certainly typical of very many non-medical patients.

These are examples of the momentum for change identified in Chapter 3, and they emphasise the need to find ways to 'knit up the ravelled sleave of *health*care' (if you and Shakespeare will forgive me!).[4] The orthodox medicine of the twentieth century has to acknowledge that it does not reflect or satisfy the healthcare aspirations of very many people. It is a limitation that paradoxically is compounded by the expectations of its power and the demand for its services that medicine itself has created.

The shape of the new model

This last part of the book looks at what a new model of medicine should look like, but takes account of what it is already beginning to look like, because a new model of medicine is already beginning to take shape. The challenge is to make sure that it is true to medicine's vocation and its proper goals; and that it really works.

What are the goals of medicine and health care? What are the principles that inform those goals? What is the process for achieving those goals? And what is the context that will determine the success or failure of that process? All of those questions have been touched upon in earlier chapters, and some answers have been suggested or implied. The aim now is to present them as a coherent whole.

The themes relate to the same three broad domains of health care that were outlined in Chapter 3 ('What sort of model?') – clinical practice, process of care, context of care. But they are not presented strictly in that order because these are not self-contained categories. Some themes recur in all of them, and a 'clinical' theme may be best understood when its 'context' has already been established.

Clinical practice concerns what goes on during or as a result of the encounter between clinician and patient. *Process* encompasses the delivery of care, the therapeutic methods available and their integration into a system of care, the education and training of healthcare professionals, research, and public health provision. *Context* encompasses political, economic, social, cultural and philosophical influences on the goals, principles and provision of health care.

Prescription for a new 'cosmology'

A paper that I have mentioned earlier and that I have found particularly helpful in thinking about 'remodelling' is David Greaves' *Reflections on a new medical cosmology*.[5] He identifies three problem areas – the structure of medical knowledge, the conception of the patient, and the organisation of practice and services. To these we should add the social and cultural milieu of medicine, which he also touches upon in his paper. Within this broad landscape of health care he points out a number of landmarks that must be present if it is to represent the new 'cosmology'. These include:

- 'Goals and values'; the vision and ideals that determine what medicine is for other than biomedical and technological mastery over disease processes.
- A better understanding of the boundaries of medicine and health care that acknowledges that these cannot be precisely defined.
- The 'reconfiguration of medical knowledge', firstly with regard to those uncertain boundaries, but also with regard to its many dimensions, from the technological to the humanistic; and to the different perspectives of those we might call its stakeholders – patients, professionals and society.

- Changes in medical education consistent with this reconfiguration; not a downgrading of factual knowledge and technical skills, but rather their appreciation within a different and wider context.
- The rehabilitation of healing as "central to any new system of medicine and health care, and seen as integral to all parts of it."
- A reappraisal of the balance of responsibility for, and participation in the pursuit of personal and communal health and process of health care, between patients (and presumably society), and professionals.

It will be evident that this schema reflects most of the themes in this book. Again it does not explicitly encompass the social and cultural issues, though they are clearly implied. If there is something wrong with the way we do medicine, and if we are to put it right, all these features of the medical landscape, these component parts of the health care system, are implicated. And the key question is 'where do we start?' Health care is so complex, and all aspects of it so interrelated and interdependent. Is there any one area where we might trigger a cascade of changes throughout the system as a whole, in the way that a small physiological stimulus can trigger a cascade of chemical changes throughout an organism?

There certainly has to be a 'critical mass' of dissident voices and paradigm pioneers willing and able to promote and work for change. It will need to include patients, health care professionals, managers, and policy makers. There undoubtedly is momentum for change, but the reasons and necessity for change need to be articulated effectively, which is the purpose of this book. And because the paradox in medicine described in the prologue to Part 2 is so keenly felt by many, and despite the resistance to change discussed in Chapter 11, it may not require a huge stimulus for the cascade to start. Unlike a physiological cascade which is very rapid, however, a cascade of health care changes of this nature will take a long time to progress. Or will it?

References

1 Schumacher, E. *A Guide for the Perplexed*. London: Sphere; 1978.
2 Greaves, D. *The Healing Tradition*. Oxford: Radcliffe Publishing; 2004.
3 Sweeney, B. The place of the humanities in the education of a doctor. *British Journal of General Practice* 1998; 48:998–1102.
4 Shakespeare, W. *Macbeth*, II, ii, 36.
5 Greaves, D. Reflections on a new medical cosmology. *J Med Ethics* 2002; 28;81–85.

15

CLINICAL PRACTICE

Summary

- The importance of the therapeutic relationship in medicine is taken for granted but too little appreciated. It must be properly understood and effectively used, not only as a vehicle for good clinical method, but as the starting point of the healing process.
- The concept of healing is central to this. It must embrace the well-being of the person as a whole as well as the disordered 'part'.
- Fundamental to all clinical practice is that care of the *person* enhances healing on every level, whatever technical skills are also required.
- Patients must know themselves to be cared for as a person with a story endowed with value and meaning, and not as a circumscribed problem.
- Practitioners will understand themselves as agents of the healing process, whatever knowledge and skill they bring to the task.
- There must be no tribalism in clinical practice, no narrow orthodoxy, no discrimination between therapeutic approaches based on their mechanism of action, explanatory model or therapeutic theory.
- The essential criterion of good medical practice is its ability to serve the goals of medicine.
- Practitioners must have sufficient appreciation of the work of other health care professions to make or advise appropriate choices of different therapeutic methods.

The therapeutic encounter

In the introduction I apologise for the book's tendency to make the doctor the focus of attention when so many other healthcare professionals have an indispensable role in medicine. In this final part, to be properly inclusive I am using 'clinician' or 'practitioner' to refer to anyone who attends another person with a heath care need in a professional capacity. Or, in the sense of my earlier, broad definition of medicine, makes disciplined use of their knowledge and skill in the service of healing.

This implies, as I intend it to, that no *clinical* activity is ever technical and impersonal. Every clinical activity involves a personal relationship which inevitably affects the 'quality and outcome' of care for better or for worse, regardless of the technical requirements of the task. Any evolving model of medicine must make the quality of that relationship and its essential contribution to a good outcome, its first principle.

This encounter between clinician and patient is the starting point for the development of any model of medicine, its key component. It focuses attention on the two core principles: the *person* in his or her totality who is ill or in distress or in need; and the opportunity to invoke their innate capacity for self-regulation and healing. All other components of the model, all other processes of care and all that shapes them must arise from it and converge upon it. For example, the dynamics of the therapeutic encounter will be the centre point of the curriculum for all medical education. Its aim will be to enable clinicians to 'come to an understanding with a patient', Kafka's hard task;[1] and to help patients to come to an understanding with themselves. So that, to paraphrase the quotation from W B Houston in Chapter 3, clinicians themselves, as therapeutic agents may be refined and polished to make them a more potent agent; to make the drug 'doctor' a more potent prescription, promoting a healing response in the patient through the consultation and the relationship, regardless of what other intervention is required.

This is not to devalue the contribution of others who are not involved in face-to-face patient-care, which may be essential to the way it unfolds. Nor is it irrelevant to students whose interests or aptitudes are better suited to non-clinical roles in medicine. It is simply to say that all other activities that are part of the process of care must be an appropriate response or adjunct to that core event. And it means that health professionals whose service to healing is in non-clinical fields will develop their skills and do their work with a clear understanding of the personal dimension of the process to which they provide essential support.

The heart of the matter

Medicine's susceptibility to social and political influence, and its responsibility to care for people whose illness stems from social circumstances or life-style choices, make it very difficult for healthcare professionals to initiate change on their own. This is a plausible argument, but one that I challenge. If the practitioner–patient relationship is at the heart of medicine, surely that is the place to start – the heart of the matter? And if the quality of that relationship is essential to the contextual healing that is such an important part of the therapeutic package there is even more reason to focus attention there.

The practioner–patient encounter is the key event in the health care process. Three questions determine the nature and content of that encounter – 'Who?', 'Why?' and 'Where?' The permutations are, of course, numerous. 'Who?' includes the individual practitioner or the care team; and the individual patient, alone, or together with or represented by a carer or advocate. The reasons 'Why?' range from an acute emergency to terminal care. 'Where?', may be the home, roadside, hospital ward, or hospice. Sometimes, often in fact nowadays, 'Who' will not be a nurse or doctor. It may be a paramedic, a speech therapist, or a complementary practitioner. The encounter may be a first contact, or one of a series of contacts with practitioners with different roles and expertise. In other words the process of care will vary greatly according to the context. The permutations of care that I describe in Chapter 16 might seem too numerous for any attempt to describe the essence of the medical encounter. But I suggest that we can identify the core principles that apply to all encounters (Box 15.1).

BOX 15.1 *Core principles of the medical encounter*

- Presence (being there for the patient).
- Attentiveness (observing, listening, hearing).
- Compassion (humaneness, empathy).
- Time.
- Knowledge.
- Competence.
- Trust.
- Integrity (honesty, humility, maturity, self-knowledge, integratedness).
- Discernment (insight, awareness, imagination).
- Interprofessional awareness.

You may place this list in a different order of priority, perhaps modify it, perhaps add to it. Its purpose is to suggest the essential ingredients of the relationship that as patients we may seek and as practitioners we should offer in any healthcare encounter.

Presence

There is a story whose attribution I have lost, but it may be from Cicely Saunders the founder of the hospice movement. It concerns a young man whose wife has just died and who is taken into the office by the ward sister. They sit there together in complete silence for some time. As the young man gets up to leave, nothing still having been said or done, he says to the nurse, "Thank you. I have never felt so consoled in my life".

This is an example of what can be achieved simply by *being* with a patient. It depends on the quality of our presence, regardless of what we are or are not doing. It is in our attitude. And it can accompany even urgent activity. It says, 'You are a person, deserving of worth-ship. I understand. I care. And I am here for you.'

Attentiveness

This is an aspect of 'presence', but is more active. Being present to another requires that we give them our whole attention. That means that we do not see them through the filter of our own assumptions or expectations. We get ourselves out of the way in order that we may be fully aware of them. Then we can make the unprejudiced observations that will tell us the 'whole truth' about the other person; or as much as we need to know or they wish to share with us at the time. By giving our whole attention we can achieve the empathy, and really hear the story, as far as circumstances demand or permit. And there are few, if any circumstances that do not demand and permit it. They include the emergency care of an unconscious patient, because we should not underestimate the subliminal communication that is possible, even then.

> Medicine and art have a common goal: to complete what nature cannot bring to a finish . . . to reach the ideal . . . to heal creation. This is done by paying attention. The physician attends to the patient, the artist attends to nature. If we are attentive in looking and in listening and in waiting, then sooner or later something in the depths of us will respond. Art, like medicine is not an arrival, it is a search. That is why perhaps we call medicine an art. (MT Southgate[2])

Compassion

This essential attribute of care has been discussed already in Chapter 8, including the question whether it is innate or can be acquired. In fact if we learn presence and attentiveness, which we can, compassion will follow. We cannot be fully aware of another person in distress, which presence and attentiveness and absence of self-interest will ensure, without responding compassionately to them: 'something in the depths of us will respond'.

Time

We know that spending time with people in a therapeutic encounter enhances contextual healing as well as allowing for activities that take time. But duration of time is not of absolute importance; quality of time is. (See 'Finding the time', later in this chapter.) Presence, attentiveness and compassion are prerequisites for quality time. But *knowledge* and *competence* must be demonstrated as well, because they are indispensable to the *trust* that is essential to the healing process.

Trust

Pellegrino and Thomasma describe five elements of trust.[3] (I have added my own interpretation of their criteria in brackets.)

- Confidence in the faithfulness to what is entrusted. (Confidence that the doctor will deal faithfully with all that is entrusted to her/him; with all aspects of the life that the patient puts into his/her hands.)
- The sense that the person trusted has promised explicitly or implicitly to act well with respect to the interests of the other person. (The understanding that all decisions made, advice given and action taken will be in the patient's best interests.)
- The belief that the discretionary latitude necessary to the trusting relationship will be used well and properly. (The belief that decisions or actions on behalf of the patient that depend upon the judgement or discretion of the doctor will be well and properly taken.)
- Congruence of understanding on those three elements. (Doctor and patient are of one mind on these three points.)
- An act of faith in the benevolence and good character of the one trusted. (The patient commits him/herself to the good intentions and integrity of the doctor.)

Trust, however, can be generated without being deserved, as the Harold Shipman tragedy amply demonstrated. Trust is only justified by *integrity*.

Integrity

Integrity assumes *honesty*. But that in turn depends upon *self-knowledge*, which requires *humility*. Humility requires acknowledgement not only of our limitations and our 'bounds of competence', but also of our strengths, the things we really are good at. It also requires acknowledgement of our *vulnerability*; the things that hurt us and weaken us. (See 'Learning to cope', Chapter 19.)

You might say that the attributes so far described are common to all really good human relationships. Of course, they are. But just as they are too seldom found in ordinary human relationships, sadly they are not necessarily common to all therapeutic relationships, where above all they belong; which is largely because there is too little room for them in the present medical model.

Knowledge and competence

We take knowledge and competence for granted as part of the qualification and professional discipline of a health care practitioner. Training, examination and regulation ensure this, where they are properly established. But in several complementary healthcare modalities they are not well established, and the knowledge and competence necessary to professional integrity may be lacking. (See 'Regulation', Chapter 16.) This lack constitutes the indirect risk, but it also prejudices the next two essentials of the therapeutic encounter.

Discernment

Discernment is often associated with spiritual insight, but has more general application in the sense of being able to discriminate between different possibilities. Discernment in healthcare is necessary to identify different threads in the tapestry of the patient's story or case history, and to tease out and follow through each thread appropriately. It requires knowledge and experience, and the wisdom that comes from experience. It also requires the integrity that does not claim ownership of any aspect of a patient's problem or story which we cannot or should not try to manage ourselves. Discernment allows us to see clearly the patient's various needs, and to identify and seek appropriate help for those to which we cannot respond adequately. To do so we must have a sufficient degree of *interprofessional awareness.*

Interprofessional awareness

Interprofessional awareness means knowing what other resources, skills or services exist that may help a patient, in addition to or rather than one's own. It means knowing enough about them to understand how and why they might do so; not a lot about them necessarily, but just enough. And it means a willingness to point the patient in the right direction. It applies to physicians in relation to other physicians with different expertise, and to physicians in relation to surgeons, and vice and versa. For general practitioners, the 'gatekeepers' to the services of the whole range of specialist colleagues, it is a *sine qua non*. It is necessary for all doctors in relation to other healthcare professions. And for all conventional health care professionals it is increasingly necessary in relation to complementary and alternative (CAM) medical practitioners, many of whom are to be found within their own conventional ranks. It is just as necessary for CAM practitioners if they are to avoid the indirect risk of neglecting to advise conventional treatment that may be needed. And it is necessary for healthcare workers in relation to the spiritual and social needs of the patient.

All this requires, of course, the knowledge and discernment that are already among this list of core principles.

Despite the increasing emphasis on interprofessional education (see Chapter 19), there is at present too little knowledge – due in part to lack of research, to unwillingness or lack of opportunity to collaborate, to the inadequacies of professional curricula, to engender this breadth of awareness. Tribalism and prejudice also inhibit effective interprofessional awareness and the interprofessional care it should promote. The rivalry between physicians and surgeons was by no means a myth.

> "Ah", said the Professor of Medicine accompanying me as a junior house surgeon to see one of our post-operative patients when a trolley spilled its metallic load at the other end of the ward, "Ah, a good surgical noise!"

Tribalism between conventional medical disciplines is by no means altogether dead. And negative attitudes towards CAM practitioners are by no means always justified by legitimate scepticism or concerns for patient safety.

Greater interprofessional awareness and better interprofessional care will be a conspicuous feature of the new model. This will be the foundation for the integrated and integrative care that is becoming something of a *cause celèbre* in medicine, but has yet to achieve any widespread coherent expression. And although, as a goal, there are many factors needed to achieve it, it has to be rooted in the interprofessional awareness within the practitioner–patient encounter. (See 'Learning to collaborate', Chapter 19.)

Implications

These core principles of the therapeutic encounter cannot be taken for granted, and other aspects of the process and context of care will need to change in the new model to enable them to be fully achieved. We will look at these more thoroughly shortly, but for example: Of my list of ten principles, only two, knowledge and competence can be assumed to have a place in the medical school curriculum. And the other eight can only be *taught* to a limited extent. They have to be *learned* and developed – by guided experience, by exposure to the riches and complexity of human nature in the study of the humanities and in real life, through reflective practice and peer group support, from the example of role models among the teachers and clinical leaders, and through good supervision. They need to become, in part, tacit knowledge of the kind that is acquired through good apprenticeship.

Another example: None of those eight principles will be helped by targets and guidelines. Even knowledge and competence cannot be replaced, but only supported by such protocols, and may be undermined by them. The other eight certainly will be undermined and inhibited by protocols that focus attention firmly on the biomedical features of 'the case'.

Thirdly: None of the ten principles can thrive in the conveyor belt system of medicine that operates in so many of our general practices, clinics and hospitals, and that is one of the reasons why CAM practitioners are so popular.

But staying with the practitioner–patient relationship, what difference will the implementation of these core principles make?

Promoting 'natural healing'

There can be no doubt that an encounter founded upon these principles will greatly enhance the natural healing discussed in Chapter 12. That is a supremely important goal of the new model, perhaps the most important. It is the answer to that question posed by W.B Houston, "How can the doctor himself as a therapeutic agent, be refined and polished to make him a more potent agent?" That was written some time ago. It will more often apply to the doctor 'herself' today, which may be reason to hope that the core principles are more likely to be fulfilled. But that goal has still to be met and of course it applies to all practitioners, not just doctors.

Making the most of the healing potential of the practitioner–patient relationship through the application of these principles is the 'bottom line'.

But their implementation will help to change one of the besetting problems of the present model – the problem of false expectations.

Managing expectations

As family doctor Tony Woolfson writes in his letter to the *British Medical Journal* quoted earlier, "Doctors often complain that patients' expectations are unreasonably high, without seeing that the medical profession has played a large part in creating these expectations".[4] Expectations that medicine can answer "the heartache and the thousand natural shocks that flesh is heir to";[5] that because medicine is able to do so much, something must be done and always can be done. Expectations that affect patients and health care providers alike.

This problem of expectations has been highlighted repeatedly throughout the book. As with all the remodelling tasks we are considering there is no easy, let alone single answer to it. A charge for GP consultations to deter attendance for trivial or commonplace ailments is recommended by some and dismissed by others. Better education of the public about appropriate use of health services is advocated by some, but again, dismissed by others as a futile exercise. But whatever else, the solution has to be rooted in the practitioner–patient relationship. And the core principles we are discussing will be essential to that solution.

Firstly, they set the practitioner, particularly the doctor, free from the immediate pressure, inner or target driven, to give undue prominence to the biomedical assumptions of the diagnostic and treatment process. Secondly, they create a relationship in which the practitioners can more confidently challenge those assumptions, and any inappropriate expectations and demands. They create a relationship in which it is possible, again in the sense of the Kafka story already quoted, to come to that understanding with the patient that is so much harder than writing a prescription;[1] and equally importantly, to help patients to come to an understanding with themselves. This understanding may be that the problem is not medical. Or that it is medical but can be tolerated or coped with without professional help. Or that there are causes or predisposing factors that the patient needs to address. Or that although the problem is medical, there is an absolute limit, for one reason or another (perhaps including cost) to what it is possible to do, or reasonable to do. Or that rather than pursuing a quick fix, a longer term and truly healing solution is worth pursuing and making the effort to achieve. The central importance of the therapeutic encounter is represented in Figure 15.1.

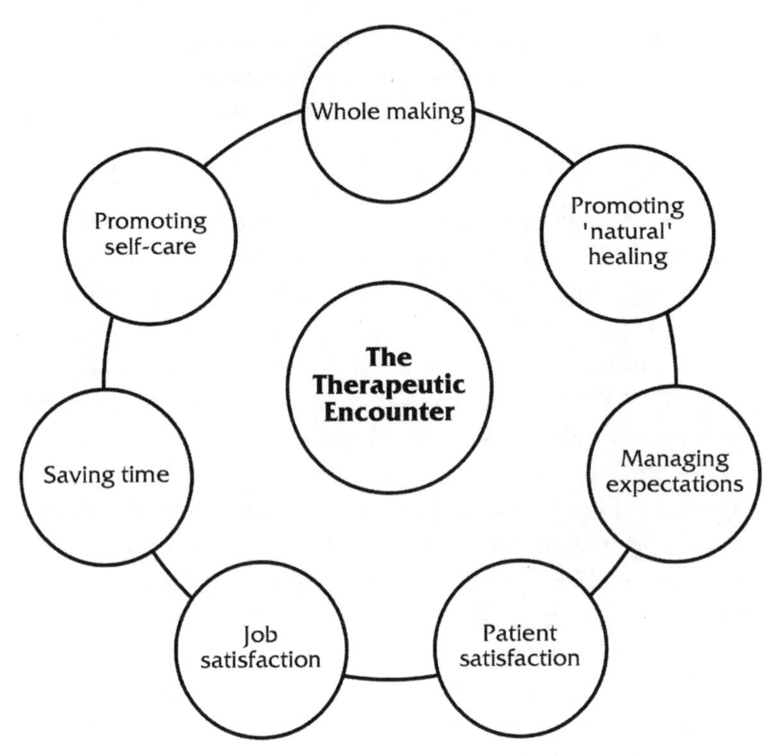

Figure 15.1 *The heart of the matter.*

Finding the time and making best use of it

It is self-evident that the more thoroughly a problem is understood or a necessary task performed at the first encounter, the more time and trouble will be saved later. A problem that is not understood, or a task that is hurried or skimped, will create a bow wave of unresolved problems and work still to be done. In fact, that is not a precisely accurate way of stating the case. The very first encounter may reveal a need for a better understanding of the problem, or for a task to be performed more thoroughly, which circumstances do not permit just then. So additional time and trouble may need to be committed subsequently, in the short term in order to save time and trouble later. Nevertheless, that very first encounter will have been critical in perceiving the immediate need and responding appropriately. If the need is not perceived, and the response is not appropriate, the bow wave of extra work will build up. The extra work may involve the practitioner who was first consulted, or another practitioner, chosen perhaps because the first did not answer to the patient's need. Or it may involve work for others, or cost perhaps, resulting from investigations or referrals, or prescriptions that would have been avoided if the problem had been more thoroughly understood and attended to in the first instance. Scottish general practitioners are clear that additional work of this kind could be avoided if they had the time necessary to work more holistically with their patients.[6]

The outcome of that critical first encounter and encounters that follow on from it may depend on the time available, but it is the use that is made of whatever time is available that matters. It may or it may not be necessary or possible to find the time, if time is needed, there and then, and the extent to which patients' expectations of the consultation are met is not necessarily time dependent.[7] But time will be wasted and the momentum of the therapeutic process lost if the time spent, however short or long, is not quality time, 'meaningful' time.[8] A critical factor in achieving that quality, and in evoking that meaning, which we know to be such an important component of the contextual healing effect, is empathy. Empathy is experienced by the patient but created by the practitioner; perhaps the most important of the core principles of the medical encounter discussed earlier.

There is a general consensus, which research supports, that longer consultations do yield benefits.[9,10] But there is a similar consensus that without an increase in effectiveness, longer consultations would reduce efficiency.[9,10,11] Empathy is the key to quality of care.[12]

Obviously some medical consultations and therapeutic procedures (disregarding inevitably lengthy surgical procedures) do require more time than others. This may depend on the technical complexity of the task, or the condition of the patient. A full neurological examination, for example, takes time if it is to provide useful information. A patient who is old, disabled, distressed or very ill will need to be given time. But the outcome will always reflect the quality of empathy in the relationship. Even the duration and severity of the common cold is reduced by a high level of empathy in the consultation.[13] And the same study suggests, as would common sense, that empathy is an all or nothing affair. You can't have a bit of empathy. Either it is present or it is not.

But its presence or absence is not wholly dependent on the innate attributes of the practitioner. Empathy can be improved and successfully taught at medical school, especially if it is embedded in the student's actual experiences with patients.[12] Which requires that it is modelled by their teachers, and the learning is supported by good supervision. There is a connection between patients' satisfaction with a consultation and their perception of how long it lasted. Patients who are well satisfied with a consultation perceive it as having lasted longer than it actually did. For patients who were not it seems shorter, and feels too short.[11] Satisfaction does not depend on the actual length of the consultation but on the content;[9,14] most important to that sense of satisfaction is that the patient's emotional needs have been met. Trust in the practitioner's competence matters, but empathy has been found to enhance diagnostic accuracy.[12]

The effectiveness of the consultation is also enhanced by the greater willingness of satisfied patients to comply with treatment and accept advice about changes in their life that will improve their health.[11] The most effective consultations are those in which doctors *most directly* acknowledge and perhaps respond to patient's problems and concerns (My italics).[9] It is empathy that will ensure that problems and concerns are acknowledged *most directly*. And there is no 'perhaps' about it – empathy requires that the acknowledgement is reflected in the active response. In short, clinical effectiveness is not primarily, dependent on the *quantity* of time committed, but on its *quality*. Increasing the quantity will not automatically improve effectiveness unless that increase in time also allows for an increase in quality. And whatever technical knowledge and skill is employed will be most effective where there is empathy.

Time is one component of the therapeutic 'black box', the complete consultation + intervention package, but it is most effectively 'activated' by empathy.

The actual length and content of a consultation within the absolute limits of workload or an appointment system, is determined by the doctor's perception of the problem. Where this is dominated by a biomedical approach, longer consultations may only provide for more technical and pharmacological management but little empathy, more control but less enablement. Understandably, a more biomedical agenda helps to avoid some of the difficult, possibly uncomfortable, emotional and often insoluble content that patients sometimes bring to consultations'.[14] But with the best will in the world, practitioners well equipped to provide it may find their store of empathy at times exhausted. As a psychiatrist colleague with whom I discussed my dwindling resources to meet the needs of a particular patient aptly remarked, "Sometimes the milk of human kindness just runs dry". Richard Stevens and Anne Mountford remind us. "Doctors have to balance competing and ever-increasing demands, and they may be 'actively trapped' and unable to make the initial investment in changing (their) consulting style. They have to hear stories of loss and even death, and contain patients' anxieties on a daily basis."[14] Which is true for other health care professionals as well, of course. Nevertheless, there is some evidence that longer consultations well used reduce the stress.[10]

So it is questionable whether the comment of some conventional doctors on the work of complementary (CAM) practitioners that 'if I could afford to spend that much time with my patients I would get the same results', is necessarily true. (Disregarding the implied admission that CAM practitioners do get good results.) The same biomedical agenda merely given more time might just get the same results as before. The nature and efficacy of the 'specific' ingredients of the CAM black box are controversial. There is no disagreement that the black box is effective, nor that its contextual components, such as those described for homeopathy in Chapter 14, contribute to its effectiveness. But it is perverse to throw away the box for that reason. All the more reason to unpack it carefully – and of course to take advantage of its effectiveness without waiting for it to be completely unpacked.

Time does permit more to be done, and to be done more thoroughly, and often with good effect. And practitioners and patients consistently desire more time. However, length of time is not the be all and end all. Finding enough time, even if it is well used, may seem impossible in the face of increasing demand and expectation. But there is good reason to believe that providing just enough time and using it competently and above all empathically, will pay dividends in terms of good outcomes, a diminishing 'bow wave', and time saved.

Holistic practice

Holism is a way of looking at people and the world, and at the way people inhabit and relate to the world. In medicine it applies to the understanding we seek of a patient's predicament – its depth and its breadth: depth in the sense of our understanding of the whole person as represented by the overlapping inner circles of Figure 1 in Chapter 12; breadth in the sense of the interplay of those 'inner' dynamics with the circumstances of the person's life represented on the perimeter, the 'outer' circle. As 'The holistic perspective' (Chapter 12) implies, holistic practice is primarily in the mind and in the intention of the practitioner, whatever his or her role or method. If practitioners are unperceptive of the *person*, unaware of the mixed dynamics of the problem, and unresponsive to them, their practice cannot be holistic. If they are perceptive, aware and responsive to this totality of the patient's need, then it will be. That is not to say that holistic practitioners need to possess some sort of omniscience; just that they will be aware of the possibilities – open to whatever aspects of the 'whole' problem a patient may express or that may be discerned as underlying the presenting problem, and willing to acknowledge and respond to these.

Those are, so to speak, the minimum of requirements for holistic practice. But in a review of the literature on holistic health care Charlotte Paterson and Nicky Britten identifies a specific set of assumptions that underpin holistic practice:[15]

1. An emphasis on the unity of mind, body and spirit.
2. A positive view of health as well-being.
3. Individual responsibility for health.
4. The importance of health education.
5. Control of the social and environmental determinants of health.
6. Low technology or 'natural' therapeutic techniques.
7. Facilitating the body's innate capacity for self-healing.
8. A relationship between the provider and the client that is relatively open, equal and reciprocal.

The extent to which practitioners are able to engage actively with these holistic principles will vary according to the circumstances, but there is no reason why they should not always be in their attitude and intention towards the patient. There are two major factors that will either facilitate or obstruct their application. One, which usually separates orthodox and complementary practitioners, is the therapeutic method. Orthodox practitioners are restricted in their ability to make effective what may be a genuinely holistic intention by the biomedical repertoire of treatment available to them. When something needs to be done, what is available to them may limit the scope of their therapeutic role to some narrowly targetted (reductionist) and mechanistic intervention. This may well be in the context of a relationship and a style of consultation that preserves the holistic intention, but it makes it more difficult and may seriously undermine it in the patient's perception. Paterson and Britten quote the survey of Scottish general practitioners already mentioned in the discussion of the holistic perspective, of whom 87% agreed that a holistic approach (not defined) was essential to providing good health care, while only 7% felt that the current organisation of primary care was conducive to it.[6] This introduces what the authors describe as a 'structural' difficulty, represented in the Scottish survey by the organisation of primary care, including, as in other NHS settings, lack of time.

Although the duration of a consultation is not in itself a determining factor of its quality, in contrast to their orthodox colleagues, complementary practitioners often do provide a generous measure of consultation time that will help to make effective the holistic intention they may hold to.

But still more important, and in contrast to the orthodox doctor's limited biomedical repertoire, is likely to be what Paterson and Britten call the 'therapeutic theory'. If this is based upon a truly holistic perspective of the person, and of the dynamics of illness and healing, and if the therapeutic method (exemplified by homeopathy in Chapter 14) requires that the 'anamnesis' embraces this broad perspective, then the content of the consultation will strongly reinforce its holistic intention. 'Anamnesis' or calling to mind, is a better term than 'case taking' or 'history taking' because it implies the narrative aspect that is essential to the holistic approach.

It is clear that patients value this 'whole person' approach, particularly if they have chronic or complex problems, even though they may not be dissatisfied with mainstream GP care.[16] But it is disappointment with orthodox medicine and/or the hope of additional health gains that leads many people to seek complementary medicine, and it is in this context that the role of the therapeutic method becomes more significant. The therapeutic method, what a practitioner *does*, neither confirms nor denies the practitioner's holistic attitude and intention. The therapeutic *theory* may certainly reinforce the holistic approach, but the *method* does not define it, except in as much as it fulfils points 6 and 7 on Paterson and Britten's list of holistic precepts; that is, to use low technology or 'natural' methods to facilitate the body's (person's) capacity for self-healing. (The word 'natural' has to carry the proviso given in Chapter 12.) The holistic significance of the method is in the clinical outcome. The changes induced in the patient may indeed involve the whole person – creativity, emotions, general body functions, and energy; and symptoms other than those for which the patient sought treatment. And the consequences of treatment may extend into their personal and social lives, and into the way they react to their environment in diverse ways that relief of the primary complaint does not account for. This 'broad spectrum' response to treatment may well exceed the patient's expectations, but it is likely to be part of the practitioner's holistic intention and consistent with the method's therapeutic theory. The patient's holistic expectations of the process might be limited to 1 and 6 in the list of precepts – to be treated as a whole person, and with 'natural' therapies.

Holistic practice, then, can be represented in various degrees and permutations by the practitioner's intention, the therapeutic theory, the therapeutic method, the outcome of treatment, and the patient's expectations. Certain forms of complementary medicine provide the most complete expression of these five components of the process. The outcomes can be excellent, and patient satisfaction high. Which you might suppose is sufficient justification for giving them an established role in health care. But orthodox medicine is broadly dismissive of such a proposition. This is because all those five components of holistic practice have powerful 'meaning', powerful contextual healing or 'placebo' characteristics. The therapeutic methods themselves, implausible to medical science, are not regarded as the specific agents of change in the manner of biomedical interventions. Their *effectiveness* is clear, but their *efficacy* is doubted. So as far as established orthodoxy is concerned complementary practices are regarded as disreputable, even though they may fulfil the ideals of holistic practice that mainstream medicine espouses.

The research implications of this are discussed later, and they are challenging but very exciting. Or they should be if medical science really wants to 'know'; to get at the truth of the matter. But in the absence of the evidence that medical science would find compelling, many mainstream practitioners nevertheless do incorporate complementary methods or concepts, either into their personal repertoire, or into their clinical team on the basis of their 'informed empiricism'. And there are areas of mainstream medicine that are conspicuously holistic in intention, theory, method and outcome, whether they include complementary methods or not; the hospice movement and palliative care are examples.

Doctors who incorporate complementary methods into their personal repertoire or clinical team may do so to extend the scope of their holistic practice. And/or they may do so for pragmatic reasons – they make life easier: shifting the burden of difficult patients, saving money (avoiding costly drug treatment, investigation or specialist referral), satisfying patient choice. But also, the doctors learn so much about human nature, illness and healing in the process; lessons that were hardly touched upon in their medical education, if at all. Writing about these advantages and how they were achieved in her general practice, Charlotte Paterson says, for example:[17]

> It is in these new ways of seeing our patient's problems that we gain the biggest benefit; the benefit of allowing ourselves to see that biomedicine, even the bio-psycho-social variety, is a very useful and cohesive healing system, but that it is not the ONLY system of medicine. Once we can see that this is so, by witnessing how other therapies can help people that we cannot, we can also open ourselves up to the multiple ways that our patients may be making sense of their illness.

She is proposing that by this expansion and fuller implementation of its holistic perspective and intention, primary care can be transformed, and she concludes:

> A health service which provides a range of complementary therapies in primary care is likely to benefit from the expanding understanding of mind-body-spirit connections, of how both individuals and society can promote health and maximise the body's natural healing ability, of safer alternatives to modern pharmaceuticals, and of the importance of multiple ways of knowing, and understanding our bodies and our lives.

A review of the provision complementary medicine in primary care for the Department of Health does not explicitly state that these benefits would be the result of the more holistic practice that would result from increased provision, but this is implied: "Patients clearly experience complementary therapies as efficacious, both in terms of ameliorating and curing conditions, including chronic problems";[18] they value the quality of the relationship with the therapist, an explanation of their problem (Paterson's 'therapeutic theory') that fits with their life story, and more active role in managing their health. Increased complementary provision would help to fulfil the promise and the potential of Primary Care and help to mitigate some of its failings. Apart from the more holistic experience for patients that they describe and the patient satisfaction that results, there are pragmatic reasons for this that reflect Paterson's experience: complementary therapies may provide more appropriate care in some instances, prove effective when conventional medicine has failed or has little to offer, compensate for lack of time in routine GP consultations, enhance personal care, emphasise self-healing and self-care, address patients' disappointment at the ability of orthodox medicine to meet their needs or their dislike of orthodox approaches, and reduce some of the general practitioner's more difficult workload.

But regardless of the possible value of complementary medicine in achieving it, the holistic approach is likely to be productive in itself. The Scottish GPs in the survey already quoted clearly believe that lack of opportunity to practise holistically leads to higher rates of prescribing – 73% agreed or strongly agreed, and higher referral rates to secondary (specialist) care – 63%. And interestingly, 57% agreed that this failure of holistic practice lead to an increased demand for complementary therapies.[6]

So, although complementary medicine may do much to fulfil the intention of holistic practice, it has again to be emphasised that its use is not a defining characteristic of the holistic approach that many doctors in conventional practice would love to provide. David Peters and colleagues explain this well in a book that deals comprehensively with the role of complementary therapies in primary care:

> For doctors seeking ways of working more holistically complementary therapies (CTs) may not be the final destination, but they can be an important signpost

> on this journey. Doctors are after all applied scientists, and there's the rub, because CTs are often based on world views quite different to those of scientific medicine. Of course, that's their attraction and possible strength too, but because they are shaped by other traditions and rooted in vitalism they illuminate an unfamiliar and alien psychosomatic territory. Entering this landscape doctors are taken to the roots of medicine, a place where they have to ask what motivates their work and must confront unavoidable issues about attitudes, ethics and diverse questions about the human condition.[19]

The authors of the Scottish survey conclude, "These results give voice to deep concerns among GPs who remain committed to a holism they are struggling to deliver."[6]

Integrative practice

> Integrative Medicine is the practice of medicine that reaffirms the importance of the relationship between practitioner and patient, focuses on the whole person, is informed by evidence, and makes use of all appropriate therapeutic approaches, healthcare professionals and disciplines to achieve optimal health and healing. (The Consortium of Academic Health Centers for Integrative Medicine[20])

Truly holistic practice will be integrative in the sense described in Chapter 12: it will be 'whole-making' for the patients, and for the people involved in their care. Bringing different practitioners together in a group, or facilitating referral between practitioners, orthodox and/or complementary in a practice area, does not in itself constitute either holistic practice or practice that is integrative as I have described it. Integrative practice requires more than the structural proximity of different practitioners, and more than a willingness to share patients.

In the book by Peters and colleagues referred to earlier there is an interesting schema (page 77) 'Defining a quality integrated therapy service', reproduced from a report from the Foundation for Integrated Medicine (now subsumed within the College of Medicine). It relates to the integration of complementary medicine (CAM) and CAM practitioners into mainstream practice. It describes practice provision in terms of *structure* (how are things organised, is proper provision for the service made), *process* (how are things done, how does it work does it work), and *outcome* (is it effective, satisfactory). These three parameters are then used to assess six key aspects of a service:

- Appropriateness.
- Accessibility.
- Acceptability.

- Equity.
- Effectiveness.
- Efficiency.

And the appropriateness of the service is separately assessed according to the degree of collaboration between the GP and the CAM practitioner. The schema is reproduced as Appendix 15.1.

This is a very useful schema as it stands in relation to the issue of mainstream/CAM integration, but what struck me was the extent to which it could be applied equally to the quality of integration of mainstream medical services themselves; and particularly to the *integrative* quality of these services. I wonder how often and how critically the questions posed in this schema are in fact asked of the integration of mainstream services? I doubt that we know. And I doubt that if we did know we would be reassured or particularly impressed. 'Integrated Medicine' is commonly taken to refer to mainstream/CAM integration. But if we are really serious about integrated medicine, let alone integrative medicine this is not the only issue. Mainstream medical services need to be better integrated, and certainly more integrative as well. It is the whole landscape of healthcare that needs to be harmonised.

In a discussion of integrative healthcare, Heather Boon and colleagues identified seven steps in a continuum of *integrated* care that ranged from parallel practice (minimal collaboration) to fully integrative practice (close collaboration).[21] Their description of these two poles of the continuum reads:

> *Parallel* – characterised by independent healthcare practitioners working in a common setting; each individual performs his/her job within his/her formally defined scope of practice.
>
> *Integrative* – consists of an interdisciplinary, non-hierarchical blending of (healthcare knowledge and skills) that provides a seamless continuum of decision-making and patient-centred care and support; based on a specific set of core values that includes the goals of treating the whole person, assisting the innate healing properties of each person, and promoting health and wellness as well as the prevention of disease; employs and interdisciplinary team approach guided by consensus building, mutual respect and a shared vision of healthcare that permits each practitioner and the patient to contribute their particular knowledge and skills within the context of a shared, synergistically charged plan of care.

I have changed a few words in their actual description of integrative care to reinforce the point in the previous paragraph. Integrative care should be the pattern for all health care; for the whole spectrum of medical practice. So in this passage I have substituted the words 'blending of health care knowledge and skills' for the original text, which reads 'blending of both conventional medicine and complementary and alternative healthcare'.

The fact that CAM is part of the reality of contemporary health care and so must be part of the integrative practice and process of care, is the primary concern of Heather Boon's paper. But the challenge of integrative care applies equally to the present state of mainstream medicine, and the CAM issue must not divert attention from that. Interprofessional care, originating in the concepts of the primary health care team and community care and their evolution since the late 1960s, has been a theme of continuing importance in primary care, and the role of interprofessional education in this evolution is discussed in 'Learning to collaborate' in Chapter 19. The success and effectiveness of interprofessional care within mainstream medicine and in relation to social care is fundamental to achieving the kind of integrative practice I am writing about here, and they are not yet fully assured.

Complementary medicine is an additional and even greater challenge to effective integrative care. It cannot be shirked because it is part of the reality of contemporary healthcare and of value and benefit to very many patients. But it is a very different 'species' of health care to the variety that most doctors are familiar and comfortable with. Part of the problem is its nebulous and unregulated nature, but this will not be solved by refusing a relationship with the vigorous, healthy and whole-making baby (albeit a centuries old baby in some instances), while properly wishing to dispose of a certain amount of bath water. That attitude is dis-integrative and does a dis-service to patients who choose the therapeutic pathways that CAM makes available. And it is actually profoundly disrespectful of their intelligence and health-consciousness.

CAM is a different species of healthcare because its therapeutic principles and methods do not conform to the biomedical paradigm, and because they are based on the precepts of self-regulation, self-healing and enhanced healthfulness rather than disease control. The methods are culturally, philosophically and scientifically alien to the formative biomedical curriculum of most Western doctors. And yet for those who are acquainted with them, or use them or work with those who use them, they have all the cultural, philosophical, clinical and scientific advantages described in the earlier quotations by Charlotte Patterson, at the end of which she affirms "the importance (and, I would add the excitement and satisfaction) of multiple ways of knowing, and understanding our bodies and our lives".[17]

The story of sickness is composed of diverse causes (a variety of contributory factors) and effects (symptoms and other consequences of the illness). Together these represent the totality of a patient's needs. The quality and outcome of care will depend upon the extent to which they are met (the therapeutic relationship). It is possible that they may be met adequately by one practitioner in one clinical setting, but it is unlikely; particularly when there are causes and effects that are social and biographical. It is possible that these needs may be met adequately within one encounter or a short series of encounters with one or more practitioners. But it is more likely that the whole story will unfold over time. It may be presented piecemeal to a number of people in different settings, and years may elapse between the first presentation of a problem and the revealing of a critical piece of the story. Perhaps even the realisation by the patient that a particular experience belongs to the story.

This, of course, is the way the story of our life unfolds, into which the story of sickness may be woven. And when this is the case it is inevitable that, to quote Charlotte Paterson again, "multiple ways of knowing and understanding our bodies and our lives" will be required if the story of sickness is to be unfolded in a way that is whole making, whether the sickness can be cured or controlled or not. And there may be multiple occasions on which this unfolding takes place.

No system of medical records, or any other kind of record, can comprehend let alone do justice to the diversity and richness that may be necessary to the unfolding of such a story in a way that is therapeutically fruitful or healing. Certain facts must be recorded and communicated, between practitioners and over time, if a patient is to be safe and there is to be continuity of essential care. Those facts may be biological or biographical or both. But those facts alone do not constitute the multiple ways of knowing and understanding that may be necessary to the therapeutic process, particularly if it is to be a truly healing process.

This is why the *principle* of integrative care needs to be properly understood if the practice is to be effective. Understanding the principle means several things:

- It means realising that healthcare can have an integrative or dis-integrative effect on people. It can be whole-making or it can be depersonalising.
- It means that healthcare professionals see themselves as belonging to a *community of care* with a common concern for the well-being of the individuals and communities they serve, however occasional the contact with particular individuals may be. They are not purveyors of separate health care commodities but members of *a healthcare partnership* with one another and with the patient.

- It means realising that if this community and partnership are to be a reality, a certain minimum of *interprofessional awareness, respect and collaboration* is essential. This 'minimum' may in some instances be considerable. For example, a neurologist may need to know a lot about and have great respect for the help that a speech therapist can offer a patient. It will be less, but must at least be sufficient for, say, a general practitioner to appreciate the added value that a homeopath, osteopath or acupuncture practitioner may bring to the understanding and resolution of a particular patient's problem; and, of course, vice versa. And that appreciation must be rooted in a sufficient awareness of and respect for the contribution that the other practitioner can make to these multiple ways of knowing and understanding our bodies and our lives.
- Finally it means realising that *the integrative process resides in the experience of the patient.* Integrative practice facilitates the process, but the whole-making experience is the patient's. In this respect patients are their own healthcare record. Each patient brings with him or her, to each encounter, not only the story of their sickness, but also the story of their previous healthcare encounters and the integrative or dis-integrative effect of those encounters. Integrative practice requires that each encounter with the same or with a different practitioner, is understood as part of a continuing integrative process or journey.

So the starting point of integrative care is not organisation but attitude. Heather Boon and colleagues described seven ways of organising care, that could be called integrated, only one of which, quoted above, is truly integrative. The service implications of integrative practice and the work needed to achieve it are considerable. It is hard enough to integrate the wide spectrum of expertise within orthodox medicine, let alone to include complementary medical disciplines. The latter task is comprehensively reviewed in the book *Integrating Complementary Therapies in Primary Care* by David Peters and colleagues, and I have already pointed out how some of the principles they propose apply to mainstream medicine as well.[19] I cannot overemphasise the fact that integrative healthcare has to take account of the whole of the actual landscape of healthcare, bringing all its elements into partnership. As in my depiction of the structure of wholeness in Figure 1 in Chapter 12, there can be no separate compartments. In a new model of medicine there can be no Cinderella services, no poor relations. All healthcare professions will collude in the hubris of their shared goal of greater well-being for individuals and communities. But it will be that paradoxical state of humble hubris.

If the starting point of integrative care is the attitude that makes integrative practice possible, then as with all other attitudes that will determine whether medicine is to serve a healing vocation it must be nurtured, which means demonstrated by education. Education is part of the process of care that enables and sustains clinical practice, the subject of Chapter 19, where the task of 'learning to collaborate' as the basis for integrative practice is discussed. Changing the culture of medical education to facilitate this will take time., but that change will progress in parallel with the developments in integrative practice that are already under way, and the two processes will reinforce one another.

In their book, David Peters and colleagues write, "British general practice at its best has pioneered a holistic approach since the 1950s: healthcare for people as minds and bodies coping with their families and jobs and culture. Its great strength and a measure of its success have been a capacity for comprehensive, continuous long-term care that reflects local need. Which is why, given the resources, GPs should be best placed to encourage more integrated holistic care".[19] That was written in 2002. Now, in 2011, it looks

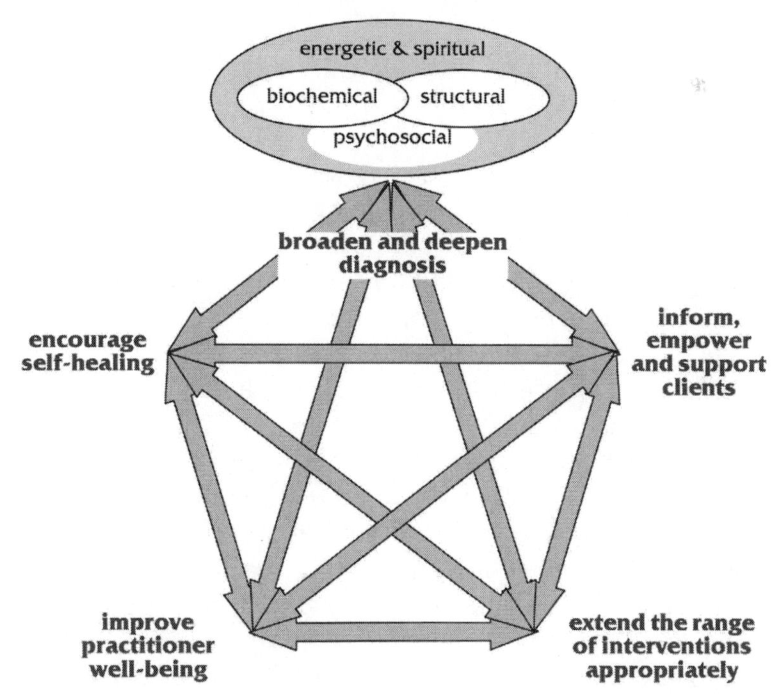

Figure 15.2 The elements of the integration process.[19]

(Reproduced with the permission of Elsevier Global Permissions).

as though GPs will be given those resources. Let us hope they will use them in that way.

Something of the integrated approach to healthcare promoted by Peters and colleagues is represented in Figure 15.2, reproduced from their book, to which they attach the following challenging and inspiring text:

> The main elements in the integration process are interconnected. If the aim is to encourage better physiological and personal functioning then a broader approach to 'diagnosis' of what has disturbed the organism's normal state of self-organisation will be needed. It may be that CAM approaches to diagnosis have something to add to conventional methods. If so then an extended range of interventions would have to follow and that could mean involving different kinds of practitioner in the care team. Because such reflective collaboration depends on professional learning and careful organisation, it requires considerable staff development. It is a challenge to work realistically and humanely in a team with a range of colleagues spanning the fields of medicine, CAM, nursing, social care and psychotherapy. Nor is the process of engaging with patients as co-workers and co-inquirers always easy or straightforward. 'Whole person' approaches to health care will call for practitioners who are prepared to become 'whole people', by cultivating their ability to collaborate, cope and care.[19]

Those three attributes will feature prominently in Chapter 19, 'Learning to do medicine'.

Health promotion

This is an area of health care that at first sight seems remote from clinical practice and from the core principles of the therapeutic encounter that I have proposed. But in fact, those principles, and the relationship of which they are part, provide the basis for any effective attempt at health promotion, and I introduce the subject here as an example of their central importance to the whole spectrum of health care.

Clean water and efficient drainage are public health measures that we take for granted and would be furious to be denied. If we can taste the chlorine and don't like it we can filter the water, but we wouldn't choose to have it left untreated. Fluoride in the water, to preserve our teeth, is another matter. Some people object, and it is alleged to be harmful. The introduction of fresh fruit and vegetables to the diet of sailors on long voyages saved them from the miseries of scurvy, and was (eventually) universally welcome. Present day exhortations to eat our 'five-a-day' fruit and veg come into 'nanny state' territory. The need for drink driving legislation is not controversial; the threshold for the blood-alcohol limit is. 'Safe sex' is common sense but some ignore it, and some deliberately flout it.

And the provision of sex education, particularly when and where to provide it, is hotly debated.

Health surveillance (screening) prevents diseases and saves lives, but creates 'partial patients' and the worried well, and subjects partial patients with false positive test results to unnecessary, distressing and possibly harmful treatment.

Education and public information cannot be relied upon to change behaviour, even when the benefits are obvious. Sixteen years of 'click clunk' advertising failed to achieve widespread use of seat belts in cars. Legislation eventually did it. It is no secret that 'tobacco kills', but many ignore the fact, or choose to take the risk, or believe the tax they pay justifies the health care they may need as a result.

And regardless of all other factors that influence or determine the health of individuals and communities it is the social circumstances of a person's birth and life that are likely to predict the quality, and inequality, of their health and health care. (See Chapters 4 and 16 for discussion of health inequality.)

And life is precarious. And the research that tells us what is necessary for a healthier or longer life produces contrary results from year to year. And doctors who care very much for the well-being of their patients are dismayed by 'the avalanche of public health rhetoric' (Chapter 5) and 'the tyranny of health' (Chapter 8).

What is medicine's responsibility towards this somewhat chaotic scenario? These tensions at the interface between clinical practice and social and public health policy are not easily resolved; particularly because they often put the well-being, aspirations or lifestyle priorities of the individual against the well-being of the community, or against some theoretical ideal norm of healthy living. If the starting point for building the medical model, the key component is the therapeutic encounter and relationship, how could the solution to this conundrum be found there?

The answer lies in the opportunity that it provides to come to an understanding with the patient, and to help patients come to an understanding with themselves. This opportunity presents itself more often than we might think because most of us consult some kind of practitioner, at least once and often a few times a year. The person we consult may just as well be a pharmacist, a podiatrist or a complementary practitioner, as a nurse or a doctor. The reason for the consultation, with any of these, might be quite circumscribed – an over the counter medicine, a verouca, a manipulation, a blood pressure check, a certificate of some kind. But any encounter allows *some* opportunity to encourage the understanding necessary to promote greater awareness, a greater desire to be well, and a greater responsibility for being well.

That may seem ridiculously ambitious and unrealistic. And of course it is – unless. Unless the medical model becomes enlightened enough to recognise and exploit these opportunities. For this to happen it has to become expansive enough and inclusive enough to acknowledge and affirm the role of all practitioners in providing the opportunity and encouraging that 'understanding'. It has to become respectful enough of insights into the dynamics of what we might call 'health consciousness' from a wide variety of practitioners from without as well as within orthodox medicine.

Health promotion and complementary medicine

Some complementary practitioners do a great deal to promote positive 'health consciousness' in their patients, irrespective of the unorthodox nature of their therapeutic method. Traditional Chinese Medicine places great emphasis on health promotion, and it is not surprising to find this confirmed in a recent study of the health promotion content of consultations with acupuncture practitioners.[22] This involved analysis of audio-taped consultations by four acupuncture practitioners with eighteen patients. The recorded content of the consultation related to symptoms, the therapy, conventional medical matters, 'social talk', and self-care. In one transcript of a 30 minute consultation, 'self-care talk' occupied more than half the time.

Appendix 15.2 is an excerpt from the newsletter of a complementary therapy clinic, and gives another simple example of self-care in complementary medicine.

A study by Faith Hill, whose particular purpose is to explore the role of complementary medicine (CAM) in health promotion, describes five different models in general use in health promotion:[23]

- The 'medical' model includes screening – 'surveillance', and the preventive procedures that result from it, and immunisation.
- The behaviour change model depends on persuasion to adopt a healthier lifestyle and assumes that individuals have the ability to control their health by making such choices.
- The education model emphasises freedom of choice based on the provision of unbiased information without indoctrination or manipulation, leaving decisions about behaviour to the individual.
- The empowerment model goes beyond the provision of information as the basis of free choice, aiming to facilitate action and raise critical

consciousness. It does so by working from the bottom up, responding to needs identified by the individual rather than the expert, and by encouraging self-esteem, a sense of having personal control over the circumstances, and a sense of self-efficacy or adequacy, of being able to take control.

- The social change model focuses on changing the social determinants of health and illness and health inequalities, rather than individual behaviour and responsibility. Which may in turn be a necessary prerequisite for empowerment amongst disadvantaged individuals.

All of these models have their part to play in promoting the better health of individuals and communities, bearing in mind though the reservations that have been expressed about surveillance medicine and public health rhetoric. But only the empowerment model provides the motivation for the individual that must justify and underpin any effective change, particularly any change that enhances wellbeing as distinct from health in the sense described in Chapter 12. This could, I suggest, include motivation for the individual to have a voice, and perhaps take action, in remedying the social factors that affect health and wellbeing; to become a participant in implementing social change. The opportunity for this empowerment resides above all in the practitioner–patient relationship and the therapeutic encounter, as we have seen in Chapter 8 ('Compassion, empathy and enablement'), and in this chapter ('Finding the time').

Because there is such diversity of practice amongst what is loosely labelled CAM it can have no clearly defined role in health promotion. But in its various manifestations, which also include elements of 'medical model' practice, it does support the behaviour change, educational and empowerment models. Some health promotion practitioners see CAM as opposed to the social change model because it caters for a relatively advantaged section of the community and is not relevant or helpful to the problems of health inequality. Others see advantages in making the insights and health maintenance possibilities of CAM more widely known and accessible. But it was in the opportunity for empowerment that the closest synergy between CAM and health promotion was found. Which is consistent with other experiences of the advantages of CAM in facilitating holistic and integrative practice that have already been discussed in this chapter.

Health consciousness

The 'health consciousness' I am describing here is not the unhealthy 'health self-consciousness' that ranges from the adoption of dietary fads to massive over supplementation or self-medication and hypochondriasis;

largely stimulated by media messages and advertising, but also by the avalanche of public health rhetoric and surveillance medicine.

'Health consciousness' means a reflective attitude to our mental and physical well-being, and informed common sense about what is good or bad for us personally. It may require special expertise to assist us in this if we have particular problems. But any practitioner, whatever the presenting problem and context has some opportunity to encourage the reflection that may help the individual to achieve insights or make appropriate choices that will benefit their well-being.

The plurality of health care resources outside the NHS as well as within it is a public health reality. They all offer opportunities for this kind of health consciousness. Cumulatively they could do more good for public health than any amount of public information, if they are all truly complementary. Which means all giving much the same basic message: that it is worth thinking about the way we live our life and the way it affects our health. This is not the same as 'the tyranny of health' because it is not coercive and it is not prescriptive. It is not preaching. It is an invitation to reflection within a relationship of trust. A relationship based on the core principles of the therapeutic relationship.

Health consciousness of this kind, fostered through the patient–practitioner relationship, will encourage us to be more discriminating of well-presented public health information, and more receptive to as much of it as is relevant to us and our situation. And if one additional minute can apparently make a difference to opportunities for health promotion in general practice,[10] surely the same can be true for other attempts to encourage greater self-sufficiency. Not every consultation will require this investment, but when it is made, and in the right manner, the bow wave of illness might diminish just a little.

The proposition that any therapeutic encounter can be a source of 'health consciousness' that promotes more effective public health presupposes complementary adaptations in other parts of the model. These will include the education and training of practitioners, and the integration necessary to achieve sufficient common understanding of what 'health consciousness' means and requires amongst all practitioners. And it will include a change in the medical culture towards a culture of inter-professional awareness and respect that both expects and acknowledges the shared goal of a common healing vocation amongst all practitioners. This also means recognising the de facto contribution to the wider landscape of public health of practitioners who are not members of the orthodox medical establishment, and valuing the insights they may be able to offer.

These and other presuppositions are explored earlier in this chapter and elsewhere. But the point is that promoting public health, other than in areas like clean water and drainage which individuals cannot provide for themselves, depends on promoting personal health. Making health a personal aspiration is best achieved through a personal relationship in the context of some therapeutic encounter. An encounter with the doctor's receptionist or the pharmacy assistant can be in some small degree therapeutic; and sometimes to a great degree.

Promoting an aspiration to personal well-being through a relationship in this way is no different from promoting other positive aspirations in life, through a good relationship with a good teacher, for example, or with our parents, or with any good mentor in any role that we may be lucky enough to meet.

The 'avalanche of public health rhetoric' is perhaps a measure of society's desperation to 'require people to do things for their own good that, they would not have chosen to do for themselves'. Exhortation seems to be singularly ineffective in achieving this goal. Effective encouragement to do things for ourselves requires the personal touch.

It might be argued that the opportunity to encourage greater health consciousness and the motivation and empowerment associated with it could be limited by the social circumstances or intelligence of the patient. My experience of health education work with teenagers from a variety of social backgrounds, including the bottom stream in a secondary modern school, does not suggest that. On the contrary, once a good rapport was established the less scholastically intelligent and less advantaged youngsters were generally more receptive to the issues and ideas being discussed than their theoretically brighter peers.

This is particularly relevant to the currently pressing problem of the increasing incidence of teenage pregnancy and sexually transmitted disease amongst the young (though not exclusively) in the UK. Where young people encounter health care practitioners person to person, the argument in these pages may apply. But this age group have few health care encounters (until one of these problems has arisen), and so opportunities of the kind I have described to encourage them 'to come to an understanding with themselves' that is proof against temptation and peer pressure are few. In this case as in others, the effectiveness of any form of health promotion will depend on the ability and willingness of the person to understand and respond. And this will depend to some extent, and in the case of young people exposed to these risks to a great extent, on the social and cultural context of their life; a theme we will return to in Chapter 17.

A proviso

> Humans qua humans are owed respect for their ability to make reasoned choices that are their own and that others may or may not share. (Pellegrino and Thomasma[3])

We look to government to encourage 'green' energy production, by the building of wind turbines for example, but may object fiercely if those turbines threaten a cherished landscape. We expect public health measures to provide a sufficiently risk free environment, clean drinking water for example, but may rebel if those measures interfere with a cherished aspect of our lifestyle, smoking in pubs perhaps. It is the responsibility of doctors to look after our health, but we do not necessarily want them to tell us how to live our lives. There may be changes to the way we live that might theoretically, or even obviously reduce some risk to health or even life but that would represent an unacceptable denial of something that for us makes life worth living, or that may be a deeply ingrained and normal cultural or social habit. Health, however we define it, and quantity of life, are not the only measures of quality of life. Surely our 'autonomy' entitles us to choices that may not, medically speaking, be good for us? Provided they do not cause unacceptable distress or harm to others, perhaps. There is a tricky balance to be struck between health promotion and life promotion.

Remember the second option that David Misselbrook proposes as the purpose of health care that I quoted in Chapter 3: "Health care exists to enable patients to live the lives that they choose, as much as possible unencumbered by, or despite, disability – to reduce suffering – and to prevent premature death – always where compatible with the patient's goals."[24] This was in contrast to "maintaining biomedical parameters within the normal range", and "controlling any aspects of patients' lives that threaten these normative measurements". Patients' goals, that make life worth living or may even represent the purpose of life for them, may simply be incompatible with those parameters; or with parameters of risk that threaten health in other ways. In which case, exercise of the discretionary latitude that Pellegrino and Tomasma advocate as an essential ingredient of trust between patient and doctor, requires almost exquisite circumspection: "We want someone who will use the discretionary latitude our care requires with circumspection – neither intruding nor presuming too much nor undertaking too little."[3] But this is just another instance of the principle task of the therapeutic encounter – to come to an understanding with the patient, and help patients to come to an understanding with themselves.

That understanding may extend to the kind of tolerance towards 'unhealthy' behaviour illustrated in the conclusion to Michael Fitzpatrick's critique of *The tyranny of health*[25] by a quotation from René Dubos:[26]

> In the words of a wise physician, it is part of the doctor's function to make it possible for his patients to go on doing the pleasant things that are bad for them – smoking too much, eating too much, drinking too much – without killing themselves any sooner than is necessary.

References

1 Kafka F. *A Country Doctor in the Penal Settlement*. London: Secker and Warburg; 1949.
2 Downie R. Introduction. *The Healing Arts*. Oxford: Oxford University Press; 1994.
3 Pellegrino E, Thomasma D. *The Virtues in Medical Practice*. Oxford: Oxford University Press; 1993.
4 Woolfson T. Integrated medicine: orthodox meets alternative. Challenge of making holism work. *Br Med J*. 2001; 332:168.
5 Shakespeare, W. *Hamlet*; III, i, 56.
6 Hasegawa H, Reilly D, Mercer SW, Bikker AP. Holism in primary care: the views of Scotland's general practitioners. *Primary Health Care Research and development* 2005; 6:320–328.
7 Jenkins L, Britten N, Barber N *et al*. Consultations do not have to be longer. *Br Med J*, 2002; 325:388.
8 Mechanic D. How should hamsters run? Some observations about sufficient patient time in primary care. *Br Med J*. 2001; 323:266–268.
9 Freeman GK, Horder J, Howie J *et al*. Evolving general practice consultation in Britain: issues of length and context. *Br Med J*, 2002; 324:880–882.
10 Wilson A. Childs S. The effect of interventions to alter the consultation length of family physicians: a systematic review. *Br J Gen Pract*. 2006; 56(532):876–882.
11 Ogden J, Bavalia K, Bull M *et al*. "I want more time with my doctor": a quantitative study of time and the consultation. *Fam Pract*. 2004; 21(5):479–483.
12 Mercer SW, Reynolds WJ. Empathy and quality of care. *Br J Gen Pract*. 2002; 52 (Supplement): S9–S12.
13 Rakel DP, Hoeft TJ, Barrett BP *et al*. Practitioner empathy and the duration of the common cold. *Family Medicine* 2009; 41(7):494–501.
14 Stevens R, Mountford A. On time. *Br J Gen Pract*. 2010; 60(565):458–460.
15 Patterson C. Britten N. The patient's experience of holistic care: insights from acupuncture research. *Chronic Illness* 2008; 4:264–277.
16 van Dulmen S, de Groot J, Koster D *et al*. Why seek complementary medicine? *Journal of Complementary and Integrative Medicine* 2010; 7(1): Article 20.
17 Paterson C. Primary Health care transformed: complementary and orthodox medicine complementing each other. *Complement Ther Med*. 2000; 8:47–49.

18 Luff DT. *Models of Complementary Therapy Provision in Primary Care*. Sheffield: Medical Care Research Unit of the University of Sheffield – for the Department of Health; 1999.

19 Peters D, Chaitow L, Harris G, Morrison S. *Integrating Complementary Therapies in Primary Care*. Edinburgh: Churchill Livingstone; 2002.

20 Consortium of Academic Health Centers for Integrative Health. Minneapolis: Available online at www.imconsortium.org.

21 Boon H, Verhoef M, O'Hara D, Findlay B. In: Parallel practice to integrative healthcare: a conceptual framework. *BMC Health Serv Res*. 2004; 4:15. Available online at doi:10.1186/1472–6963–4–15.

22 Evans M, Paterson C, Wye L *et al*. Lifestyle and self-care advice within traditional acupuncture consultations: a qualitative observational study nested in a co-operative inquiry. *J Altern & Complement Med*. 2011; 17(6):519–529.

23 Hill F. Towards a new model for health promotion? An analysis of complementary and alternative medicine and models of health promotion. *Health Educ J*. 2003; 62:369–380.

24 Misselbrook D. *Listening to Patients*. Newbury: Petroc Press; 2001.

25 Fitzpatrick M. *The tyranny of health*. Abingdon: Routledge; 2001.

26 Dubos R. *Mirage of Health*. London: Allen & Unwin; 1960.

APPENDIX 15.1[1]

DEFINING A 'QUALITY' INTEGRATED THERAPY SERVICE FOR COMPLEMENTARY THERAPIES (CT) – 1

Structure	Process	Outcome
	APPROPRIATENESS	
Are CT practitioners (CTPs) appropriately trained, supervised and supported?	Do teams allocate CT appropriately to meet patient needs?	Do GPs successfully identify patients appropriate for CT?
	ACCESSIBILITY	
Are the CT services suitably located and available to all who might need them?	Are the waiting times for CT within the practice's Patients Charter guidelines?	Do CTPs enhance accessibility by detailed feedback to GPs?
	ACCEPTABILITY	
Do the CT services available reflect local needs?	Are patients satisfied with procedures for accessing the CT services?	Are patients satisfied with the results of the CT services?
	EQUITY	
Are minority groups catered for?	Are procedures applicable to all minority groups?	Are outcomes equitable in relation to other CT services?
	EFFECTIVENESS	
Do intake procedures make maximal use of resources?	Do CTPs establish and maintain 'allied' relationships within the CT field	Are the results of CT clinically effectives?
	EFFICIENCY	
Are resources allocated to monitoring, and reducing non-attendance?	Do the CTs provided optimally balance treatment with need?	Is the allocation of CT and its uptake cost effective?

DEFINING A 'QUALITY' INTEGRATED THERAPY SERVICE – 2

The importance of GP collaboration to the appropriateness of CT

With collaboration	Without collaboration
STRUCTURE	
1 CTPs are supervised managerially in the practice	1 There is no contact or management
2 CTPs have training funding to develop services	2 The practice accepts no responsibility for professional development of CTPs
3 CTPs are appointed with the necessary skills to deliver the proposed service	3 The CTP is appointed with no job description or adequate training to deliver the planned service
4 The practice has a clear idea of what they want, and make sure they get it	4 The GPs don't know what the CTP is doing apart from an annual report
PROCESS	
1 CTPs and GPs have agreed to target particular patient groups (e.g. high users) and work together to manage them	1 GPs refer patients without discussion or planning of aims and expectations
OUTCOME	
1 GPs correctly identify patients for CT using agreed protocols and guidelines	1 CTPs feel expected to accept all comers and cope – who else will otherwise?
2 CTPs are able to assess patients' suitability for treatment, refer back accordingly, and measure outcome	2 GPs expect CTPs to manage all referrals, with no review of the service provided

Maxwell's criteria for service quality on which the above schema is based

Criteria	Questions	Methods
Acceptibility	Which conditions are poorly managed by conventional methods? Are there categories of patient who find CTs particularly acceptable?	*Practice review* What do doctors say they need? Have they used CTs previously? How? What do other practitioners need? What do patients think?
Appropriateness	What evidence is there for using a range of CTs in these conditions and categories of patients?	*Assessing the evidence* Review various evidence bases. What do CTPs and GPs believe works? What is their experience? What do patients say?
Accessibility	How could access to potentially effective CTs be organised?	*Designing the service* Which therapies to include? Selecting coworkers. Structured collection of data: referrals, treatment, and outcomes.
Effectiveness	Does access to a range of CTs improve clinical outcomes in the patients and conditions treated?	*Delivering the service* Action research on structures and processes. What do patients say about the process? Reflection on reports of clinical activity.
Efficiency	Does access to a range of CTs improve the practice's use of resources, to produce individual or population health gain?	*Monitoring service outcome* Analysis of resource use: GP time, prescribing costs, referrals outside practice. (Plus epidemiological studies and comparative trials.)

Criteria	Questions	Methods
Equity	Is a range of CTs available to all who might benefit?	*Modifying the service* Review access criteria and outcomes. Adapt service and intake accordingly.

Reference

1 Peters D, Chaitow L, Harris G, Morrison S. Integrating Complementary Therapies in Primary Care. Edinburgh: Churchill Livingstone; 2002 (Reproduced with the permission of Elsevier Global Permissions.)

APPENDIX 15.2

Two simple examples of health and self-care promotion from a Complementary perspective. Reproduced from the January Newsletter of the Nine Springs Clinic, Yeovil.[1]

How to walk on ice!

I am writing this just as we emerge from the great December 2010 freeze-up. Being an avid follower of weather patterns, an early cold spell usually predicts another cold spell later, so be prepared for it. And on this note, here is a little bit of advice of how to walk on that treacherous ice.

We can learn something here from Tai Chi (and most of the martial arts). It teaches us to keep our weight centred in the 'Dantien' – that is, the area below our navel, which is the natural centre of gravity of the body.

When we tense up, or become fearful, our energy naturally rises up the body, mainly to the chest and shoulders, which causes us to be ungrounded on our feet. But if you shift your attention to the Dantien it can make a considerable difference to your balance and 'sure footedness'. Here's how you do it:

1 Stand with your feet hips width apart. Make sure your feet are well connected to the ground, as if they have roots going down into the earth.
2 Put your hand on your Dantien (the area below your belly button) in order to remind yourself where it is.
3 Now allow your knees to bend very slightly, feeling as you do so, how your pelvic area drops a little. Now just pretend that your legs are springs, giving yourself a little bounce from your feet to your pelvis. Really get a sense of your centre of gravity being lower.
4 Now start to walk, keeping your attention on your Dantien. It is best to start by practising walking quite slowly in order to get the feel of it.

If you are doing it right you will experience that you are walking in a much more grounded and rooted way, and that you feel more relaxed and confident.

I have had to walk quite considerable distances on the ice recently and find this invaluable, with no slips to date. However I do have to keep reminding myself to 'keep my weight down', as it is only too easy to become distracted and forget! It is important to practise it on a daily basis in order to make it more automatic, which will help you to keep calmer as you go about your daily life as well.

In China they have carried out research which showed that amongst the elderly, those who do Tai Chi are not nearly so prone to falls as those who do not, a testament to how it makes one more sure-footed by being more balanced. None of us need the pain or inconvenience of broken bones.

If you wish to explore this further we have several Tai Chi and Qi gong classes at the clinic. Please see the classes timetable for more details.

And a further note about the cold. Remember that the place your body loses heat from most is the head – develop a new trend – wear hats in the house to save on fuel bills!

Dance and movement for energy, expression and well-being

We are pleased to welcome (HL) who will be running a weekly Dance class from January 13th. She will help to guide you through basic dance techniques and exercises and to express yourself creatively.

The class will primarily draw on contemporary dance, an accessible, graceful form of dance that works with core stability and alignment, gravity, balance, co-ordination, flexibility and extension.

A one-hour window in your day. A lovely way to begin your Thursday evenings.

Reference

1 Robinson J. How to walk on ice. *Nine Springs News* 2010 January; Hendford, Yeovil: Nine Springs Clinic.

16

PERMUTATIONS OF CARE
The process of care

Summary

- The permutations of care that any one of us may need in the course of our life and available within the health care system as a whole are numerous.
- They include the reason or need for care, the time-scale of need, the goal of care, who provides it and where; and the social, cultural, economic and political factors that affect the experience of health care.
- Care may be formal or informal, appropriate or inappropriate; and will depend upon availability, accessibility, and cost, interprofessional awareness, communication, collaboration and continuity of care.
- These permutations of care must take account of the place of complementary medicine in the landscape of health care.
- Greater interprofessional awareness and respect, and better management of the permutations of care could save time and improve quality.
- The fragmentation of care is detrimental to patient care. Reconciliation and closer integration is essential and achievable.

The many dimensions of care

The permutations of care that any one of us may need in the course of our life are numerous, and the permutations of care theoretically available within the health care system as a whole, formal and informal, conventional and unconventional, even more so. The elements of the care process listed here (see Box 16.1) reflect its complexity and its diversity. Separate items in a column are not necessarily mutually exclusive. Some, such as 'treatment' and 'healthcare professional' are themselves large categories. Others, such as 'education' and 'reassurance' belong in more than one column. But the lists give a fair impression of our various experiences of health care, and of how our health care needs are woven into the narrative of our lives.

BOX 16.1 *Elements of the care process*

Need for care (Why?) (of body, mind or spirit)	*Time scale/course* (of illness or of care)	*Goal of care* (intended outcome)
Trauma	Mild, moderate, severe	Cure, resolution
Collapse	Acute, sudden	Palliation, amelioration
Pain, distress	Episodic, recurrent	Maintenance, coping
Disability, incapacity	Chronic, persistent, relapsing	Education, insight
Malaise, dysfunction, dis-ease	Self-limiting, remitting	Reassurance, comfort
Lumps and lesions	Progressive, terminal	Quality of life
Worry, uncertainty, fear	Prophylactic, preventative	Well-being
Susceptibility (genetic, environmental, etc.)		Healing

Provider of care (Who?)	*Place of care (Where?)*
Us, ourselves	Home, domestic
Passer by	Public place
Friend, family, neighbour	First aid post, ambulance
Volunteer, amateur	Clinic, surgery, consulting room
Health care professional	– NHS, private
– generalist, specialist	Hospital ward, hospice
– orthodox, complementary	Nursing home
– NHS, private	Pharmacy, 'natural' health store
Priest, chaplain, etc.	Bedside, office, home, etc.

The various permutations that all these elements of the care process make possible and that the precariousness of life may require, cannot be reduced to any tidy model of care. And running through them and connecting them are other factors that will determine the actual quality and effectiveness of care (see Box 16.2).

BOX 16.2 *Determinants of care*

- Social, cultural, religious context and circumstances.
- Availability and access.
- Interprofessional awareness.
- Patient choice.
- Cost of care, payment for care.
- Communication and collaboration between carers.
- Continuity of care.
- Standards of care, regulation.

Broadly speaking, healthcare is either informal, amongst friends, neighbours, family and community, or formal, provided by those with a defined commitment or responsibility.

Informal care

The quality of informal care depends upon a number of attributes that are not necessarily easy to define or quantify: the common sense, compassion and generosity of spirit of individuals; the strength and cohesion of families or communities; courage and selflessness. Education helps, but not necessarily formal health education or first aid training or a particular level of intelligence. Knowledge that is local, domestic, vernacular, or 'folk' may be invaluable.

Informal care will also be affected by the wider health care culture and the attitude of professional carers. A culture that encourages, respects and facilitates informal care, and gives positive messages and useful information, one that enhances the willingness, confidence and competence of individuals and communities to look after themselves and each other, will enhance the well-being of all concerned and reduce the burden on formal service providers. Whereas a health care culture that creates the belief and the expectation that the professionals, the health service, will and should meet every need will have the opposite effect.

The extent, the scope and the quality of informal care will be determined by the culture of the society as a whole and of the health care culture in particular. Recognising the appropriate limits of informal care, the point at which formal care should take over, will depend upon the way that formal carers and care services are integrated within communities and integrative of them. By encouraging, facilitating and supporting informal care, formal carers will develop an understanding of when transition from one to the other, informal to formal and vice versa, is appropriate and necessary, and how it should be done. This is a reciprocal learning process. It will happen most effectively through the relationship between practitioners and providers of formal care and people in situations where informal care is being provided, or where informal care could or should be the appropriate alternative to formal care.

Informal care may be the natural, sensible, appropriate response of people to a health care need, or it may be the outcome of enlightened negotiation between formal providers of care and the people on the ground. It is the job of health care professionals to empower and enable people to care for themselves and each other and to make appropriate decisions about care. This will happen most effectively where the principles of holistic practice are accepted, and where the multiplicity of factors that affect health and illness is understood and is a normal part of the conversation between practitioners and patients. This approach is known to increase people's sense of control over their own health care needs, which in turn will increase their resources for informal care.

Informal carers

These remarks apply to all informal care, but informal care of a particular kind is completely indispensable to the UK health care system. A recent review reports that each year, 2 million people move in and out of unpaid caring for a sick, disabled or older relative or friend who is unable to manage on their own. There are around 6 million carers in the UK at any one time and 1.2 million of those are caring for over 50 hours. Of that particular group, 72% report adverse effects on their health. A meta-analysis of 23 studies across 11 health categories of family caregivers of persons with dementia concluded that caregivers had a 23% higher level of stress hormones, and 15% lower level of antibody responses.[1]

There are even 175,000 children, aged between 5 and 18 years, in substantial caring roles, among whom a worryingly high level of self-harm and other emotional health problems has been recognised. Family carers are estimated to save the NHS £67 billion (€78.3bn, $103.5bn) or more per annum.[2] These carers represent the largest health and care workforce in the UK, and are of central importance to any discussion of permutations of care.

Self care

Minor illnesses account for 18% of general practitioner workload. But unless or until there is no improvement, or patients becomes too anxious, or children are involved, or family or friends persuade them to consult, most people treat themselves (52%) or do nothing (22%). This overall pattern has not changed for 20 years, although consultations for particular categories of minor illness in the UK, such as acute respiratory tract infections, have decreased.[3] Promoting more and better self-care must be a priority for the NHS. That eighteen per cent is an extravagant use of GP services, bearing in mind the unsustainable growth in demand. Average GP consultation rates increased from 3.9 per person per year in 1995 to 5.3 in 2006. Simply providing information has little effect on changing patient self care behaviour. Effective change implicates the individual, the immediate family or social circle, and society in general. And the direct

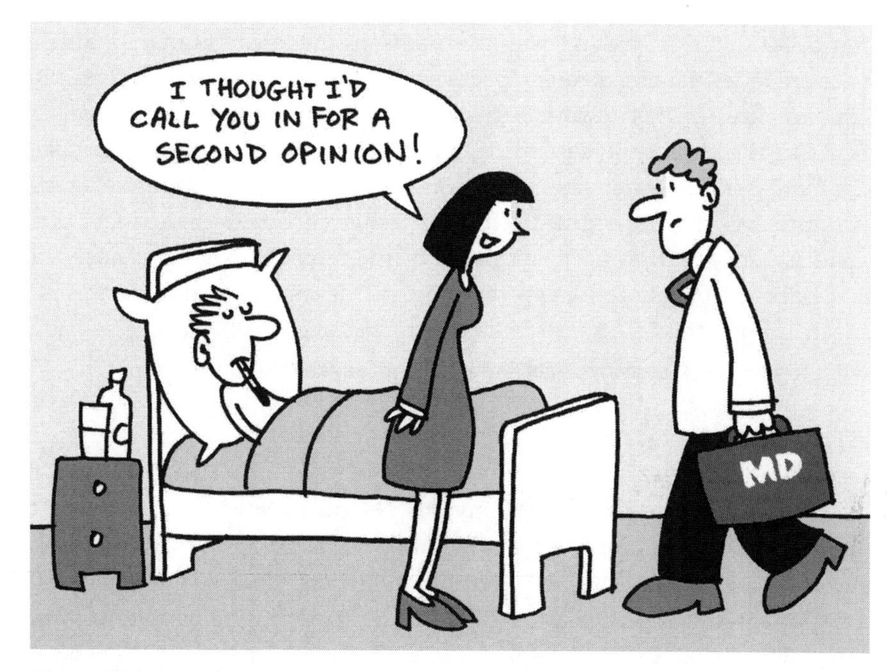

Figure 16.1 *Formal support for informal care!*

involvement of health care professionals in conversation with patients is key to this.

Formal care

Supporting informal care

So a first principle of formal, professional health care is perhaps to recognise its responsibility to encourage and strengthen the resourcefulness of individuals and communities for informal care. This aim is exemplified at one level by the steadily increasing provision of NHS support for the family carers who make such an extensive and demanding contribution to care in the community.

But the process of professional encouragement for self care needs to be much more widespread, and more enlightened if it is to impact upon that 18% GP workload. For example, the prescribing habits of doctors are powerfully influential on how patients regard their ailments. The review I have quoted reports that of patients who received a prescription for a previous minor ailment 62% visited the doctor at the next occurrence of the same complaint. Refraining from prescribing antibiotics when not clearly and immediately indicated can lead to a small but significant reduction in future consultation rates for similar conditions. Actions that make a difference include: helping people to develop accurate knowledge about the consequences of their health behaviour; enhancing self-efficacy (people's belief in their ability to care for themselves effectively); enhancing social approval for self care; and promoting concrete plans through action planning. All these are most likely to be achieved within the context of a good patient–practitioner relationship in the immediate circumstances of a therapeutic encounter; a central point of the argument in Chapter 14, 'Health promotion'.

Appropriate care

The first question to be asked of any possible permutation of care is – is it appropriate? Is the goal of care, the pattern of care, the provider of care, the place of care, and other determinants of care (see Box 16.3), really appropriate to this particular need? You will remember the quotation from David Haslam at the very beginning of the book: "We use the medical model because the medical model is what we use, even though it may not be *appropriate.*"[4] (My italics.) This is an admission of a kind of tunnel vision, or conditioned reflex that can affect medical thinking, decision making or behaviour in many situations. Any practitioner may be blinkered by the limits of their own knowledge, skill, attitudes or personality if they are not sufficiently self-aware. A doctor's biomedical filter may exclude explanations of a patient's illness or possible solutions that do not fit that framework of knowledge. But so may any therapeutic theory, and a complementary practitioner may be similarly blind to other diagnostic and therapeutic possibilities. We cannot know what may be appropriate if we are not aware of the alternatives and of the limits of our own repertoire.

On the other hand we may be aware of the possibilities, aware that another explanation or course of action may be more appropriate, but lack the opportunity or resources (personal, clinical, technical, social, economic, etc.) to pursue it. The survey of Scottish general practitioners that has been mentioned elsewhere demonstrated the extent to which the doctors aspire to provide more holistic care, and to be more attentive to psychological aspects of patients' problems, but are unable to do so because of the way that general practice is organised, particularly because of lack of time.[5] We have seen how complementary practitioners well integrated into a care team can mitigate this problem.[6] The wider dimensions of people's needs may or may not be taken into account. Some practitioners are aware of the spiritual needs of patients and that these may play a significant part in the story of sickness, and that meeting them may make an important contribution to the recovery of their well-being. For others this is a no-go area, even those for whom faith or spirituality is important in their own lives. Hospital chaplains may or may not be regarded as part of the care team. Proposals to reduce their numbers in the NHS have been a cause of controversy.

BOX 16.3 *Patterns and determinants of care*

Patterns of care
- Self-care.
- Informal care.
- Professional care.

Determinants of care
- Choice.
- Appropriateness.
- Access.
- Cost.
- Time.
- Interprofessional awareness.
- Collaboration.

The patient's role

For any particular health care need, appropriate decisions about formal care – the goal of care, the type of care and who should provide it, the time and the place, depend on

- Understanding the problem.
- Awareness of the possibilities, including awareness of and respect for what other practitioners can offer.
- The willingness, determination, opportunity and resources to do what is appropriate.

But increasingly patients are deciding for themselves, at least initially, what is appropriate care. The decision may range from going to the GP for an antibiotic or a sick note, to seeking a private operation, negotiating residential care for an elderly relative or consulting a complementary therapist. In any situation of this kind the attitude of the health care professional concerned is all-important. This must be respectful of the patient's intentions and perceptive of the reasons; they may well be right and good for that patient, even if the practitioner does not share them. The right attitude may be to support and guide, and maybe help to shape those intentions, but it is not necessarily to be acquiescent where there is doubt or obvious error, or perhaps where there is unjustifiable demand for a form of care that is potentially harmful or unnecessarily costly. What a patient desires or decides may not be in their best interests, or the best interests of the one for whom they seek it, or for others implicated in the decision. Coming to a different understanding with patients, and helping them to come to a different understanding with themselves, may be the practitioner's proper responsibility.

Availability of care

The preferred course of action may be appropriate, but it will not be possible if the necessary resources are not available. Eighty seven per cent of the Scottish GPs see a more holistic response to be appropriate to their patients' needs and would prefer to offer it.[5] But the constraints of general practice do not permit it. The holistic response might be to help the patient understand that an antibiotic is not needed for a self-limiting viral pharyngitis, or it may be to explore the possibility that the recurrent sore throat is a symptom of the patient's life situation rather than some underlying disease. But if the time, mental energy or even the moral courage is lacking it will not happen.

If a patient wonders whether skilled homeopathy might reduce his dependence on inhalers for his asthma, or whether acupuncture might reduce the pain of her arthritis, and the doctor agrees that this might be an appropriate course of action, it will not happen if there is no skilled practitioner available, or if the patient cannot afford to pay for it and the health service does not provide it. It would be possible to create a long list of appropriate health care decisions and choices that cannot be pursued or implemented because the necessary willingness, opportunity or resources are not available.

The current financial crisis in the UK is likely to mean that certain healthcare options will not be so readily available through the NHS. This has already caused clinicians to consider critically whether they were appropriate in the first place (see Chapter 9 'A crisis of cost'), and raised questions about the quality and consistency of clinical decision making as one of the factors that determine the widespread variations in permutations of

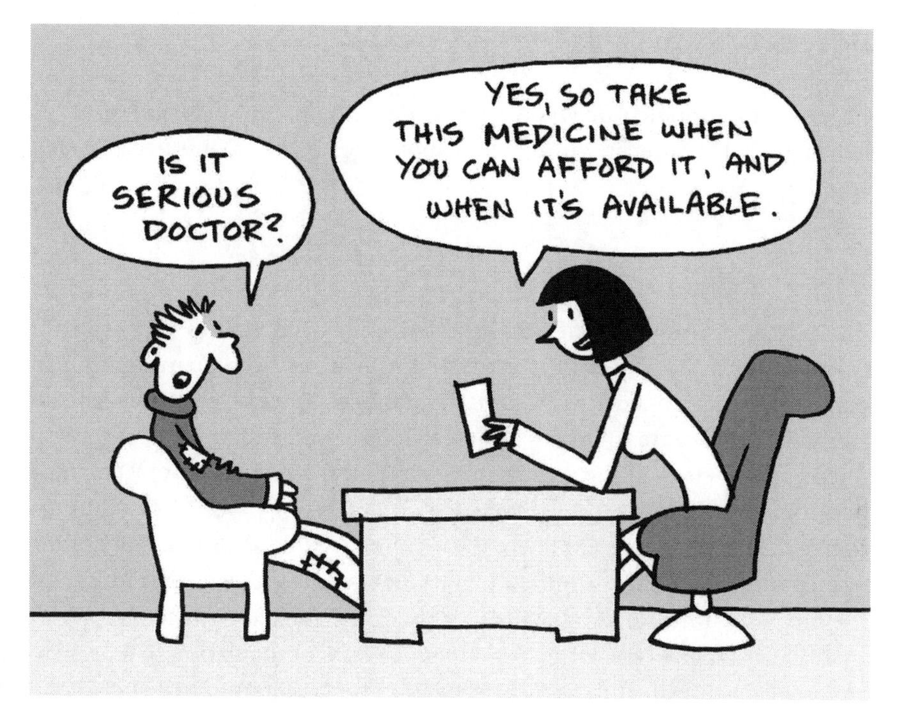

Figure 16.2 *Healthcare can be a bit of a lottery.*

care that are known to exist. These considerations highlight the uncomfortable fact that in the UK, and elsewhere, what is appropriate is not always available, and what is available is not always appropriate. Or, to paraphrase slightly a recent commentary on variations in clinical practice and their cost implications, 'When we fail to reduce bad variation, which reflects the limits of professional knowledge and failures in its application, while preserving the good variation that makes care patient centred, we provide services to patients who don't need or wouldn't choose them while we withhold the same services from people who do or would, generally making far more costly errors of overuse than of underuse'.[7]

Remodelling medicine requires that we achieve a far more perceptive and determined correspondence between what is appropriate and what is available. This must include a far broader, more eclectic understanding and acceptance of what may be appropriate care that lies outside the present framework of mainstream medicine, particularly some complementary therapies. This will in turn require sufficient provision of those therapies to make them actually available, and the reconfiguring of knowledge, attitudes and interprofessional relationships that the earlier discussion of holistic and integrative practice implies, and that the discussion of what 'learning to do medicine' (Chapter 19) proposes.

Access to care

Access to appropriate care will obviously depend upon its availability in the first place. Thereafter it will depend upon two things – who decides, and who pays.

Who decides?

At present, decisions about access to NHS care (the goal of care, type of care, provider, place and time of care) are made by some permutation of patient, doctor, appointments officer, manager or administrator. Patients are involved because, theoretically, decisions are made in partnership with them. The doctor's clinical judgement is central to the decision, but may be subordinated to or even dictated by a variety of political or administrative decisions. These are likely to be influenced by issues of availability, particularly where this is limited by lack of resources, especially money. Or they may be influenced by evidence-based decisions about the validity of a particular type of care; either its validity overall, or in relation to a particular health care need, and possibly in relation to its cost. And evidence-based decisions may be influenced by attitudes and beliefs.

The exception to this rather convoluted decision making process in NHS care is patients' complete freedom (subject to the availability of appointments) to see their general practitioner or a member of the primary care team, or to attend a drop-in centre, or to turn up at an accident and emergency department, entirely on their own initiative; a decision that may or may not be appropriate.

Access to private health care, paid for directly or through insurance, is usually a patient's decision, except when the health service buys private care to meet its targets. Many patients buy time. Conventional biomedical time can be bought, from doctors and physiotherapists in private practice. This is money spent to get things done quicker and/or to ensure a more leisurely consultation. But whether it buys better quality time, with all its attendant benefits, or just more time with the same outcomes as routine waiting list consultations and procedures is another matter.

Unless a patient seeks a second opinion privately on their own initiative because of some doubt or dissatisfaction about their care, the decision whether treatment is necessary and what needs to be done is just as likely to be made by a doctor in consultation with the patient when resorting to private care as when using the health service. Most decisions about access to conventional care are made by or influenced by doctors or other conventional health care practitioners. This is inevitable when in conventional practice the problem is construed in biomedical terms, and the knowledge and skills required for its effective management on those terms are the preserve of the bio medically trained practitioner.

There is wide variation in clinical practice in the UK (and even wider variation in the USA), and this variation is reflected in variations in the cost of care, some of which are wasteful of resources. This is not just a consequence of strategic financial decisions by health authorities, but of variations in clinical decision making – decisions by doctors about what to do. A report from the King's Fund that addresses the need to increase productivity in the NHS in the light of the current financial crisis emphasises the need and the opportunity that this presents to provide *better* quality care with the resources available, not the *same* quality of care for less money – "getting *better* value for patients from the resources available to the NHS". This will depend on improving clinical decision making.[8] It depends on "doing things right *and* on doing the right things" (My italics). The editorial commentary on this report in the *British Medical Journal* spells out the problem that variety in permutations of care presents: "All measures to tackle practice variation have proved inadequate. The lessons from these failures relate to the complexity of clinical decision making and the need to improve the quality of decisions. They are also about the power relationships among clinicians, patients and the public, and those who pay for health services, including government. But deciding what is the right thing to do is complex because of uncertainty about the health outcomes that will follow an intervention and the variable assessments that different patients make of the same outcome. Evidence and professional knowledge about the likelihood of different benefits and harms can contribute to better decisions but it is not enough. Patients' concerns about what matters to them are also relevant when there are trade-offs to be made".[7]

Even in conventional medicine where there may be ample research into the treatment of a particular condition, the choice of the best method may still be uncertain and contribute to variations in practice. Decisions about access to complementary medical care are still more complicated. Quite apart from the influence of variation in attitudes of conventional practitioners, there is little if any clear understanding of which complementary therapy is most appropriate for a particular condition. There is little to guide a decision between say, acupuncture, homeopathy or cranio-sacral osteopathy for a particular condition, other than common sense, hearsay, instinct, chance or the personal appeal of the therapy or therapist. Sceptics will say that it makes no difference anyway because they all depend on contextual or placebo factors rather than the specific effect of the therapeutic method. Those who are convinced of the specific effects may nevertheless agree that the choice of method is not necessarily critical because they all eventually stimulate a common pathway of self-regulation and self-healing. And who is to say that a patients' own judgement about the complementary treatment best suited to their constitution and their need, their 'concerns about what matters to them', is unreliable?

Understanding the appropriate use of complementary medicine and how to make appropriate decisions about access to it is not a trivial matter because it constitutes a very large part of the landscape of health care; very many people use it, and very many people benefit from it. And, of course, they pay a lot of money for it, whether directly or through the few health insurance schemes that covers it.

Questions about the appropriateness and availability of different kinds of care, conventional or unconventional, and of access to it will benefit from research. But in the first instance and more importantly they have to be addressed by collaboration between practitioners of the same and of different disciplines to provide the empirical experience that will in itself inform clinical decision making, and that will generate the questions that need to be and can be resolved by formal research. (See 'Research' in Chapter 18, and 'Learning to collaborate' in Chapter 19.)

The cost of care

The cost of health care and how to pay for it are familiar hot topics. But if we think about it, and as the report and commentary that I have quoted imply,[7,8] these are not primarily questions of the funding of health care. They are questions about the provision of *appropriate* care. The success of the biomedical model has seduced us into a ready acceptance of a great deal of inappropriate care. It has blinded us to possibilities of other more appropriate forms of care, or inhibited us in pursuing them and investigating their potential for more cost effective health care. It has resulted in the paradigm paralysis and scientific tunnel vision described in earlier chapters. And it has inhibited the holistic practice that general practitioners, as suggested by the survey from Scotland, believe would not only benefit patients but would be cost effective.[5]

Unfettered access to biomedical health care and all its technological possibilities is unaffordable. The better solution is not to ration it, but to develop permutations that make better use of it, or that are effective alternatives to it, or that avoid the necessity for it.

The first of these is the basis of the response to the unaffordable cost of Western medicine that the financial crisis has thrown into sharp relief. It seeks 'productivity plus' – more productive use of health service resources through better quality of care. Permutations of care that avoid the need for costly biomedical and technological solutions certainly include better quality of more appropriate care, including better use of biomedical care, but also better 'health consciousness' and effective health promotion (Chapter 15), more and better informal care and self-care, and more discriminating use of formal care.

The second part of the solution, making better use of alternatives among existing permutations of care include the use of complementary medicine either instead of biomedical treatments, or together with biomedical treatments to enhance their effectiveness or mitigate costly side effects. Research to investigate the actual cost effectiveness of complementary medicine's contribution to health care is scarce and slowly progressing, but attracts too little investment – and presents formidable challenges. David Peters and colleagues describe these in discussing the delivery of complementary therapies (CTs) in primary care:

> Whereas reductions in drug costs, referral rates, revisits to the GP and adverse events can be costed, many of the benefits that CTs are commonly declared to produce cannot easily be measured. The latter, including patient preference, patient empowerment, the process of the consultation, lifestyle changes with delayed health benefits, quality of life including improved stress management, the value of having other options for help available when orthodox treatments have failed, and the preventive aspects of the therapies themselves.[9]

The Glastonbury Health Centre project, running since 1992, which is described in Peters' book, is a well studied experiment in providing complementary therapies integrated within UK primary care (www.integrated health.org.uk). A subsample of 41 patients with long-term problems studied over one period of the project showed a marked reduction in the use of other health services for the problem referred, particularly amongst the heaviest users of other services prior to referral. GP attendance dropped by a third. There was an even greater reduction in the number of prescriptions, and a similar reduction in further referrals, test and other treatments in this group, particularly referrals for physiotherapy and X-rays. Overall, there was an estimated reduction in costs for such services after treatment for this group of around £2,500 (€3,000, $3,900) a year. In one year alone (1995/96) there was an estimated saving in costs for secondary referral of £18,000 (€21,000, $28,000). And the service as a whole has been consistently cost-effective. This is not conclusive of what could be achieved by the wider integration of complementary and mainstream medicine, but it is suggestive, and justifies serious investment in further studies.

According to the Glastonbury study complementary medicine accounts for 30% of primary interventions in the UK, in other words the first port of call for patients; a very significant component of the actual permutations of care that the population of the UK uses. It will be inexcusable if the exploration of 'getting better value for patients from the resources available to the NHS', by 'doing things right and doing the right things', does not take this into account. We need to know to what extent the resistance to the possible benefits of complementary medicine within a more effectively holistic and integrative model of care reflects 'the limits of professional knowledge and failures in its application', and restricts 'the good variation that makes care patient centred'. Failure to understand this, and to remedy it where it proves to be a 'bad variation' in clinical practice, will be one reason why we continue to provide some services to patients who don't need or wouldn't choose them while we withhold others from those who do and would. One of the costly mistakes we can no longer afford.

Who pays?

Although I did not work within the NHS for the whole of my medical career I have been a committed supporter of its principles throughout. I have used homeopathy both within the health service, in the NHS outpatient clinic at Bristol Homeopathic Hospital, and outside it as a private practitioner. In the latter role, with my background in general practice, I found it uncomfortable requiring patients to pay for my services. I would allow concessions, or charge virtually nothing to people on low incomes. But the poorer people were almost always keen to pay something. And sometimes people who could well afford it would try to avoid paying the full rate. I never completely got over this discomfort at being paid directly, but I knew it was a hang up. Even in NHS general practice there are items of service that patients pay for. And people spend large amounts on over-the-counter medicines, or nutritional supplements, or other self-help health products; and spend extravagantly on other commodities and activities that are not only of far less value to them than their health and well-being but may be positively harmful. Cost should never be a barrier to a real need for care, but I suspect that my hang-up is not just personal but a characteristic of our NHS healthcare culture as a whole.

It is right that taxation should ensure that appropriate healthcare is available when it is really needed regardless of cost at the point of need. But I suspect that people will never fully appreciate the value of health care, nor fully recognise their own responsibility to care for their own health, while the health (or sickness) service is seen as completely 'free', as of right. Taxation subsidises public transport, but we still have to buy a ticket, unless we are entitled to free passes or discounts by virtue of age or disability. What is not acceptable is the wasteful use of taxation on services that are inefficient, unproductive or inappropriate; all of which apply to some aspects of healthcare; as is now generally acknowledged, and for which remedies are being sought.

The Glastonbury project has been subsidised by various means throughout its existence, but patients have still paid something towards their complementary therapy, even those with the greatest burden of need. In 2010 this was £14 (€16, $22) per session.[10]

Patients (that's all of us) do want to be participants in the process of care, and a willingness to participate more directly in meeting the cost of it is consistent with this desire. It should not require a huge shift in the culture of healthcare, and in the wider culture of which it is a part, to negotiate a fair and acceptable shift in this aspect of the relationship.

Interprofessional awareness: collaboration, continuity and communication

Appropriate decisions about care can only be made if practitioners are clearly aware of the limitations of their own diagnostic insight, therapeutic repertoire and personal competence, and equally aware of what others have to offer to complement their knowledge and skills or to compensate for their limitations. Appropriate permutations of care will only be worked out and implemented where this awareness is developed through active collaboration between practitioners from different disciplines. And they will only be safe and properly effective when there is good communication between all concerned and continuity of care for the patient is assured. Good awareness, collaboration and communication must be rooted in good medical education – 'learning to do medicine' (Chapter 19). And for that learning experience to lead to better permutations of care, the culture and curriculum of all aspects of medical education, conventional and unconventional will have to evolve and converge. But the process can start now; in fact has already started and could progress more rapidly. Effective collaboration, communication and continuity are best practice in mainstream medicine, although not always found there. (See 'Continuity of care' in Chapter 8.) And as the discussion of holistic and integrative practice in Chapter 15 has shown there are good examples of interprofessional care involving conventional and complementary practitioners.

Nevertheless, lack of interprofessional awareness and respect, failure of collaboration and communication, and the failure of continuity of care that results harm patients. They are dis-integrative, compound indirect risk, waste resources, and undermine care. They are a problem that does arise in mainstream medicine and that is routinely deplored. They are even more of a problem in the relationship between conventional doctors and complementary practitioners. This can be a problem even for conventional doctors providing complementary medicine. The largest group of these comprises doctors using homeopathy. (See Chapter 14, 'Experimental model'.) Those who provide NHS inpatient and outpatient services can expect to engage in the usual communication with general practitioners and other consultants – referral letters and progress reports. But because of the scarcity of NHS services for homeopathy in relation to the demand, many also work independently of the health service. Here, communication with patients' other doctors is more of a problem. Patients often take the initiative for the consultation without formal referral from their GP or consultant, but the homeopathic doctor will, or should, write to that colleague about it nevertheless. The purpose is to elicit important information about the patient's history, or insights into their problem; to share insights and information gained through the homeopathic consultation that might be helpful to the other doctor; and to explain the rationale of the treatment, its intended outcome, its interaction with other medication or treatment, difficulties that might be encountered, and so on. This is partly common good practice, and partly to help the other doctor to be aware of the different perspective on illness and healing that the homeopathic approach provides; and to invite feedback on the patient's progress from the other doctor's perspective. But a response is rarely received, despite the homeopathic doctor's conventional medical credentials. This is obviously to patients' disadvantage because it limits or even denies them the reassurance and confidence that collaboration and continuity of care between the two doctors would provide, and because it deprives both doctors of information that might have a significant influence on their respective roles in managing the problem.

This is the common experience of many practitioners of complementary medicine, whether they have conventional medical qualifications or not, who wish to collaborate with patients' doctors. Some feel too diffident or marginalised to communicate at all. Some give up because there is no response; some persist in their one-sided attempt at interprofessional care regardless.[11]

The problem is exemplified by the experience of The Nine Springs Clinic (formerly The Avenue Clinic) in Yeovil, western England. At its inception in 1980 the clinic provided acupuncture, osteopathy, homeopathy and herbal medicine. It now provides 26 therapies and 19 well-being and self-help classes. In an average week 165 patients attend for treatment and 92 for classes. Collaboration with local doctors is minimal, but this reluctance is not due to the therapists. A recent invitation to all GPs in the district, at a convenient time of day, to attend the launch of a new low-cost acupuncture clinic elicited one reply, and other than the GP giving the introductory talk only one other doctor, already using complementary medicine, attended.

Conventional medical education (the medicine taught in medical schools) may now acknowledge that there are various therapeutic methods to which students' future patients may resort. But it does not encourage serious reflection, or constructively critical thinking about the actual contribution that these may make to patients' health and well-being, and particularly to patient *care*. Individual medical schools do make various kinds of provision for this, but it may be superficial, or optional, and in any case a side show to the biomedical curriculum. However well these matters are presented to the students who avail themselves of them, as with the place of humanities in the curriculum, they are seen as incidental to and subordinate to the real business of medical qualification, which is the control of disease rather than to the care and general well-being of the person. And this may also be true of the scanty knowledge that doctors in general gain of the work of allied professions, such as Speech and Language Therapists or Occupational Therapists, on whom in fact the well-being of patients may absolutely depend.

It is probable that most non-doctor therapists, complementary as well as mainstream, know more about what doctors do and how they think than vice versa. Moreover, non-doctor therapists, mainstream and complementary, are more likely than doctors to be in tune with how patients think and feel because they are closer to the patient's illness narrative, more aware of the story of sickness. This is a generalisation, and the truth of the matter depends of course, on the quality of therapeutic relationship. But it is a proposition that needs to be taken very seriously. Because as we saw in the discussion of consultation time ('Finding the time', Chapter 15), being aware of how a patient thinks and feels, and responding appropriately to that, makes a real difference to the outcome of the transaction as a whole, whatever the specific technical component of the therapeutic black box.

It is not possible for every practitioner to be intimately acquainted with the narrative of every patient's illness and how she or he thinks and feels about it. And that is precisely why interprofessional awareness is so important; and of course interprofessional respect, and good communication. Without it, the opportunity to share our different insights to the overall benefit of the patient is lost; interprofessional *care* fails.

One of the regrettable and potentially harmful consequences of the present situation of complementary medicine is that patients sometimes do not want their doctor to know about their complementary treatment. This may be because they fear the doctor will be dismissive. Indeed some doctors will decline to continue to provide conventional care to a patient receiving complementary treatment. This forces the patient into a completely 'alternative' framework of care and denies any possibility of a complementary and integrative process of care. The reluctance to let the doctor know may reflect the patient's concern, or even certain knowledge that the doctor will not take seriously the story the patient wants to tell. The doctor may already have been dismissive of symptoms that matter to the patient but do not fit the doctor's biomedical framework. We have seen that this is a limitation acknowledged by many doctors themselves. Or patients may doubt the doctor's willingness or ability to understand why they believe that acupuncture, osteopathy, homeopathy or whatever is well suited to the way that they construe their problem. Patients may sense that a conventional biomedical response to their problem is not appropriate, or not sufficient in itself. It is certainly truly hubristic of conventional medicine to assume that the patient is wrong. And it is deeply ironic and a very serious matter that this dismissive attitude from doctors towards complementary medicine may exacerbate the indirect risk incurred when patients that have been alienated by it do not pursue conventional options that may be really important;[12] a category of risk associated with complementary medicine of which doctors often complain.

There is a somewhat impolite word that describes the attitude of those in medicine who are unwilling or unable to see beyond the frontier of the biomedical paradigm and to engage in the traffic in truth across it that is essential to interprofessional awareness: 'obscurantism'. It means to oppose enquiry, enlightenment and reform (*Concise Oxford Dictionary*). This attitude is not exclusive to doctor's attitudes to complementary medicine. It seems to be a long-standing endemic trait within the established medical profession, as the discussion of 'bad medicine' and institutional inertia in Chapter 11 suggests. Enlightened inter-professional awareness will depend in large measure on professional self-awareness.

Time, again

The one commodity necessary to every permutation of care is time. The one commodity always in short supply in the health service is time. No one working in the NHS has enough time. As we have seen in Chapter 15

('The heart of the matter', and 'Finding the time'), the effectiveness and outcome of medical consultations depend, unsurprisingly, on their quality. A number of factors determine that quality, and the length of the consultation is only one of them. But it very definitely is one of them, and is often insufficient.

Many years ago I came across the proposition in a medical journal that if ever effective methods of treatment were developed that depended on time, the NHS would collapse overnight. If that meant simply spending longer with every patient it would certainly be true. But if we learn to make best use of time, and how best to provide time, the reverse might be true – an effective health service no longer confronted by an insurmountable bow wave of unresolved illness and cost.

The problem of lack of time, particularly lack of quality time would be solved if:

- The demand for time was less.
- Available time was used more productively.
- More people were available to provide more time.
- Providing better quality time under less pressure.

All four of these possibilities would be mutually reinforcing. Do away with the bow wave of inadequately managed problems and the demand will be less. Remove the organisational constraints on the use of time, and it could be better used and more productive. Provide more people to manage the problems and more time could be made available.

The diversity of permutations of care that were mapped out at the beginning of the chapter is inevitable because many problems will require a variety of expertise and resources. This need is met within the health service by referral between conventional medical specialities and agencies. But the process can be thoroughly unproductive. It may mean that the patient is seen more *times*, but without benefiting from any more quality *time*. It can lead to what the psychologist Michael Balint who did so much to promote a better understanding of the dynamics of the doctor–patient relationship called 'the collusion of anonymity'.[13] This is a situation in which no doctor takes ownership of the problem, and more importantly, primary responsibility for the care of the *person* with the problem who becomes anonymous, vanishing from the medical gaze. The old adage about rearranging the deck chairs on the Titanic comes to mind. Certainly patients may often feel rather like a constantly rearranged deck chair as they pass from one professional or one department to another.

If all that has been said about the central importance of the therapeutic encounter, and about the characteristics and benefits of a good quality encounter is accepted and applied – in other words if time is better used – the burden of insufficient time will be less. But it will not be resolved. In addition, time must be invested in appropriate activities that will achieve the greatest health gains. This is part of the challenge of overcoming the 'bad variation' in health care that was discussed earlier in this chapter that depends on improving clinical decision making, doing things right and doing the right things; providing better quality care with the resources available, not the same quality of care for less money, getting better value for patients from the resources available to the NHS.

This process must include the provision of sufficient time of sufficient quality. More flexible, enlightened and discriminating use of the diversity of therapeutic methods available to us would help to distribute the workload so that this can be achieved. And as has already been implied, amongst the diversity of therapeutic methods available to us, and in fact heavily used though rarely included in the resources available to the NHS, are complementary therapies. Their flexible, enlightened and discriminating use within an effectively holistic and effectively integrative health care system offers one solution to the vexed problem of time for care, as well as a solution to much else that is wrong with the present system. In recent years, too, some conventional practitioners have been willing for their patients to use complementary therapies, and may have encouraged them to do so, or even adopted the therapy themselves. But this pluralism, which is discussed later in this chapter, is often not enlightened or discriminating, and certainly not integrative. There is a great deal we do not know, and need to know, about the best use of the diversity of therapeutic methods available to us.

Doctors working in the NHS are often envious of the amount of time that complementary practitioners spend with their patients. Ironically it sometimes seems that the more sceptical doctors are of complementary practitioners' methods, the more envious they are of their time; even that the more jealously they assert their professional superiority the more envious they are of the complementary practitioner's opportunities. That is a pejorative statement, I know, but it serves to highlight a sheaf of related ironies, which are that:

- We know the outcome of therapeutic encounters is enhanced by the quality of the time spent with the patient.
- Quantity of time is not always a critical factor for quality, but lack of time is often a constraint on quality.
- Orthodox practitioners deplore the lack of quality time with patients.

- Lack of quality time generates a bow wave of unresolved, poorly resolved or mismanaged problems.
- Orthodox practitioners disparage complementary practitioners, whose popularity and success they attribute to the provision of quality time.
- Lack of quality time makes the delivery of holistic care impossible.
- Holistic care improves clinical outcomes and reduces demand for other services.
- GPs observe that lack of opportunity for holistic care increases patients' use of complementary therapies.
- GPs find that the integration of complementary therapies reduces their burden of care.
- Whatever the nature of their effects, patients find complementary therapies effective.
- Doctors who use complementary therapies find them to be an effective addition to their conventional repertoire.

If patients using complementary medicine do well, conventional medicine has something to learn from complementary colleagues about their use of time, or about their techniques, or, and most probably, both.[14] Understanding the appropriate use of complementary therapies, and being willing to use them has a great deal to commend it, including a solution to the problem of time.

Pluralism, integration, or 'transcendence'

A key question for the remodelling process is the relationship between its different elements. The relationship between the different planets, stars and galaxies in the new 'medical cosmology' of David Greaves's vision.[15] I have, for example, suggested in the Introduction that the model of allied professions being in a planetary relationship around a doctor-inhabited sun is wrong, and will be different in a new model. In Chapter 11, I discuss 'border disputes' between different methodologies and paradigms; the fruitless controversy between biomedical and human perspectives; the possibilities and difficulties of rapprochement, of extending boundaries without abandoning fruitful territory already occupied. I question whether paradigms that are not commensurable, that is measurable by the same standard, may nevertheless be commensurate, or coextensive. I have talked about achieving a better 'balance' between the biomedical and holistic perspectives of health, discuss the proper meaning of 'integration', and suggested a common vocational purpose (healing) and vocational framework for different inhabitants of the medical cosmos. And I argue repeatedly that complementary medicine is *de facto* a member of this cosmos. But what is its relationship with its fellow members to be?

The argument that even with the best will in the world radically different approaches to the practice of medicine cannot be effectively integrated, in other words that methods and paradigms that are incommensurable cannot be made commensurate, is exemplified by Ted Kaptchuk and Franklin Miller in their discussion of the relative merits of opposition, integration or pluralism in the relationship between mainstream and alternative medicine.[16] Opposition and frank hostility were once the norm in this relationship, succeeded by a state of more peaceful coexistence and tolerance. But that hostility has never altogether subsided and erupted in 2010 in the libel case brought by the British Chiropractic Association against a journalist who criticised the validity of its treatment claims; and in the vote by British Medical Association (BMA) representatives to exclude homeopathy from the NHS, and the designation of homeopathy as 'witchcraft' by one of those representatives, despite its regulated use by many of their fellow BMA members.

Despite this simmering hostility, however, it is probably true to say that integration of many complementary and alternative (CAM) therapies within mainstream medicine is a *fait accompli.* This includes long established therapies like homeopathy and acupuncture, but also more recently established treatments like aromatherapy and reflexology which have found a place in palliative care. This statement needs to be qualified by my earlier comments about the limited nature of some programmes of integration. And by the exclusion of therapies sometimes lodged under the umbrella of CAM and characterised by Kaptchuk and Miller as 'overtly supernatural', such as crystal therapy, from any such framework. Some sceptics, however, would characterise the healing stimulus claimed for homeopathy, acupuncture or reflexology to be as 'supernatural' as crystal therapy. (The language of almost superstitious fear that crops up in some references to CAM is interesting, and indicates the difficulty that some critics who challenge the rationality of CAM have in engaging with it rationally.)

Pluralism allows for irreconcilable differences between systems of thought and practice, but respects patient choice in the matter, based on frank discussion of the difference, and on the implications of the choice. For example, a mainstream practitioner would explain the risk of foregoing a conventional treatment of proven efficacy in favour of an alternative treatment of unproven efficacy and uncertain effectiveness. A homeopath would explain that a conventional drug might suppress or modify the body's natural healing response to an illness.

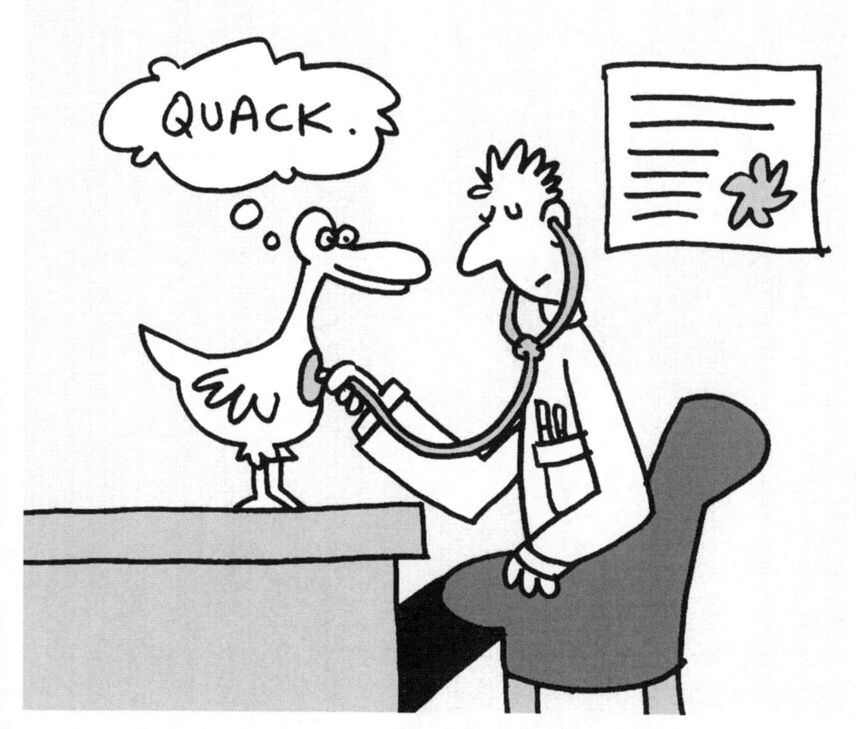

Figure 16.3 CAM practitioners are still regarded with some scepticism.

This is the relationship favoured by Kaptchuk and Miller, because:

- Diverse medical systems, based on fundamentally different medical theories and methods of validating treatments inhabit the medical landscape.
- Despite many irreconcilable epistemological (theories of knowledge) and practical differences, mainstream and alternative medicine share the goals of promoting health and relieving suffering.
- Both mainstream and alternative medicine should respect the autonomy of competent patients to make therapeutic choices in consultation with mainstream physicians or alternative providers.

The integration model does not work, they argue, because it does not offer a coherent medical framework. The epistemological, philosophical and practical differences defy coherent integration. And integrative practitioners will be unable to give patients a consistent and clear rationale for therapeutic options.

This is a very helpful analysis, although I don't agree with it and have proposed a different framework for this kind of relationship. What is

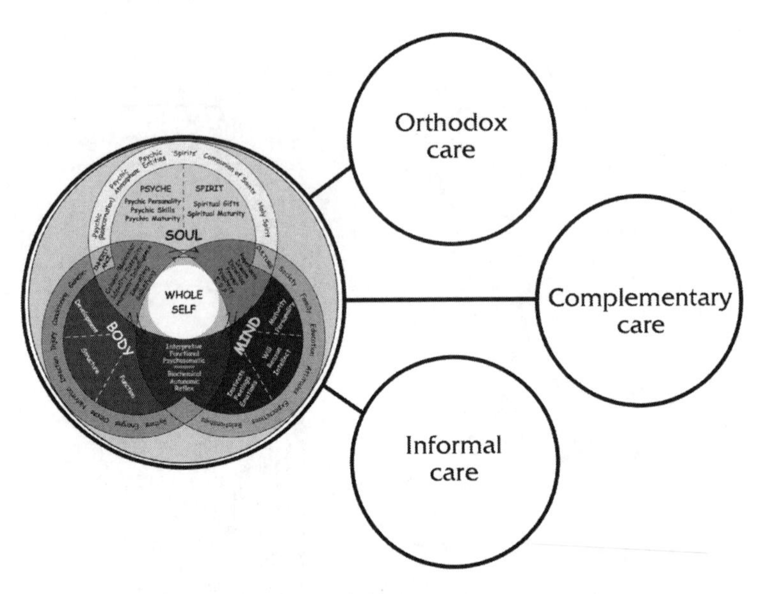

Figure 16.4 *Pluralism. (See also Figure 12.1.)*

particularly helpful about it is that it applies to different diagnostic and therapeutic perspectives *within* mainstream medicine as well. There has always been an element of disagreement and competition between different schools of mainstream thought and practice; between medical (non-surgical) and surgical treatments, or psycho-dynamic and pharmacological approaches to mental illness for instance.

Different views of the degree of integration of the care process are shown in Figures 16.4–16.6.

I have recently become acquainted with the world of pain medicine. Chronic pain is a very difficult clinical challenge. Approaches to pain management range from the narrowly biomedical and mechanistic to the broadly holistic; the latter represented by the British Pain Society's philosophy and ethics special interest group. There is a comparable spectrum in Psychiatry represented at what I suppose cynics might call the supernatural end of the spectrum, by the Royal College of Psychiatrists' Spirituality special interest group.[17] It will be evident from the whole tone of this book that my own philosophy of medicine attracts me to both these special interest groups. But I have also been immensely grateful for the anaesthetics and analgesics used in my own medical care, and respectful of the value of psychotropic drugs in my practice.

The point is that medicine cannot be segregated into different territories with clear-cut boundaries. There are tribal districts for sure, whose inhabitants defend themselves aggressively, often on the principle that the best

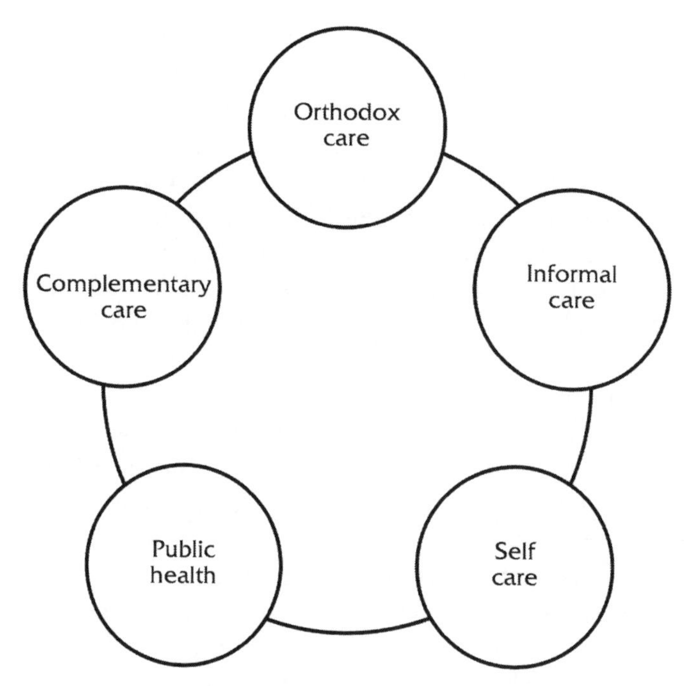

Figure 16.5 *Integration. All a part, but often apart.*

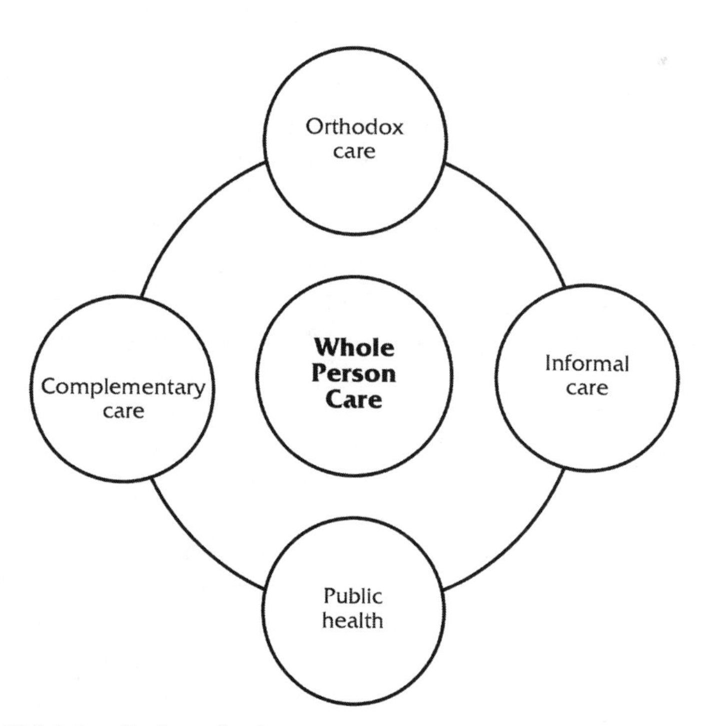

Figure 16.6 *Integrative 'cosmology'.*

form of defence is attack. But a large part of the population of the medical landscape is relatively undogmatic, eclectic and pragmatic with regard to what makes sense to their patients and what 'works' for them. This eclectic approach can be likened to the attitude of many good contemporary musicians to the different musical styles and idioms which can attract somewhat dogmatic attitudes amongst their adherents – classical v. pop, for instance. These more eclectic musicians argue that the idiom is not the issue; there is only good music and bad music. There are certain principles of musicality and musicianship that distinguish the one from the other. Good music can be played on a variety of instruments and in a variety of styles. The same may be true, metaphorically, for medicine.

I have mentioned David Greaves' appealing use of the concept of 'cosmology' to represent a coherent structure for the diversity of medical thought and practice.[15] It is a broader concept than paradigm, embracing the moral and cultural aspects of medicine as well as the scientific and the technical, the practical as well as the theoretical. And a cosmos doesn't shift, it evolves; which, although I have suggested that a minor revolution of a Kuhnian kind may be necessary, is more in tune with the picture of evolution and struggle, and metamorphosis that I have also described. David Greaves also introduces the concept of 'transcendence' as part of the evolution of the new medical cosmos. This implies that those parts of the old cosmology that are fit for purpose will occupy their appropriate orbit in the new, and those that are not will be subsumed or will not survive.

In other words, this is a process of *reconciliation,* whose definition in my *Concise Oxford Dictionary* has elements of friendship after estrangement, healing, and harmonisation. As in the reconciliation of parties to any relationship, it requires the surrender, the letting go of attitudes and behaviours that inhibit the fruitfulness of the relationship and the acceptance of differences that are valuable to it. This is not to diminish the special qualities that each brings to the relationship but to enhance them in the creation of a partnership that is greater than the sum of the parts.

Another, more obscure concept that I find helpful in exploring the ideal relationship of the elements of a new model is *co-inherence.* This term was coined by the poet, novelist, theologian and literary critic Charles Williams (1886–1945), a friend and colleague of C.S. Lewis and J.R. Tolkien. It is primarily a theological concept, but has the more general sense of relationship within a union; things that exist in essential relationship with one another, as innate components of one another. For example, people living together through the sharing of tasks and responsibilities, as in a community. For me the concept of co-inherence has a quality of intimacy within a common purpose that cosmology lacks, but not the sense of structural relationship that cosmology implies. The pluralist model is unsatisfactory because although it proclaims mutual respect and patient choice it retains the competitive element of the present model. It risks complicating rather than facilitating choice, and is likely to continue the dis-integrative trend in modern medicine.

From this variety of concepts and metaphors we can derive a set of principles for a new model of medicine that will work:

- The goals of medicine are the service of healing and the relief of suffering.
- Medicine is the disciplined use of human knowledge and skill in pursuit of these goals.
- Many human skills and attributes contribute to this task, but it is fulfilled and made effective through a personal relationship between practitioners and patients.
- This diversity of knowledge, skills and attributes has common ground in their common purpose and values.
- These common principles constitute an essential relationship between the varieties of medical practice.
- In this relationship varieties of medical practice are united by shared tasks and responsibilities as members of a health care community.
- Distinctions such as orthodox/unorthodox and mainstream/alternative misunderstand and misrepresent this essential relationship.
- There is only good medicine and bad medicine.
- Good medicine fulfils its goals and observes its values.
- Good medicine is defined by the 'musicality' and 'musicianship' of its practitioners rather than the instruments they play.
- Medicine's tasks and responsibilities are moral and cultural as well as scientific and technical.
- Medicine is deeply implicated in the life of the society of which it is a part in fulfilling these responsibilities.

It is obvious that to build a model of medicine on these principles that really works will require a lot of effort. They will have to be worked on. There is little sense of the cohesion that they imply in contemporary mainstream medical practice; let alone of the co-inherence. And even less in its relationship with unorthodox practice. This is inevitable because there is too little exploration of common goals and values.

There is no coherent health care community. We are too much preoccupied with differences in instrumentation and musical idiom, and too little concerned with musicality and musicianship, the counterpoint, syncopation and harmonies that make for good music and good medicine.

Cross fertilisation between musical idioms occurs when musicians listen to one another and play together, transcending their stylistic and technical boundaries, and this is commonplace nowadays. Cross fertilisation between medical idioms does occur, when practitioners listen to each other and work together, and with good results. There are health care teams that are truly integrative, and forums for exploring shared tasks and responsibilities where differences and boundaries are transcended, for example in cancer care.[18] But this quality of teamwork is not guaranteed by bringing people together, and "there is, however, anecdotal evidence of professional enmities, autocratic practice, and hierarchical boundaries making teams dysfunctional and participation stressful". Such forums for developing a sense of community in care are not commonplace, and they should be – from an early stage in the education of all health care practitioners, whatever their preferred idiom. (See 'Interprofessional education', in Chapter 19.) I was 30 years into my medical career before I gained any real insight into the work of Occupational Therapists and Speech Therapists (Chapter 13) – their particular understanding of illness and disability, and of the means of mobilising the resources of body and mind to overcome or cope with these; experience gained fortuitously as part of a project to develop a shared terminology for electronic medical records.[19]

But the variety of therapeutic methods and insights that comprised my training and experience as a general practitioner was actually no less diverse. The care of women before, during and after childbirth, the care of people with cancer, and the care of people with psychological illness are just three examples of the diversity of routine general practice. The insights that each provides, and requires, into human nature and into the way the human organism works, and the dynamics of health, illness and healing, and the skills developed to go with these insights, have many differences; the 'management' of birth and death being perhaps the obvious extremes. But they are co-extensive, they have an essential co-inherence. They represent a common purpose and common values. To express and fulfil that purpose and those values properly they must be rooted in the ten core principles of the therapeutic relationship that I have proposed (Chapter 14, 'The heart of the matter').

But this diversity of skills and insights, the often unexplained complexity that they reveal, and the common ground of purpose, values and relationship that they share, is mirrored in many varieties of clinical experience. The Occupational Therapist, the Osteopath and the General Practioner all occupy the same medical 'cosmos'. Their work is co-extensive, and there is a co-inherence of principle. They are members (potentially) of a health care community with inter-related and interdependent tasks and responsibilities. They share, we hope, a vocation to whole-making and healing. They are all an integral part of our culture and the fabric of our society.

There is no reason or excuse for segregating the different therapeutic modalities in our medical cosmos. The explanation for it is medical tribalism, scientific tunnel vision, and paradigm paralysis. There is more than enough common ground to allow the 'traffic in truth' that will render existing border disputes obsolete, transcend the differences, and enrich our understanding of human health and healing.

Regulation

All health care professionals and all services within the mainstream UK health care system are statutorily regulated one way or another and established informal volunteer organisations such as St John Ambulance have required programmes of training and certification. Registered health care professionals using complementary medicine are regulated by their professional body (e.g. the General Medical Council for doctors) in association with the organisation responsible for standards in their complementary discipline (e.g. the Faculty of Homeopathy for statutorily registered health care professionals using homeopathy). Osteopaths and Chiropractors are now statutorily registered and regulated, and other leading complementary therapies are on the path to regulation. But some complementary practitioners are resistant to such formal control of their practice, reluctant to subordinate themselves to a system that is so closely associated with the orthodox medical establishment and the biomedical model.

The fact that there is a large part of the landscape of healthcare occupied by practitioners of therapeutic methods loosely described as complementary which are wholly unregulated, other than under common law, creates problems. There is obvious risk to patients from therapists whose professional and ethical standards and competence are uncertain. The appropriateness or effectiveness of the therapy they offer may also be uncertain. That risk may only be to the patient's pocket, but much more serious is the risk that more appropriate or more effective treatment that the patient badly needs may be neglected.

It is arguable that no-one should be able to promote their activities as being in the service of health or healing without submitting to some kind of regulation that ensures the integrity and safety of what they do. For example, there is currently discussion within the Christian Healing Ministry about the need for some kind of certification of members of parish teams that offer the ministry. There is concern among some involved in the ministry that it may attract people whose primary motive is self-aggrandisment. (This is a temptation that is not unknown among some members of the medical profession.)

It is difficult to know whether, where and how to draw an absolutely rigid line between activities that should be regulated and those that need not be. There are people of great integrity with a genuine vocation to help others and the personal gifts and attributes necessary to do so, and people practising traditions of folk medicine within their community, whose activities would not be susceptible to regulation or for whom it would not be appropriate. It is probably reasonable that such people should be judged on the basis that 'by their fruits you shall know them'. But those who promote themselves publicly, and for gain, as in any way offering better health or healing should be willing to submit to scrutiny and regulation appropriate to what they do. Perhaps the Trade Descriptions Act has something to offer where such activities are clearly on 'the fringe'?

An essential ingredient of the solution to achieving appropriate regulation of all who offer healthcare will be a change of attitude among the health care elite – the orthodox professionals – to those outside the mainstream. The best way for the regulated professions to encourage similar standards in other practitioners, to recognise where such standards actually already exist despite their misgivings, and to encourage them where they do not, is to engage with the practitioners concerned. This would also serve to identify those whose work is plainly undeserving of any credibility or trust. If this implies a 'holier than thou' attitude, it is not meant to negate all that has already been said about the substantial and very real benefits for orthodox practitioners in learning from, and learning to collaborate with the best of their complementary colleagues. I'm referring to a section of the complementary 'field' whose practitioners are not willing to engage in that way. The majority of established complementary practitioners are only too keen to do so, if they are made welcome.

Unfortunately the plethora of unregulated alternative practitioners, dubious practices and over-the-counter health care products alienates many doctors towards all forms of complementary therapy. Doctors who are well aware of the limitations of the biomedical model and the vagaries of the U.K. health service and who desire change, refuse any closer rapport even with the best complementary medical practice because of the activities of what they see as its lunatic fringe. For some doctors all complementary medicine is tarred with the brush of its most worrying manifestations. Nevertheless, it is by extending dialogue and improving rapport that a clear understanding of the need for whatever regulation is appropriate will emerge, and an effective system of regulation will develop.

References

1 Vitaliano PP, Zhang J, Scanlan JM. Is caregiving hazardous to one's physical health? *Psychol Bull.* 2003; 129:946–972.

2 Fox AS. Carers and the NHS. *Br J Gen Pract.* 2010; 60:575;462–463.

3 Nazareth I, Murray E. Promoting self care for minor illness: worthwhile but hard to achieve. *Br Med J.* 2010; 340 c2913:262–263.

4 Haslam D. Who cares? *Br J Gen Pract.* 2007; 57(545):987–993.

5 Hasegawa H, Reilly D, Mercer SW, Bikker AP. Holism in primary care: the views of Scotland's general practitioners. *Primary Health Care Research and development* 2005; 6:320–328.

6 Paterson C. Primary Health care transformed: complementary and orthodox medicine complementing each other. *Complement Ther Med.* 2000; 8:47–49.

7 Mulley A. Improving productivity in the NHS. *Br Med J.* 2010; 341 c3965: 213–214.

8 Appleby J, Ham C, Imison C, Jennings M. *Improving NHS productivity: more with the same not more of the same.* London: King's Fund; 2010. Available online at www.kingsfund.org.uk/publications/index.html.

9 Peters D, Chaitow L, Harris G, Morrison S. *Integrating Complementary Therapies in Primary Care.* Edinburgh: Churchill Livingstone; 2002.

10 Welford R. Personal communication.

11 Swayne J. Homeopathy in the NHS: a holistic and interprofessional challenge. *Journal of Interprof Care* 1985; 9(1):53–59.

12 Smithson J, Paterson C, Britten N *et al.* Cancer patients' experiences of using complementary therapies: polarization and integration. *J Health Serv Res Policy* 2010; 15 Suppl 2:54–61.

13 Balint M. *The Doctor His Patient and the Illness.* London: Pitman Medica; 1968

14 Doherty M, Dieppe P. The "placebo" response in osteoarthritis and its implications for clinical practice. *Os Car.* 2009; 17:1255–1262.

15 Greaves D. Reflections on a new medical cosmology. *J Med Ethics* 2002; 28;81–85.

16 Kaptchuk TJ, Miller FG. What is the best and most ethical model for the relationship between mainstream and alternative medicine: Opposition Integration or Pluralism? *Acad Med.* 2005; 80(3):286–290.

17 Timms P. editor. Help is at Hand series of leaflets. *Spirituality and Mental Health.* London: The Royal College of Psychiatrists; 2010. Available online at http://tinyurl.com/yfnuo4c.

18 Taylor C, Munro AJ, Glynne-Jones R *et al.* Multidisciplinary team working in cancer: what is the evidence? *Br Med J.* 2010; 340 c951:743–745.

19 Swayne J. A common language of care? *J Interprof Care* 1993; 7:29–35.

17

MEDICINE, CULTURE AND SOCIETY
The context of care

Summary

- Real change requires a change in the cultural context that influences the way we do medicine and that is powerfully influenced by the way we do it.
- Medicine is susceptible to cultural beliefs about what it means to be human, to be a person; and about the values and virtues that define our shared humanity.
- It is not alone in this, but has a special responsibility because of its privileged place in human affairs. It must have the 'humble hubris' to engage with the mystery of human nature as it is expressed in health, illness and healing.
- Medicine has the opportunity for leadership in respect of social issues, and has a responsibility for advocacy that can promote social healing.
- This responsibility requires diligent attention to 'the virtues in medical practice' and medicine's own moral standards.
- Personal care and advocacy will quite often require that clinicians resist inappropriate expectations and demands.
- Medicine is inescapably implicated in the whole mystery of the human condition and the meaning of life.

A push-me-pull-you relationship

Whatever the implications of political change, I have no doubt that it is from within clinical practice that real change must come, and that the therapeutic encounter is the key. But the role of clinical practice has cultural significance that needs to be clearly understood. Real change requires a change in the cultural context within which we do medicine that

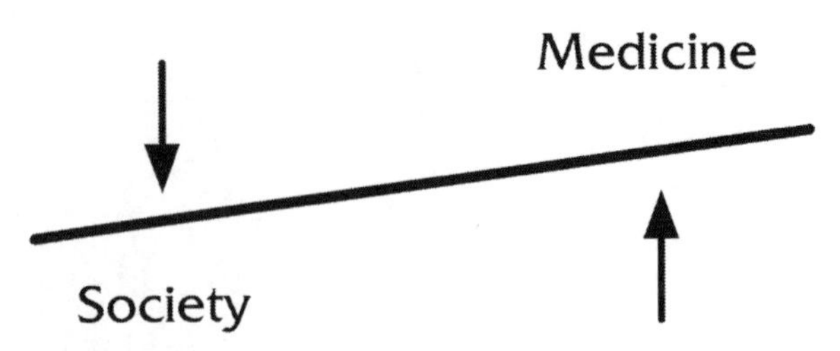

Figure 17.1 *A push-me-pull-you relationship.*

powerfully influences the way we do it and that is powerfully influenced *by* the way we do it. It is a 'push-me-pull-you' relationship.

The closeness of the relationship between medicine and society inevitably means that the remodelling of medicine has implications for the remodelling of society. This is not a radical statement. This medical shaping of social attitudes happens all the time. Whenever a general practitioner declines to give an expected but unnecessary antibiotic for a self-limiting viral illness and explains why and is understood, she is promoting a small scale change in the model of health, illness and healthcare held by the individual who previously expected it, and possibly their family, and even their friends and neighbours. When the members of the British Medical Association vote for or against assisted suicide they are influencing or responding to social attitudes. They are debating the goals of medicine and the working of the medical model. In earlier chapters we have looked at other examples of medicine's influence on society and the social and political control of medical practice. So we are entirely familiar with the fact that people's values and aspirations – personal, communal and political – influence medical thought and practice, and vice versa (Figure 17.1).

Medicine is susceptible to cultural beliefs about what it means to be human, to be a person; and about the values and virtues that define our shared humanity. And because of the closeness of the relationship with society and the intimacy of its relationship with the individual patient, medicine has a responsibility for forming those values and virtues and an opportunity to do so. And its responsibility is to do so in a way that is creative, healing, whole making and integrative.

Of course medicine is not alone in this. The teaching profession has a responsibility for education that is creative, whole making and integrative; the legal profession for justice; politicians for social cohesion; and so on. It is a common responsibility of our shared humanity, individually or as a member of an organisation or institution.

A special relationship

> The principles of medical ethics are statements of the right and good that derive from the ends and purposes of medical activity – healing, helping and caring in a special kind of human relationship. (Pellegrino and Thomasma[1])

But medicine, I suggest, has a special responsibility because it has a special relationship. It touches people, literally and metaphorically, at many points in their lives, from the cradle to the grave. And these points are often moments of intimacy; vulnerable moments, moments of uncertainty and introspection, moments of loneliness, fear and hope; times of crisis in the best sense – times of decision, turning points. (The point we are at in the evolution of Western medicine.) In the past, when medicine's power to control events was limited, the 'crisis' in the course of a disease was the point at which the body's natural healing resources would prevail or fail. That drama of natural healing is rare in modern medicine in the developed world, but there are still many critical moments at which those natural resources can be invoked, or, unfortunately, neglected and ignored.

This special responsibility and special relationship implicates medicine deeply in shaping a healthy society and in resisting cultural tendencies that pervert its goals and undermine its healing vocation. Tendencies that devalue the person, that are de-meaning, are prevalent in our culture and reflected in the way we do medicine. This is why David Greaves seeks a more pervasive influence of the study of the humanities in medical education. Its aim, he suggests, should be "a permeation and change of orientation of the culture of medicine, which will transform not only clinical practice but also the theoretical basis and social structures of medicine and healthcare". The aim is not only the humanising of practitioners, but the humanising of medicine.[2] My argument, too, which Pellegrino and Thomasma proclaim, as we shall see, is that this reorientation both requires and can promote a similar reorientation within society itself.

Humble hubris

In his book *Medical Hubris*, a reply to Ivan Illich's *Medical Nemesis*, David Horrobin suggests that the medical profession needs to exercise 'controlled hubris', using its authority to influence people, to persuade or require them to do things for their own good that they would not otherwise do for themselves.[3] At the end of Chapter 5, I develop this idea in a different direction, suggesting that because of its privileged place in human affairs medicine must have the hubris that dares to engage with the mystery of human nature as it is expressed in health, illness and healing, but that this must be a 'humble hubris.' Medicine must aspire to a quality of service and relationship that affirms the unique value of every person it meets in the therapeutic encounter. We clinicians must presume to know enough about human nature to be able to make that affirmation; must assume responsibility for encouraging an equal self-affirmation in the patient; and must be courageous enough to do so. That is hubris; a promethean task, stealing fire from the gods for the well-being of humanity, and seeking to imbue each patient with that fire.[i]

It must be a humble hubris, rooted in the awareness that we are not omniscient or omnipotent. The awareness that there will always be a gap between what we know and what there is to be known; awareness of the limits of our discernment, empathy and skill, and of our own vulnerability.

Even if we have a strong vocation to medicine these qualities do not come easily. Nor are they easily developed in the course of our medical education; nor easily preserved amidst the pressures of everyday practice. Medicine remodelled must allow for their development and make space for them.

These are somewhat pious sentiments, but they are not platitudes. They need to be spelt out because if medicine is to fulfil its role in society, and have a salutary influence on its culture, it must demonstrate authority. Not the authority of power, but of wisdom, discernment and integrity. This 'natural' authority can only be learned, earned and demonstrated through our relationships – with our peers and teachers during our education and training, with our colleagues in practice, with other organisations and institutions that we deal with, and above all with our patients. Our authority to comfort, counsel and heal, our authority as advocates, and where necessary as leaders, will not be earned by knowledge and skill alone but by the way we demonstrate these qualities of relationship. In Chapter 15 I propose ten core principles for the therapeutic encounter, the starting point for the remodelling process. They are not only essential attributes for patient care, but the foundation of medicine's wider authority in the community.

Proper hubris

Medicine shows strong leadership in confronting a number of social ills. A good example is the problem of social and health inequalities described in

---

i Prometheus was a demigod who stole fire from Olympus for the benefit of humankind and as punishment was chained to a rock to be preyed upon by vultures.

Chapter 4. Medicine has been forthright in its analysis of these problems, for example in the Black report (1977).[4] This was commissioned by a Labour government but sidelined by an incoming Conservative government that was "distinctly cool on the subject of health inequalities".[5] This brief quote is from an editorial in the *British Medical Journal* introducing a new report, the Marmot review, published under the title *Fair Society, Healthy Lives*.[6] The authors of the editorial hope that more public debate about the sort of society we want to live in might provide a context for greater political courage, in contrast to the poor record of policy success in this area in the past – because we are all adversely affected and our lives diminished by the growing gap in health status between the poorest and the richest in our society. Michael Marmot, was chair of the World Health Organisation Commission on the social determinants of health and author of the new report that proclaimed, "Social injustice is killing people on a grand scale", and asked the question "Why treat people . . . without changing what makes them sick?" Its report has had a powerful impact around the world, and it is chastening that the criticisms and challenges it presents should be as pertinent to the state of the nation's health in the U.K. as anywhere else.

The Black report, the WHO Commission report and the Marmot review collectively are an example of the proper controlled hubris advocated by David Horrobin, and are good examples of medicine seeking to fulfil its responsibility for advocacy. They represent just the right mixture of science with wisdom, discernment and integrity that makes for true authority. Even so, lamentably little has been achieved in the UK, particularly by comparison with the Nordic countries and Japan, as a review in the *British Medical Journal* of two books on the subject reveals.[7] The reviewer offers the chastening observation that, "The health professions, which for the last 30 years have had excellent evidence about the importance of inequality to health outcomes, have not offered the leadership to combat the problem". Despite a general increase in life expectancy, inequalities in premature mortality between different geographical areas and between the poorest and richest in our society are still increasing.[8]

Social healing

Fairness, equality, social justice are big themes. They featured prominently in the 2010 UK general election, and are a proper target for medical advocacy. Medicine can make the diagnosis, and suggest a treatment strategy, but it can't deliver the solution because "the key drivers of health inequalities lie outside the healthcare system";[9] particularly the physical, social, emotional and educational environment in childhood. Medicine can and must, however, reflect those principles in its determination to behave accordingly towards everyone in its care. It can encourage the public debate, and help ordinary folk who are the 'victims' of these circumstances to be part of the debate, and the solution, by making those circumstances and the need for change and the possibilities of change part of the therapeutic conversation. (See 'Health promotion', in Chapter 15.) This means that the conversation within the therapeutic encounter must include the 'story of sickness', because those circumstances are part of the story. It requires compassion, and at least a degree of empathy, which we know can empower patients to take more control of their lives (Chapter 8). In the book *A guide for the perplexed* that I quoted in the introduction, Schumacher also writes about three ingredients necessary for this kind of empowerment, and for promoting change.[10] They are faith, awareness and adequacy: faith that change is possible, which encourages awareness of what is preventing change and what is conducive to change, which develops adequacy – the capability to do something about it. Fairness, equality and social justice will require top down solutions, but they also require a bottom up momentum. And by encouraging faith, awareness and adequacy in its everyday conversation with patients, medicine can help to promote this, and to make the 'victims of circumstance' agents of change. This is the social equivalent of illness as the agent of healing.

The gradient of the virtues

In the prologue to this last part of the book, and earlier in Chapter 9, I suggest that the minor revolution that is required to achieve the remodelling process includes a minor revolution in medical morality. This, perhaps startling claim does not mean the institution of some kind of medical puritanism. Most health professionals will still drink alcohol, make love, and enjoy a good comedy. But it will probably require that they take a stand against some of the moral attitudes of our present medical, social and political culture. Let me explain. Or rather, let me call upon the work of authors who have examined this question in depth to help me explain. In *The Virtues in Medical Practice*, Edmund Pellegrino and David Thomasma, whom I have quoted already, question the reliability of the profession's moral compass.[1] The challenge they offer is very clear:

> Should the health professions . . . reshape our ethical codes to conform to the ethos of the market place, which legitimates self interest over beneficence and makes vices out of most of medicine's traditional virtues? Or should doctors stand

> firm in their belief that being a physician imposes specific obligations that forbid turning oneself into an entrepreneur, a businessman, or an agent of fiscal, social or economic policy?

They highlight the influence of technology, and the changing roles of the medical profession in response to public and private expectations. They remark how policy makers want physicians to be gatekeepers of society's resources and instruments of the bureaucratic 'apparatus'; while 'patients want absolute autonomy and see health professionals increasingly as instruments of their wishes.' They talk about the 'consumer model' and the 'negotiated contract' model of health care. They are concerned about the 'industrial model' of medical research that makes research a commodity, product oriented rather than truth orientated.

They are writing about the U.S.A. where some of these issues are magnified, but they are not so different in the UK. We have discussed instances of them in earlier chapters. And they all undermine medicine's moral obligation to place the best interests of the individual patient at the heart of the healthcare process. They refer explicitly to a moral malaise in medicine. Some other instances (some theirs, some my own) include:

- Decisions based on fear of litigation.
- Co-operation with early discharge policies contrary to best practice.
- Denying patient choice on financial grounds.
- Submitting to policies contrary to clinical judgement.
- Colluding in medical entrepreneurism.
- Colluding in the marketing of treatments or tests of dubious necessity or validity.
- Tolerating the level of serious adverse drug reactions.
- Failure to take risks on behalf of the patient.

The common excuse for health professionals failing in their duty of trust within the therapeutic relationship, they say, is legitimate self-interest. And that is unacceptable.

But is this criticism fair? Surely medicine has shown great moral leadership in promoting many changes of benefit to society? Certainly it has. Medicine's longstanding condemnation of health inequalities is one still topical example of medicine providing powerful advocacy on behalf of the sick, and seeking to fulfil its moral responsibility towards the society in which it is embedded. (Bearing in mind the reservations about the quality of the profession's leadership in this respect, quoted earlier.) It remains to be seen whether and when new initiatives will lead to effective change, but the 'campaign' has two clear advantages. These are a blatant social ill to challenge, and a strong professional consensus about the need for change.

It also represents a high point on a not altogether admirable gradient in the moral relationship between medicine and society. It is difficult to know how to describe this gradient, but I think it is best described as a gradient of 'the virtues in medical practice'. To give a simple indication of what this means: if medicine's advocacy in pursuit of a remedy for social inequalities that are at the root of much sickness and suffering represents a high point on the gradient, then medicine's complicity in torture and the medical atrocities of the Nazi regime represent its lowest.

It may be something of a shock to you, as it was to me when I first read *The Virtues*, to be asked to think of medicine like this. But its harsh analysis of the potential moral failings in medicine does put many of the remodelling issues in an uncomfortably clear perspective. Because if medicine is to look different in the future, the implications of its social and cultural responsibilities have to be addressed.

Key 'bands' in the spectrum of relationship between medicine and society, in addition to advocacy, include:

- People's respect for medicine.
- Its role in ethical controversies.
- Its influence on life styles.
- Its role in shaping and implementing public health policy.
- Its role in occupational health and health and safety regulation.
- Its role in shaping and responding to expectations of health care.
- Its role in shaping attitudes to life and death.

This is a very broad spectrum. It reflects both the high degree of medicine's responsibility towards the society and the culture to which it belongs; and it reflects its vulnerability to social and cultural trends and influences that may not be consistent with its virtues, vocation and goals. The way it copes with these – the responsibility and the vulnerability – determines its place on the 'gradient of the virtues' in any particular instance.

Issues raised by this entanglement of medicine with society are sometimes straightforward, sometimes impossibly difficult, and sometimes very subtle. Where there is an obvious social ill to be challenged and a common will to do so, as with health inequalities, the responsibility is clear, and the issue of vulnerability arises only in respect of medicine's subordinate role to government. Either it prevails in its campaign or it fails.

In the UK this issue is clear as far as medicine is concerned and there is broad consensus, whatever the political will or resources available to effect the necessary changes. In America, where the debate about healthcare reforms has been fierce, the situation is more difficult because of the lack of consensus. In the UK the medical profession is at a high point on the gradient of virtues in this regard. But in America its position is much more ambivalent because of the degree of medicine's collusion with the status quo that deprives millions of health care. In respect of the social determinants of health, and public health policy, medicine in the USA is some way down the gradient of the virtues.

Abortion is one of the impossibly difficult issues. It is doctors, usually, who perform abortions, but others who provide support for the patient. It is a procedure that carries physical and psychological risk and requires professional care and support. Abortion is a legal procedure in the UK. But the legislation is controversial, and the range of ethical opinions extreme, depending on different understandings of the value of the life of the embryo, the stage at which it becomes a person, the 'right to life', and the freedom of the mother. Some doctors and nurses will have nothing to do with abortion because it conflicts with their belief in these matters. Some see participation in abortion as wholly consistent with the goals of medicine and high on the gradient of the virtues; others quite the contrary. This is just one area where clinical, ethical, social and political factors interact in very complex ways, and there are no right answers; except, of course, in the judgement of those who hold strongly to one particular point of view. But there is no escaping medicine's role in all this.

Acquiescence or resistance

A difficult issue of quite a different kind arises when local or national management or policy decisions direct or constrain the actions or decisions of clinicians in everyday practice. Very often this has to do with the cost of a particular drug, service or procedure; perhaps in relation to the number of people who will benefit from it, or the evidence for its efficacy. Inevitably this often limits the freedom of the patient to receive the treatment of their choice, as well as the freedom of the clinician to do what he or she believes is best for the patient. Recent examples range from the provision of certain expensive drugs for 'minority' diseases, through the closure of some small hospital units, to the availability of homeopathy on the NHS.

Many consequences of the frequent 'redisorganisation' of the health service have made it difficult for doctors to exercise clinical freedom and for patients to feel valued. To be treated like an item on a conveyor belt in order to comply with a bureaucratically acceptable transfer time in an accident and emergency department, may provide *efficient* care but it does not provide *humane* care, as Nigel Rawlinson explains so eloquently (see the end of Chapter 4). Another consequence has been the emergence of new risks – susceptibility to hospital acquired infection due to rapid turnover in bed occupancy, inadequate out-of-hours cover in primary care, poor clinical outcomes in NHS treatment centres.

Organisational problems like this might be variously attributed to collusion, acquiescence, inertia or a feeling of impotence on the part of health professionals. Whenever they result in a diminished quality of care they constitute, to some degree, the 'moral malaise' that Pellegrino and Thomasma describe; they allow medicine to slip down the gradient of virtues. This is a harsh thing to say, but whenever a practitioner follows the path of least resistance when facing a decision on behalf of a patient when another course of action would be better, he or she is moving down the gradient. This includes failure to take risks on behalf of the patient.

The respect in which the healthcare professions are generally held by the public in the UK would seem to reflect their high position on the gradient of the virtues. The great majority of people are immensely grateful for the skill and the care they receive, and rightly so, and are likely to blame errors and failings on the system rather than on the individuals who work in it. But this respect imposes great responsibility to promote and preserves essential virtues within society. Health professionals seem to have become pawns on an organisational chess board. They have also become trapped within a biomedical framework that has narrowed the focus of patient care, greatly to its detriment, as this book has been at pains to demonstrate and explain. This is not the way it should be, and medicine's acquiescence reflects a failure of its social and cultural responsibility, a vocational failure, in fact; partly despite and partly because of the respect in which it is held. It is an example of a subtle failure of advocacy that it allows a 'system' to operate in which these organisational problems and vocational lapses have been able to arise.

Pellegrino and Thomasma state the problem unequivocally:

> The physician – and the nurse and other health professionals as well – are at the moral centre of health care. They are society's delegated advocates for the sick. Ultimately they are the instruments through which health policies are implemented. They are the final common pathway through which all that happens to patients must go. They have enormous moral power if they choose to exercise it. No one can make health professionals do what is thought to be harmful to patients. As long as the reasons for resistance encompass the good of the sick, doctors can prevail against unethical practices and policies, and win public support for their resistance. Unfortunately, their collective professional societies are often so patently self-serving that they lose all moral credibility.[1]

Medicine aspires to bring relief from suffering and better quality of life where there is illness, disease or disability; or where there is the threat of these. Its first responsibility is towards the person affected or threatened in this way. Its second is for advocacy on their behalf. That advocacy may concern those involved in the personal life of the patient, the family perhaps. It will require a variable mix of sensible science, psychological insight and pastoral and interpersonal skills. At the other end of the spectrum of responsibility that advocacy will concern policy makers at various levels of government – to represent and inform; and sometimes to resist.

Personal care and advocacy will quite often require that clinicians resist the expectations and demands of others that disadvantage, disenfranchise or de-mean their patient. Those others may include family members, the local community, and perhaps the government. The expectations and demands will range from inappropriate medication to the imposition of targets or restrictions that compromise clinical judgement. Clinicians are better at the kind of advocacy that promotes enlightened health care, than at the advocacy that resists unenlightened care. In fact, they are often acquiescent in health care policy of that kind, even while lamenting it. Why is this?

Recently I was part of a small group of university contemporaries meeting informally to reflect on life at retirement. They all had considerable responsibility and influence in their various roles and occupations, and all identified areas in their respective fields of experience where creative change was badly needed, but where inertia and resistance to change prevailed. The reasons they gave were primarily bureaucracy and fear; fear, often within a bureaucracy as well as on the frontline – of rocking the boat, of loss of job security, of litigation perhaps. A third constraint in some instances was ideology, or the impasse created by competing ideologies.

Perhaps medicine's acquiescence in policy and practice that it distrusts or deprecates has similar causes? Which may not be so different from those attributed to the resistance to innovation and institutional inertia discussed in Chapter 11 in the context of David Wooton's *Bad Medicine*.[11] All these traits are part of the picture of moral malaise that Pellegrino and Thomasma allege afflicts modern medicine.

By these standards, we have to admit that medicine has slipped somewhat down the gradient of the virtues. It has failed to exercise the moral power that Pellegrino and Thomasma attribute to it. It is not showing the moral leadership that they claim could make it a model and an inspiration within our society and our culture.

There are other subtle but profoundly important ways in which medicine has the opportunity to influence social and cultural values and attitudes for better or for worse. One of these is the way that medicine conveys a mechanistic biomedical message or a humanistic person-centred message in conversation with patients. Or the way that it achieves a healthy, whole-making balance between the two; the extent to which, as my GP put it to me once, medicine treats the patient not the numbers. The numbers matter. But when they become, or seem to be, the object of the exercise, and the *person* ceases to be the focus of care, medicine has failed. The ten core principles of the therapeutic encounter (Chapter 15) are the antidote to such failure, and the core principles of the whole medical endeavour.

The example of complementary medicine

It is worth reflecting on the respect in which unorthodox, complementary practitioners are held and the reasons for it; degree of respect in which some are held not only by the public but by some of their orthodox medical colleagues, because there has been a de facto integration of conventional and complementary medicine, particularly in general practice for a long time.[12] Complementary and alternative medicine (CAM) is a fact of life; a fact of medical life and a fact of our cultural life. Its best established and most reputable practitioners are respected for many of the same reasons as conventional practitioners – intellectual ability, professional integrity, caring qualities. But they are respected, too, for some things that in conventional practice are in short supply. I emphasise 'in short supply'. I am not saying that they are not to be found in conventional practice, nor that conventional practitioners are not keen to supply them. They are to be found. And many practitioners would like to supply more of them – if the system, the model, provided for it. What are they? Well, they are the things we have touched on already: a concern for the person as a whole, and interest in the story of sickness, a belief in the ability of body and mind to regulate and heal themselves to a greater extent than conventionally understood, a belief that these properties can be stimulated by subtle means with less direct risk, a belief that individuals can be more in control of their health.

There is nothing controversial about these; nothing 'unorthodox' at all, in fact. They are simply attributes of all good medicine that are more clearly evident in some CAM practice than in some conventional practice. And that is the reason why conventional practitioners in many disciplines integrate CAM concepts and methods into their repertoire. To put it simply, these attributes are 'whole making'. Whatever is whole-making for the individual – whether good medicine, good education or good parenting – is by extension whole-making for society. Medicine is a social and cultural phenomenon because it reflects and shapes attitudes and values. If a new model of medicine is to emerge that transcends the limitations of the present model, this role needs to be clearly understood and acknowledged. And a truly integrative relationship between orthodox medicine and CAM, supported by a greater freedom of scientific thought and enquiry, will be fruitful both therapeutically and culturally.

Medicine's cultural influence

In drawing out this common yet contrasting theme between orthodox and CAM practice we begin to see the subtle but powerful influence that medicine can exert on the way people live their lives and think about life. The messages that medicine gives may echo the prevailing culture, the prevailing world view, for better or for worse, or it may challenge it. A narrowly biomedical perspective reflects and reinforces a materialistic world view. A holistic medical perspective that emphasises our unique personal value, our common humanity, and our dependence on one another and our environment, challenges such a world view.

It is not medicine's job to tell people *what* to think or what to do. But it is medicine's job to *encourage* people to *think*. To think about the things that may make for greater well-being, for themselves or others. It is not medicine's job to decide whether we become a person, a unique life, at conception or at 14 weeks of life. But it is medicine's responsibility to help people to understand the implications of any decision about terminating that life, and to be their advocate and to care for them whatever that decision may be. It is not medicine's job to tell us what to eat or what not to eat, or whether to leave a stressful job or a destructive relationship. But it is medicine's job to help us to think these things through, in as much as they impact upon our health and well-being.

It certainly is not medicine's job to collude in *sustaining* damaging social structures or cultural attitudes by medicating for the consequences. It must challenge those structure and attitudes while it cares for those who suffer them.

> It is now difficult to be honest with patients. We say nothing when patients assert their inability to work, even when our inner voice is telling us differently. We accept the misuse of the benefits system which has generated a culture of worklessness, wasting millions of lives and excluding large parts of the population from society. We know that patients abuse insurance claims by

> exaggerating symptoms, which we don't challenge. We acquiesce to demands for drugs, referrals and investigations when patients refuse to accept our opinion.
>
> Many social and personal problems have been brought under the medical umbrella instead of being taken up by broader civil action and debate. Confrontation leads to complaints, which are difficult, time consuming and undermining, so we avoid them, however unreasonable the patient. 'Patient centredness' often gives patients what they want but not what they need, and this undermines society. Sometimes we need to be doctor centred when it is wrong to do what the patient asks. We need to return to honesty, to professional discretion, and to a profession that stands together over hard choices. This is not about professional power but for the sake society and above all to help patients. (Des Spence[13])

Medicine has to be immensely careful about the messages it gives that have to do with the value of life and the quality of living; that have to do, for example, with expectations of cure and survival at all costs, as against expectations of care and worth-ship at all times. There is no formula that medicine can offer or apply to calculate the 'therapeutic ratio,' that balancing act of pros and cons, for every health care decision. But it can insist that those decisions are made within a personal relationship that fulfils the ten 'core principles' of the encounter (Chapter 15) . And that they are based on absolute respect for the person who is the subject of that decision; bearing in mind the earlier remarks about the limits of autonomy *vis-à-vis* justice, for example, limits that can only be negotiated within the sort of relationship that allows the clinician to come to an understanding with the patient, and the patient to come to an understanding with him or herself.

Every decision in medicine is subject to a therapeutic ratio, not only in terms of its clinical consequences, but in terms of the statement it makes about the relationship between medicine and society. If I give an inappropriate prescription because a patient asks for it, or because of a sense of pressure to *do something*, I not only risk causing harm if it is not well tolerated, but I am giving the message that 'anything goes'. I am reinforcing the cultural concept, which is very prevalent, of medicine as a commodity.

If any remodelling of medicine is necessary, and I hope by now you are persuaded that it is and if any remodelling is to succeed, then the complexity of the relationship between medicine and the society and culture of our day must be recognised, and its problems addressed.

The meaning of life

Medicine is inescapably bound up with the meaning of life. Medicine meets with birth, death and dying on a daily basis. Pain, disability and suffering, doubt and fear, hope and courage, anguish and joy, fecklessness and nobility, are its common currency. Even the petty bodily and emotional inconveniences that people take to doctors are episodes in the story of that person's life. Even these say something about the meaning of that person's life. Every medical encounter is an encounter with meaning.

We have seen how every medical transaction is loaded with meaning; and that the meaning of the transaction significantly affects the outcome.[14] The meaning may reside in many different aspects of the transaction – the colour of the pill, the newness or strangeness of the treatment, the size of the dose, the expectation in the mind of patient or practitioner, and so on. And it is the quality of the relationship that is the vehicle for the transaction that conveys the most powerful message about the meaning of the encounter for the people involved. A message – in words, touch or attitude – that may be positive and whole-making, or that may be de-meaning.

Literally everyone engaged in any activity that contributes to the medical endeavour is implicated in formulating and expressing the statement that medicine makes about the meaning of life. This applies to the researcher, the pharmaceutical industry, the technician, the administrator and the politician as much as to the practitioner engaged in day-to-day face-to-face encounters with patients.

Medicine is inescapably implicated in the whole mystery of the human condition. By virtue of its role in the lives of men, women and children, and of the intimate and personal nature of that role, it is constantly helping to define, for better or for worse, what it means to be human. That is a fact of life that it may ignore but that it cannot escape.

This fact places an enormous responsibility on medicine. In its collective relationship with society and its personal relationship with individual patients, medicine is engaged in evaluating and negotiating what life is all about, what really matters. The use of technology, the rationing of treatment, end of life care, fitness to work, the willingness to make a home visit, the courtesy and thoroughness of a physical examination – you name it. Every action we perform and every judgement we make in health care is an evaluation of 'the life in our hands'.

Not everything that can be done should be done. Things that should be done may perhaps not be done, because we are too busy with all the things that can be done. Medicine teaches people to believe that what can be done should be done. Not everything that theoretically could be done, actually can be done. People know, or think they know, what medical science could do for them and assume that it can and should be done. But as Michael Fitzpatrick wrote, "When health becomes the goal of human endeavour it acquires an oppressive influence over the life of the individual. If people's lives are ruled by measures they believe may help to prolong

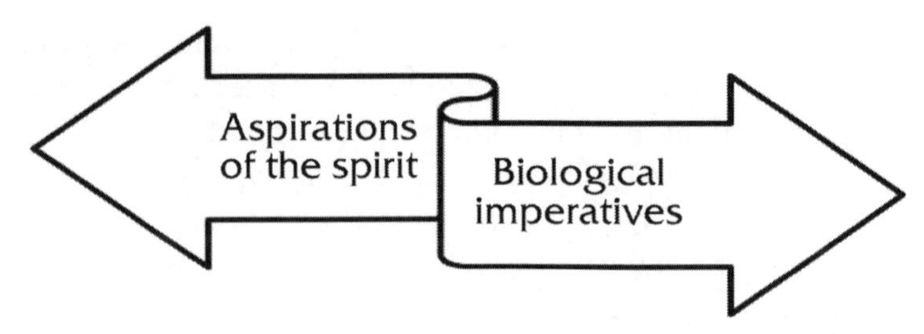

Figure 17.2 *The central dilemma.*

their existence, the quality of their lives is diminished".[15] Numerous other references throughout the book have made the same point.

This is the nub of the healthcare dilemma (see Figure 17.2) – to reconcile medicine's struggle with the precariousness of existence with the affirmation of meaning in life that transcends the precariousness and the pain; to manage the biological precariousness of existence without diminishing the biographical significance of life. Medicine must be responsive to need but discourage dependence, be an enemy of disease but a respecter of persons, a friend of hope but a manager of expectation, an enabler as well as a controller, an interpreter rather than a manipulator, a seeker after truth but at home with uncertainty. There is a tension between the contrasting elements of these contrasting pairs which may sometimes be impossible to resolve. But the only possibility of resolving them as best we can will lie in keeping them in the forefront of the discourse of medicine from the very start of the educational process that leads to any career in medicine and throughout that career, and in the forefront of all discourse concerning the role of medicine in society. Openness and truthfulness in these matters will make it at least less difficult, if never easy to resolve those tensions within the individual practitioner–patient relationship, where ultimately they have to be resolved. The quality of that personal relationship, and its ability to fulfil the sort of core principles that are 'the heart of the matter', will be critical in informing and facilitating the wider discourse within medicine. And that discourse will play a part in the still wider discourse within society about its values and priorities, and the cultural trends and forces that shape it.

References

1 Pellegrino E, Thomasma D. *The Virtues in Medical Practice*. Oxford: Oxford University Press; 1993.
2 Greaves D. *The Healing Tradition*. Oxford: Radcliffe Publishing; 2004.

3 Horrobin D. *Medical Hubris – A reply to Ivan Illich*. Edinburgh: Churchill Livingstone; 1979.
4 DHSS. *Inequalities in Health (The Black Report)*. Unpublished; 1980.
5 Hunter D, Popay J, Tannahill C, Whitehead M. Getting to grips with health inequalities at last? *Br Med J*. 2010; 340 c684:323–324.
6 Marmot M. *Strategic review of health inequalities post 2010. Marmot review final report*. London: University College London; 2010.
7 Stott R. How can we rediscover the magic of more equal societies? *Br Med J*. 2010; 341 c4155:304.
8 Thomas B, Dorling D, Davey Smith G. Inequalities in premature mortality in Britain: observational study from 1921 to 2007. *Br Med J*. 2010; 341 c3639:291.
9 Kmietowicz Z. Great expectations. *Br Med J*. 2010; 340 b5558:340–41.
10 Schumacher E. *A Guide for the Perplexed*. London: Sphere; 1978.
11 Wootton D. *Bad Medicine: Doctors Doing Harm Since Hippocrates*. New York: Oxford University Press; 2007.
12 Wharton R. Lewith G. Complementary Medicine and the General Practitioner. *Br Med J*. 1986; 2:57–58.
13 Spence D. From the front line: Doctor centredness. *Br Med J*, 2010; 341 c3755:154.
14 Moerman D. *Meaning medicine and the 'placebo effect'*. Cambridge: Cambridge University Press; 2002.
15 Fitzpatrick M. *The tyranny of health*. Abingdon: Routledge; 2001.

18

THE PROBLEM WITH SCIENCE
The context and process of care

Summary

- The goal of science is truth through knowledge. But medicine's truth is not altogether the same as science's truth.
- Science works with ideas, imagination and intuition, but essentially has to do with facts. Medicine has also to deal with meaning.
- This is not an argument for less science in medicine, but for more and better science; better in the sense of better attuned to 'the rest of life'.
- Truthfulness is a core principle of medical practice and medical science. But a kind of untruthfulness is common in day-to-day clinical practice.
- The fundamental untruth is the illusion of certainty.
- The inexcusable untruth is to reduce the patient's problem to it to its narrow biomedical parameters and to allow the patient as a person to vanish from our gaze.
- Science fails medicine by the narrowness of the scope of things it is willing to investigate. Important areas of medicine have been neglected as a consequence.
- The medical research culture must change if it is to promote science for understanding alongside science for manipulation. We need to be unsparingly critical of the distinction between useful science and wasteful science.
- "Medical knowledge is not knowledge acquired primarily for its own sake (but) for a specific purpose – the care of the sick."[1]

Scientificism

William James (1842–1910) was an American psychologist and philosopher best known for the series of Gifford lectures delivered in Edinburgh in 1901 and later published as *The Varieties of Religious Experience*. His work was reviewed in the BBC Radio 4 programme 'In our time' on the 13th of May

2010, when he was judged by one expert to have been the greatest philosopher ever! He did not draw any firm conclusions about the existence of God from his research, whose purpose was psychological rather than theological, and he was open to the possibility that some or all of those varieties of experience might be eruptions from the individual's subconscious. But he was insistent that they should be taken seriously, and was critical of the scientific attitude towards such phenomena, though he was primarily a Darwinian scientist himself who turned to philosophy in later life.

One of his criticisms is particularly pertinent to the problem of science in relation to medicine. He said that the worst thing about science is 'the religion of scientificism' – which induces a kind of fear. He said his fellow scientists crippled themselves by the fear of doing something that might be regarded as unscientific, and so they closed their minds. This is reflected in quotations from Kuhn and Polanyi in Chapter 11. James's view, consistent with Darwin's open-minded scientific attitude, was that we have to be open to the thought that what seems intellectually absolutely unavoidable today may seem really stupid to us tomorrow. So we should never close down on any intellectual possibilities whatsoever. The quotation from George Engel that introduces Chapter 6 that the scientific attitude can permit no restrictions as to the category of natural phenomena investigated echoes the same conviction. The discussion on the radio went on to reflect on the ascendancy of Bertrand Russell's philosophy, and the triumph of what James would have regarded as an over-investment in logic and a lack of interest in the diversity of human experience. This sentiment is echoed in the quotation from Mary Midgeley at the end of Chapter 6, which concludes, "We do not need to esteem science less. What we need is to esteem it in the right way. Especially we need to stop isolating it from the rest of life".[2] One of the speakers on the radio suggested that James' continuing importance is that he represents a struggle in his period and our own to reconcile naturalism, the understanding that human beings are the product of nature, with humanism; the struggle to find a place for human values in a world of nature. Which today might be represented as the question – in a world of particles, what place is there for values?

Scientific truth in medicine

> The good internal to the practice of research is truth, an understanding of what is really real about some aspect of the world we inhabit. (Pellegrino and Thomasma[1])

The goal of science is truth through knowledge. Thus, the role of science in medicine is to get at the truth. But medicine's truth is not altogether the same as science's truth. Science works with ideas, imagination and intuition, but essentially has to do with facts. Medicine has also to deal with meaning. In this, medicine comes close to theology. Science and theology are both exploring reality; different but inseparable aspects of reality. Medicine somehow has to accommodate the patient's whole reality. The truth we seek is "to understand things as they really are, knowing that in its fullness it will always be beyond us".[3] But if we abandon it we abandon our patient. And medicine's truth has to accommodate the diversity of human experience that an over-investment in logic may disregard. It has to accommodate 'the rest of life' of which our biomedical condition is only a part and a reflection. It has to accommodate the values that give meaning to the particles.

Medicine's problem with science has been a recurring theme throughout this book – a problem born out of success. The programme on William James also touched upon the fate of movements, of the spirit or of the mind, that become codified and institutionalised and suffer a loss of the life that inspired and motivated them. This is true of medical science to the extent that it has become increasingly concerned with manipulation rather than understanding; increasingly focused on the particles, and less on the rest of life. Our gratitude for the success of medical science in what it has been able to do for us need not be diminished by suggesting that it is seeking increasingly sophisticated answers to the wrong questions. Or rather that it is failing to address the right questions with the same degree of sophistication and commitment.

This is not an argument for less science. On the contrary, it is the same argument that David Horrobin made 30 years ago for more and better science.[4] That does not mean 'better' in the sense of more skilled or sophisticated, but in the sense of better attuned to 'the rest of life'. In Horrobin's terms it means making science more humane; more concerned, as he puts it, with the extraordinary potency of the control mechanisms that maintain the constancy of our physico-chemical equilibrium, without which we would never remain well. He is highlighting medical science's surprising lack of interest in this 'evolutionary imperative'; its preoccupation with learning to control the processes that go wrong at the expense of learning to enable the processes that help to put things right. And its lack of interest in learning to exploit them; even though they are integral and indispensable to every therapeutic process.

This is an argument that medical science needs to be better directed; better attuned to the humanistic rather than the mechanistic goals of medicine. It is a huge challenge to the culture of medical science; and to the culture of medicine in general. And to the culture of the society that medicine serves and helps to shape, and in turn is shaped by.

The wider cultural implications, such as medicine's role in creating the kinder, more imaginative, more generous world', 'the more just and sustainable world' envisioned in the quotations in Chapter 4, are employed in Chapter 17. The essential cultural reorientation that is required of medical science is that it should 'frame its understanding of the world to understand the world truly rather than in order to control the world easily and cheaply.' That is a crude paraphrase of a quotation from an essay on medical knowledge by HT Engelhardt that is used by David Greaves in his analysis of the problem with science in *Mystery in Western Medicine*, which I warmly recommend.[5] The quotation is crude not only in the way I have rephrased it, but in the aspersion it casts on the goals of medical science; whose application in the real world is in any case seldom easy or cheap. But it makes the point yet again that the role of science is to understand the world *truly*.

Truthfulness, I have suggested, is a core principle of medical practice and medical science, and I outline my reasons in Chapter 10. But in fact, untruthfulness is common in day-to-day clinical practice.[6] It arises, when medicine only acknowledges part of 'the story of sickness'. A diagnosis, for example, is only part of the story; a description of what is going on, rarely an explanation of why a thing is as it is, but often presented as if it defines the whole problem.[7] Untruthfulness arises when a doctor gives an antibiotic for a self-limiting illness, or another inappropriate prescription (though possibly with significant 'placebo' effect); or offers a diagnosis when the truth is 'I don't know'; or tells an ill patient there is nothing wrong because the tests are all normal.

Untruth is introduced when "the dogma of technological medicine ignores the therapeutic effect of the doctor and the self-healing powers of the patient";[8] when "doctors expect to find an answer to every problem if only they look hard enough with the right instruments".[9] It happens because although technology allows us to practise with ever greater precision and is a powerful tool for understanding, it also creates powerful misunderstanding when unwisely applied.[10]

In a great deal of medical practice, often with the best of intentions and to good effect, there is an element of deceit. This inherent untruthfulness is not necessarily to be condemned so much as to be acknowledged and reflected upon; sometimes to be corrected, sometimes to be accepted when there are mitigating circumstances.[11] Deceit and consent to deceit are inevitable in medical practice whenever we imply, and quite possibly believe, that we know the truth of the matter when all we really know are some of the facts of the matter. We are victims of the success of biomedicine because of the expectation it encourages that we have the answers; whereas we are always dealing with a high degree of complexity and uncertainty. The inherent truth of the patient's experience will often be beyond us. But that does not absolve us from the responsibility to be open to it, and faithful to it – as best we can be and as fully as the patient invites us to be.

The fundamental untruth is the illusion of certainty. The inexcusable untruth is to reduce the problem and our response to it to its narrow biomedical parameters and to allow the patient as a person to vanish from our gaze. We can have no certainty about all that determines the course of illness and healing in any individual. We have to explore constantly and courageously that penumbra of uncertainty that surrounds our presumed certainties. This attitude does not displace, but assumes and comprehends proper respect for evidence and scientific method, clinical knowledge and skill. But it leaves room for the flexibility of mind that is essential if we are to know the world truly; especially if we are to open to the inherent truth of the patient's experience. This flexibility is not scientific *laissez-fair* but an honest acknowledgement that, to paraphrase John Polkinghorne, on the one hand the physical world is too surprising to allow any a priori concept of what is reasonable, and on the other, the actual character of our encounter with reality must be allowed to shape our knowledge and our thought.[12]

The limitations of science

Science fails medicine not through lack of competence – it is able to do and to discover amazing things, but through lack of vision. Not for want of curiosity, but for the limit of things it is curious about. Not for any lack of the ability to investigate, but for the narrowness of the scope of things it is willing to investigate. The weaknesses of science are its strengths: its preoccupation with the things it does well and with the tools it knows how to use best. The opportunities of science to explore novel conceptions that do not sit comfortably with its contemporary paradigm seem to be regarded almost as threats; stifled by the fear that once a new framework is accepted it will lead to conclusions that have been hitherto, rightly or wrongly, abhorred (to paraphrase the quotation from Polanyi in Chapter 11); stifled by the quasi-religious fear of William James's 'scientificism'.

In short, science must be true to its traditional vocation to the systematic pursuit of knowledge that permits no restriction as to the category of natural phenomena investigated. The cultural and structural problems that contribute to this loss of vision are explored in the Introduction and in Chapters 10 and 11. The areas of medicine that have been neglected as a consequence, though not quite ignored, include the following:

Healing processes

We know a great deal about the causes of disease and the mechanism of the body's response to insult and disorder of various kinds; causes as precise as our genetic susceptibility; mechanisms analysed down to the cellular and intracellular level. We know a great deal about the detailed mechanics of bodily self-regulation. We know a certain amount about the influence of psychological and environmental factors on these processes. We can describe the healing of a wound by first and second 'intention', the restoration of biochemical measurements to 'the normal range', the change in certain pathognomonic symptoms (symptoms characteristic of a specific disease). But our understanding of the correlation of these factors with the well-being of the person as a whole is more uncertain. Remember the quotation from Roy Porter:

> In myriad ways, medicine continues to advance, new treatments appear, surgery works marvels, and (partly as a result) people live longer. Yet few people today feel confident, either about their personal health or about doctors, healthcare delivery and the medical profession in general. (Porter[13])

For example, we know perfectly well that the 'placebo' effect and contextual healing happen. We know that various factors can promote these effects. And we know that they account for a significant part of even the specific efficacy of treatments demonstrated in controlled trials, as well as their actual effectiveness in practice. But we have a very poor understanding of these fundamental dynamics of healing processes; let alone how to make best use of them.

We know very little about the natural history of these effects in the person as a whole. We know that placebo can induce relief of presenting symptoms, measurable physiological changes, and changes in brain chemistry. But the more general effect of these reactions in the person as a whole, and the effects over time are not known. We do not know anything much about the time scale of onset or duration of placebo responses, or their permanence or transience. We do not know to what extent they are usually limited to the target symptom or condition. We do not know whether and to what extent they have incidental effects on aspects of well-being other than the presenting problem. Bearing in mind that 'placebo' responses 'work' by mobilising resources for self-regulation and self-healing, we do not know whether these resources are thereafter enhanced to the benefit of longer term healthfulness. The only context I know, and to which I can find reference, in which detailed observations of this kind are made is the the homeopathic method that I describe in Chapter 14 and Appendix 14.1.

A piece of research begging to be attempted, for example, is suggested by the short notes on 'Healing processes' in that chapter. The detailed observation of changes in response to treatment by the homeopathic method provides a well documented account of the dynamics of self-regulation and self-healing across a wide range of morbidity. These clinical observations, described in the appendix, are valid whether the agent of the healing process is the contextual or 'placebo' effect of the method, or the homeopathic prescription itself, or a combination of the two. A similarly detailed and documented account of placebo responses, in conventional trial situations perhaps, would permit comparison between the two sets of observations. Firstly, both would be descriptions of 'natural healing', providing invaluable insight into that process, because whatever they do homeopathic medicines cannot have pharmacological effects. And secondly the comparison would cast light on the similarity or difference of the process in the two clinical situations, allowing us to draw inferences about the similarities or differences between the effect of the homeopathic medicines and the inert placebo agents used in trials.

Illness

We know a great deal about disease processes, but we do not know much about the poorly defined state that we call illness, and out of which disease arises; or from which medicine has to 'create' a disease in order to explain it. Actually, that is not quite true. It is more accurate to say that we do know a fair amount about the things that make us ill, but we can't do much about it, unless and until it becomes a disease, or unless we can turn it into a disease we do know how to treat, or at least how to control. We know, for example, that exams, bereavement and moving house, and other critical or traumatic situations in life affect our immune system and our adrenal function. We know that poverty and social deprivation make us ill; not only when there is actual lack of essential food, accommodation, hygiene, education, etc., but also where there is relative lack of material well-being compared to wealthier sections of society. And the medical and social sciences do develop or advocate the means to remedy or mitigate such problems. But there is an inevitable element of mystery to personal illness, and to the challenge of meeting the needs of a particular individual who is ill.

It may be beyond the scope of science to analyse every facet of the mystery of personal illness. But at least it must not encourage us to neglect the mysterious in favour of the measurable – the McNamara fallacy again (Chapter 10). The science that permits us to define illness in terms of precise biological disorder must not distract us from the importance of the biographical diagnosis, the story of the sickness. But more importantly it must take account of that broader diagnostic perspective, explore it, and help us to understand and manage it.

However, there are questions that may shed light on aspects of the mystery that medical science can, and to a limited extent does answer:

- *'Why me?'* Why do/did I become ill when others in similar circumstances did not?
- *'Why this?'* Why did I develop *this* illness/disease? Why do I react to anxiety/hot weather/a virus with headache, when X gets diarrhoea and Y gets eczema?
- *'Why now/then?'* Why did it happen when it did – not six months ago, or next week? What were the factors/circumstances that determined the time of onset?

The limited extent of medical science's exploration of these questions is illustrated by contrast with the particularly detailed case taking necessarily employed by doctors using the homeopathic method. This is a clinical process of a wholly conventional if unusually comprehensive kind that yields an unusually versatile and comprehensive synthesis of biological and biographical data from which, by contrast with a more conventional approach, a more complete understanding both of the evolution of the illness in that person (the story of sickness), and of what needs to be healed as well as treated can emerge.[14] This not only facilitates the therapeutic process, but also reveals the possible scope of detailed epidemiological enquiry.

Treatment – The Black Box

For a period during my GP career my surgery was in our home. My consulting room was our sitting room out of hours. Patients would often sit on the sofa. The waiting room was a small room immediately adjacent where the receptionist sat with the patients, and the atmosphere was intimate, welcoming and cheerful. The sound of laughter filtering through the door into the consulting room, unusual in the average doctors' waiting room, was not uncommon. I provided routine fifteen minute appointments, but the patients were often and evidently feeling better by the time they came in to me because of the warmth of their 'reception'. They did then get the benefit of my repertoire of clinical skills, and whatever personal qualities I brought to the relationship. This, at the time, was my therapeutic 'black box'. It would be quite difficult to itemise all of its component parts. And impossible to be sure which component made what contribution to the patient's subsequent well-being and clinical outcome. A GP colleague of mine identified 35 separate components of the therapeutic encounter.

All treatment, every medical encounter is a therapeutic black box. The workings of the black box in conventional practice, we like to think, are less of a mystery because we know what the specific component, the drug or procedure is meant to do. The workings of the black box in complementary medicine are often represented as a sort of confidence trick because we are sceptical that it has a specific component that does anything at all. In either case the result may be effective or ineffective, safe or unsafe. But the medical model justifies the use of the black box only if it has a specific component whose efficacy can be 'proved'.

One approach to the black box is to unpack it, isolate that specific component, and submit it to 'destructive analysis'. Another approach is to say that we must not attempt to unpack the black box because to try may destroy it, and deprive it of its practical effectiveness.

Science has a dual responsibility towards the understanding of human wholeness and the healing vocation that is expressed beautifully in an essay by George Orwell on *The Meaning of a Poem*:

> I have tried to analyse this poem as well as I can in a short period, but nothing I have said can explain, or explain away, the pleasure I take in it. That is finally in explicable, and it is just because it is inexplicable that detailed criticism is worthwhile. Men of science can study the life-processes of a flower, or they can split it up into its component elements, but any scientist will tell you that a flower does not become less wonderful, it becomes more wonderful, if you know all about it. (George Orwell[15])

Science must combine a humility and sense of awe in the face of the wonderful and inexplicable, and in the face of irreducible uncertainty, with a scientific passion and insatiable curiosity to know all about it. It will never fully explain, and must never seek to explain away, the mystery of life, but the mystery itself makes critical analysis worthwhile.

Medical science must accept that there is always a black box that operates between every practitioner and every patient in every therapeutic encounter. It has many components and many dimensions, and the permutation of these will vary from one encounter to another. The complete and precise operation of the black box, the outcome of its operation, its effectiveness, the human consequences, will always, ultimately defy analysis. That finally is inexplicable, and it is just because it is inexplicable that detailed criticism is worthwhile.

Medical science must not make the mistake of confusing the question *whether* the black box 'works', with the question *how* it does it. Both are valid questions, and both have valid answers. Both are worth exploring. But the answer to one does not depend upon the answer to the other. We would like to know how our black boxes 'work', and we will try to find out. But what matters more is that they do work. If we are honest, and admit, as research into placebo effects increasingly reveals, that all our therapeutic activities are effectively black box operations; and if we were to abandon all treatments in which we do not fully understand how the black box works, we would give up medical practice altogether.

Useful science and wasteful science

Useful science enables us to do things that are really worth doing. The question of what is really worth doing is an ethical and cultural question that is profoundly important to our conception of the goals of medicine and the model we devise to serve those goals. But we have seen in Chapter 9, when exploring the crisis of cost in the health service, that when challenged to reduce cost there is a considerable number of activities that clinicians consider are not worth doing. Medical science has made it possible to do them and provided the technology to do them. This bears out Lyng's suggestion quoted in the earlier discussion of the problems of technology in Chapter 11, that technology encourages 'the interventionist thrust' of modern medicine. This appetite for and tacit dependence on the necessary 'instrumentation' is fed by medical science, and rather than serving the goals of medicine simply 'creates the space for possible medical events.'[16] David Horrobin characterised this over-use of technology as "The application of a technique to a situation, without any critical consideration of whether the outcome is likely to be favourable or not".[4] We might restate David Haslam's observation that "We use the medical model because the medical is what we use, even though it may not be appropriate",[17] as 'We use medical technology because medical technology is what we use, even though it may not be appropriate.'

Science wastefully applied, because it is not really useful, is of course science harmfully applied. Every intervention carries some risk; is potentially iatrogenic. An intervention that is not really useful is one kind of medical untruth. And a wasteful intervention costs money that could be better spent.

In May 2010 the *British Medical Journal* published a 'head to head' debate, 'Is modern genetics a blind alley?'[18] "Yes", says James le Fanu. "Modern genetics has become the largest single research field in the history of biology, driven forward by the expectation that 'like a mechanical army (it will) destroy ignorance . . . promising unprecedented opportunities for science and medicine'. And yet for all this cornucopia of new facts and knowledge, its influence on everyday medical practice remains scarcely detectable." He quotes the chief executive of Genentech as saying that all this effort amounts to "the largest money losing industry in the history of mankind". He speculates that the complexities of those methodologies might explain in part the paucity of original ideas in medicine, diverting attention and resources from more fruitful forms of clinical research. Le Fanu regards it as "highly improbable that the future of medicine might lie in understanding disease at (this) most fundamental reductionist level".

D.J. Weatherall argues that on the contrary genetic research promises real benefits and is already delivering some. He points out that genetic research is a young discipline and that it would be short sighted to view it as a blind alley, considering the complexity of the subject it has to explore. But his contribution to the debate does not inspire confidence. He acknowledges the extraordinary complexity of biological function in health and disease that modern genetics continues to unearth. He compares this phase of its exploration to the endless, and some might argue similarly fruitless search in modern physics for a grand unifying theory. He acknowledges that most common diseases "seem to reflect the action of many different genes with small effects, presumably combined with environmental factors and the biology of ageing".

Research like this is presumably driven by scientific passion, and does increase our wonder at the beautiful intricacy of life, even if ultimately what makes us tick remains inexplicable. But having read this debate, I wonder to what extent the research will prove to be practically useful. Nevertheless, it is reassuring that this debate, and the ethical debates about embryo research and the like, are happening.

But science has a huge responsibility to be sure that its passion and the seductive power of what it can do, do not lead us up blind alleys, at the end of which nothing really useful is achieved; particularly if our essential humanity and wholeness is diminished in the process.

Research

Perhaps the most serious revolution that remodelling medicine requires is in medical research. There are many challenges (see Box 18.1). The predominant thrust of research programmes is to isolate a problem from its 'confounding variables' (all the other things in life that bear upon the health and well-being of the afflicted person), and then to reduce the problem to its most fundamental biological component (genetic, biochemical, functional, anatomical) so that this can be managed or manipulated. The test of the ability of any treatment that results from this process to do what is expected of it (its efficacy) requires that the measurement of this outcome is similarly isolated from the effect of confounding variables.

BOX 18.1 *Research challenges*

- The dynamics of illness.
- Healing processes.
- Enabling self-regulation.
- Context and meaning.
- 'Subtle' therapeutic effects.
- The therapeutic 'black box

This is a generalisation that is not true of all research methods, but it does represent the principal focus and predominant thrust of medical research. It is brilliantly successful in what it sets out to do. It does make it possible to manage or manipulate particular components of disease processes. But it provides a very partial solution to the whole complex spectrum of illness–disease–sickness. I have hyphenated the three words to emphasise that medicine is concerned with a complex phenomenon of which the pathology, which is what we usually mean by disease, is only a part. The illness–disease–sickness triad, whose various meanings are discussed at the beginning of Chapter 8, involves the person as a whole *and* is contingent upon a multiplicity of circumstances in the person's life. What is more any medical intervention affects the person as a whole, not just the part that it acts directly upon, and has consequences for the circumstances of the person's life. And lastly, no actual medical intervention is simple or circumscribed. As we have seen it is always a 'black box' procedure.

The narrow focus of biomedical research, for all its achievements, cannot do justice to this complexity. In fact it really has nothing to say about it. This is not to disparage biomedical science. It is not an argument to esteem science less, but 'to esteem it in the right way', in Mary Midgeley's words; 'especially to stop isolating it from the rest of life'. As Iris Bell and colleagues put it in a discussion of the research relevant to a new model for primary health care – "The reductionist approach to science is valuable (but) it fails to reflect the way the real world operates".[19] Which is perhaps why as Roy Porter reflected in the quotation in Chapter, despite the myriad ways in which science continues to advance, "Few people today feel confident, either about their personal health or about doctors, healthcare delivery and the medical profession in general".[13]

The medical research culture must change if it is to promote science for understanding alongside science for manipulation. Medical scientists might argue that the myriad advances in science do allow us to understand; to understand what goes wrong when disease affects us, and what to do about it. But it is probably fair, and more accurate to say that science allows us to *describe* what goes wrong so that we may do something about it, but not necessarily to *understand* it. It allows us to know what to do to correct the fault, but it does not help us to understand the mixed dynamics of the illness–disease–sickness process, nor of the healing process.

A change in the medical research culture that promotes this level of understanding and the health care practices that it permits will not come easily. The biomedical paradigm is so powerful and the model so successful that it is almost impervious to change. The plausibility construct or world view that sustains them is not conducive to change. Its materialist perspective encourages mechanistic solutions. "World views and the values placed on different health outcomes are closely related. Thus the values that underlie medical care shape the scientific questions that researchers ask, the health outcomes they measure, and the interpretation of the results" – Iris Bell and colleagues again, reflecting the discussion in Chapters 10 and 11.

To develop research methods that study healthcare processes that are holistic and integrative is even more difficult than studying diseases and treatments that are isolated from the rest of life. This is because, by definition they concern illness–disease–sickness that has multiple determinants (predisposing and causative factors), that affects the person as a whole (all aspects of their well-being), that has multiple outcomes (physical, psychological and social), and that involves a number of interventions (either as ingredients of the 'black box' or as separate and distinctive processes), which are individualised to the needs of the patient.

It is obvious from this scenario that research of this kind is asking far more profound questions than 'what is wrong?', and 'what works?' It is asking questions about the whole phenomenon of illness–disease–sickness within the narrative of human experience, of life. It is exploring new ways of thinking about disease and therapeutics. This may sound idealistic and impossibly challenging. It is challenging, but it is not impossible. And to a limited extent the challenge is being met, the methods are being explored, and it is beginning to happen.

This is too big a subject for me to do more than offer a few examples to illustrate it. General readers who do not have an interest in research may find the next few pages heavy going, and may prefer to skip to the Conclusion at the end of the chapter.

1. Research policy

Based on work by Trisha Greenhalgh, Professor of Primary Care Research, University College, London, writing in the *British Medical Journal*:[20]

The narrow focus of research policy and research commissioning is manifestly inadequate and inappropriate to health care in the real world: "Research policy is currently powerfully shaped and constrained by talk of the knowledge based economy and the contribution of high technology innovation to UK plc. This discourse has repositioned the core business of primary care research as running a 'population laboratory' for large scale epidemiological studies, preferably with a pharmacological component. Such studies are important but they are not the whole story." Research initiative in general practice (which might reveal more of the story) is burdened by "the creeping institutionalisation and regulation of research. Epidemiology's unanswered questions demand large scale collaborative studies that can be undertaken only within a complex research infrastructure. Non-epidemiological questions relevant to primary care (for example, on the humanistic and social dimensions of illness and healing) are currently defined as a lesser form of science for which only B-list funding and publication outlets are available".

2. Exploring illness: interpretive medicine

These quotations are taken from a paper by Joanne Reeve proposing 'interpretive medicine' as a better framework for the generalist care that must be the foundation of good clinical practice. It is "the critical, thoughtful, professional use of an appropriate range of knowledge in the dynamic, shared exploration and interpretation of individual illness experience, in order to support the creative capacity of individuals in maintaining their daily lives".[21]

The holistic and integrative ideal in medicine is best, if imperfectly, represented by general practice. Other disciplines, such as geriatric medicine and palliative care and some aspects of mental health care, also represent this generalist ideal. But it is threatened by the evidence based approach which has strayed from its founders' intention that evidence should be submitted to the judgement of clinical relevance, and become focused on "hierarchies of evidence (that) privilege knowledge from what some consider to be a narrow methodological perspective". The effect of this is to narrow the scope of the generalist's perception of the patient. "The disadvantages of constrained protocol-driven care are recognised by the profession; but still form a new formative normative framework for clinical practice." This militates against generalism, which "is more than disease-focused care delivered in a community setting. It is a different approach to understanding and addressing health and illness. (It) describes a philosophy of practice which is person, not disease, centred; continuous, not episodic; integrates biotechnical and biographical perspectives; and views health as a resource for living and not an end in itself". The generalist approach is essential to address growing concerns about the inefficiency, ineffectiveness and inequity of fragmented health care, and to promote an understanding of "specific events in their broader context, integrating biomedical evidence with a reflexive and interpretive approach that acknowledges, the complexity of individual human experience".

3. Setting research priorities: a layman's experience

This is a personal view published in the *British Medical Journal*.[22] The author, Lester Firkins, is a former banker who became involved in the world of medical research, specifically clinical trials, because of his role in a patients' charity concerned with Creutzfeldt–Jakob Disease (CJD) which had claimed the life of his son. When he attended a consumer workshop on clinical trials for CJD he "assumed that this was what always happened in planning clinical research; it seemed natural and made sense". He was surprised to discover however, that "the views of patients, their families and even clinicians are rarely sought when research priorities are being decided", and that his later involvement as co-chairman on the steering committee for a CJD research project was "an example of 'cutting edge' involvement of lay people in clinical research". Whereas to him it had seemed "a normal and sensible thing to do: who else other than someone closely involved with the disease could help with some important elements in the design of the trial?" In banking an attempt would automatically be made to research customers' needs before packaging a new product.

His experience taught him that unpleasant competition for academic status and fiefdoms must not be allowed to override patients' interests in research planning and funding: and that involvement of patients and their professional and lay carers should be normal and welcome in the shaping of clinical research, and knowledge about and participation in good clinical trials should be a normal feature of citizenship.

4. A circular model for research

Presumably the kind of participation described above would be a component of the circular model of evaluation of complex interventions recommended by Harald Walach and colleagues.[23] This is proposed as an alternative to, and an improvement upon the 'hierarchical' method for evaluating complex interventions. All medical interventions when they are applied in the real world are in effect, as we have seen, complex interventions; if only because they inevitably include contextual and placebo effects, even when they involve only one specific procedure, which is seldom the case anyway. The hierarchical research model has at its base descriptive case studies, but at its apex, and as the final arbiter of efficacy, the blinded randomised controlled trial. This depends upon the assumption that only the specific effects of a treatment or procedure, attributable to an understandable mechanism are of clinical value. This we know to be a false assumption.

The circular model described in that paper is derived from the evolution of evaluation methodology in the social sciences "which has reached the consensus that only a multiplicity of methods used in a complementary fashion will eventually give a realistic estimate of the effectiveness and safety of an intervention. Rather than postulating a single 'best method' this view acknowledges that there are optimal methods for answering specific questions, and that a composite of all methods constitutes best scientific evidence. Experimental methods that test specifically for efficacy have to be complemented by observational, non-experimental methods that are more descriptive in nature and describe real-life effects and applicability". The authors quote the synthesis of different ways of knowing described by Gabbay and le May as the 'mindlines' used in decision making by general practitioners, as an empirical example and justification for this model.[24] (See Chapter 10, 'Ways of knowing'.) "Many patients recover because of complex, synergistic or idiosyncratic reasons that cannot be isolated in controlled environments (trials).... By conceptualising evidence as circular we can highlight the fact that sometimes the 'best' evidence may not be attributional, objective, additive or even clinical."

5. Evaluating large scale and complex interventions

In fact it is not unusual that large scale healthcare interventions are introduced without clear evidence that benefits outweigh costs and harms. This was pointed out in a debate about the merits or otherwise of such a process in the *British Medical Journal*.[25] Bernard Crump argues that it can be appropriate to do so when explicit evidence is hard to come by; particularly in complex interventions that involve the behaviour of people and systems and that are just not susceptible to evaluation by the yardsticks that have been developed for narrower biomedical interventions. He, too, argues, as do Walach and colleagues *vis-à-vis* the social sciences, "We need to learn from other scientific sectors to broaden our understanding of evidence". He is not suggesting an uncritical approach to such interventions, far from it, but a process for developing programmes of improvement that "builds on feedback on intermediate outcomes and will allow for adjustment of the intervention as the implementation takes place". He recommends combining this with the 'generative' approach that takes account of the mixed dynamics of the therapeutic process and requires a deep appreciation of contextual factors, using a combination of qualitative methods (descriptive, observational, narrative) and quantitative methods (measuring what it is possible and appropriate to measure).

The other protagonist to this debate, Seth Landefeld, argues that on the contrary the evidence should be compelling if well intended interventions are not to fail, perhaps cause harm, and cost dearly. He is doubtful that observational studies provide sufficient justification. But he warns that evidence should only be accepted, and interventions put into practice "carefully, because the effects of interventions may vary among patients, providers, and medical care environments, which often differ from those in studies that establish efficacy". Which actually seems like an argument for the circular, iterative and generative approaches that others recommend.

6. Multi-disciplinary integrative care

In a study from Denmark five conventional practitioners (neurologist, occupational therapist, physical therapist, psychologist and nurse) and five complementary practitioners (acupuncture, nutritional therapy, classical homeopathy, craniosacral therapy and reflexology) explored the possibilities of collaboration in the care of patients with multiple sclerosis (MS).[26]

The project's core question was – 'Is it possible to improve treatment outcomes in people with MS by developing a model for bridge-building between conventional and alternative practitioners, and thereby facilitate and integrative treatment process at the patient level?' The study is particularly interesting, and ambitious, because it brings together practitioners with, effectively, ten different theoretical and practical approaches to patient care. The basis for the dialogue (IMCO) was the four parameters – Intervention (what does the practitioner do together with the patient?), Mechanism (how do the process and context of treatment achieve the outcome?), Context (the motivation, attitudes, personal resources, insights and expectations that the patient brings to the process), and Outcomes (what physical, emotional, psychological and social benefits are expected and achieved by the intervention?). The definitions in parenthesis are my paraphrase.

The study did not set out to evaluate the outcome of multidisciplinary integrative care of this kind, but to explore its feasibility and the means by which it can be achieved. The study process (four seminars with preparatory work) was not easy, and common objectives in terms of outcomes were very difficult to agree. But eventually the ten practitioners "developed a mutual understanding of the different treatment models; began to think as a team; developed a mutual communication platform based on trust; and developed a platform for collaboration with the researchers".

The authors conclude, "Creating bridges between fundamentally different ways of conceptualising diseases, curing and healing, simply takes time. However, collaboration *is* possible when focusing less on singular treatments and more on the primary target of optimising the treatment of each unique individual."

7. Investigating 'whole person' approaches

Iris Bell and colleagues emphasise as I have done that Integrative Medicine is not the same thing as complementary medicine (CAM) but "a comprehensive primary care system that emphasises wellness and healing of the whole person".[19] Nevertheless, they go on to say that, "As it evolves, truly integrative medicine also depends for its philosophical foundation and patient-centred approach on systems of CAM that emphasise healing the person as a whole (e.g. Traditional Chinese Medicine, Ayurvedic Medicine, and classical homeopathy). These CAM systems diverge the most in philosophy, diagnosis and treatment from conventional medicine, and thus remain marginalised. – As a result, clinicians and researchers often break off parts of these CAM systems from their original contexts to fit a few of the smaller pieces into the dominant model of conventional care and medical research. For example, numerous studies have investigated the efficacy of acupuncture for various Western disorders, but virtually no studies examine the effectiveness of the sum total of Chinese medicine as practiced. – It is a testable hypothesis that the effect sizes of the full treatment program could be much larger and more clinically significant if the entire Chinese medicine treatment program were studied as used".

A thought experiment

Only two of these examples of lateral thinking around the subject of research are directly related to complementary medicine (CAM), but they are all relevant to the particular challenge that is presented by the role of CAM, and any expanded role for CAM, within integrative health care. Here is a thought experiment that supposes the large scale introduction of a potential health care improvement for which there is not compelling evidence (example 5), but which could generate, or of course fail to generate such evidence.

The 2010 UK coalition government proposed that an £80 billion (€94bn, $124bn) budget should be entrusted to general practitioners to commission services from other health care providers. Suppose that all 500 of the GP consortia expected to manage this budget, if it is equally distributed, were required to commit 0.1% of their share of the budget to integrating complementary medicine into primary and secondary care. Or if that seems too extreme, suppose that 0.0002% of the total budget is allocated to a 20% cohort of consortia, 100 of them, for that purpose. In either case each consortium committed to the task would have £160,000 (€187,000, $247,000) to spend per year. The object of the exercise is to improve the health and well-being of their patients and to reduce the burden (of time, cost and stress) on themselves and their practices and the other services they would normally commission by the informed and discriminating use of complementary medicine; a similar exercise to that undertaken in the Glastonbury Project (Chapter 16). It would be a new exercise in interprofessional care. It would require consortia:

- Get to know the complementary practices in their area.
- Understand and appraise their potential contribution to patient care – but not to learn their therapeutic methods (example 6).
- Learn from patients' experience of using complementary medicine (example 3).

- Select therapists (Chapter 19).
- Learn to collaborate (Chapter 19).
- Negotiate payment.
- Establish proper communication and continuity.
- Audit the process and its outcomes.
- Apply all appropriate ways of knowing (Chapter 10) to inform and develop their practice 'mindlines'.
- Incorporate research from formal trials with these other sources of knowledge in a circular process of evaluation (example 4) that comprehends the effectiveness of the complementary approaches as a whole rather than isolated bits of their respective black box (example 7).

This need not actually be a hugely time consuming or demanding task. It might even be enjoyable and liberating.

Conclusion

> Medical knowledge is not knowledge acquired primarily for its own sake (but) for a specific purpose – the care of the sick. (Pellegrino and Thomasma[1])

Medical science and the study of health care delivery are already developing methods of enquiry and suggesting outcomes that justify a radical reappraisal of medical thought and practice. Subtle therapeutic methods that stimulate self-regulation and self-healing, and the contextual and 'meta-organic' factors that contribute to these have already achieved significance and importance in our understanding of the dynamics of health care. And their application is a widespread and insistent reality of contemporary medicine. Wider and more formal and systematic adoption and integration of these methods and of the precepts they exemplify promise health gains and economic benefits that are too great to ignore. If the promise is to be fulfilled, and it must certainly be tested to be sure that it can be, medical science must redirect its biomedical gaze towards these more holistic horizons. And that redirection of its gaze will require that it is more willing to adopt ways of looking at illness–disease–sickness, and at health care and healing that are far more flexible and versatile than the 'hierarchy' of evidence has hitherto permitted. Medical science must acknowledge that there are ways of knowing and things to be known that exceed the scope of its presently dominant paradigm. The examples given in these pages point the way.

Science, the systematically organised expression of our desire to know the world truly, admits to no boundaries. But medical science is an applied science. As a doctor I am guided in my practice as much by an awareness of what I should *not* do as of what I should do. There are questions that I must ask, and questions that I must not ask unless the patient invites them, at least implicitly. There are insights that I must not offer unless and until the patient is ready to receive them; things I must not say because they would be inappropriate, impertinent or unkind. There are procedures I must not perform without the patient's consent; prescriptions I must not make unless they are really needed and will be tolerated. This often requires great sensitivity, discretion and restraint. In other words I have a repertoire of knowledge and skills, and personal attributes, which must always be subordinated to my compassionate understanding of the person in my care and the context of that particular therapeutic encounter. It must be appropriately applied.

The application of science in medicine must be similarly discriminating, and always have a *person* in its gaze, even when it is a molecule that is the precise focus of attention. This is a shared responsibility between the clinician and the scientist. Scientists must fully understand the implications that the application of their science will have for the therapeutic process, the healing relationship. They must not promote its application simply out of their scientific enthusiasm for its possibilities, just as I must not impose some treatment on a patient simply because of my enthusiasm for that particular drug or procedure, or therapeutic theory. And the clinician must not adopt a scientific advance just because it becomes available. It must never be true, to misquote David Haslam again, that we use the medical science because the medical science is what we use. We must never be tempted to use a laboratory test just because it has become a cheaper and easier way of managing a patient if it does not help us to understand that patient's predicament truly; particularly if it becomes a substitute for listening to the patient carefully. And I mean *care*-fully. Clinicians must never succumb to the lust described by D.H. Lawrence and quoted by David Horrobin:[4]

> "When I went to the scientific doctor
> I realised what lust there was in him to
> wreak his so-called science on me
> and reduce me to the level of a thing.
> So I said: Good morning! And left him."

There must be a dialogue between clinicians and scientists that ensures that what clinicians *really* need to know, or *really* need to have available to them, is translated into an agenda for the scientists. And that what scientists have to offer can be *really* usefully applied in clinical practice. The same principle applies to other fields of applied science, of course. And it begs the question – When should this dialogue begin? I suspect that to be truly fruitful it must begin at quite an early stage in a common educational pathway.

References

1 Pellegrino E, Thomasma D. *The Virtues in Medical Practice*. Oxford: Oxford University Press; 1963.
2 Midgeley M. *Science as Salvation*. London: Routledge; 1992.
3 Ward K. *In Defence of the Soul*. Oxford: Oneworld; 1998.
4 Horrobin D. *Medical Hubris – A reply to Ivan Illich*. Edinburgh: Churchill Livingstone; 1978.
5 Greaves D. *Mystery in Western Medicine*. Aldershot: Avebury; 1996.
6 Swayne J. The truth the whole truth or anything but the truth. *Consent and deceit in pain medicine* The British Pain Society: Special interest group for philosophy and ethics. London: British Pain Society; 2009. pp28–43.
7 Rosenberg C. The Tyranny of Diagnosis: Specific Entities and Individual Experience. *The Millbank Quarterly* 2002; 80(2):237–260.
8 Dixon M. Sweeney K. *The Human Effect in Medicine*. Oxford: Radcliffe; 2000.
9 Spiro H. *The Power of Hope*. New Haven & London: Yale University Press; 1998.
10 Engel G. The need for a new medical model. *Science* 1977; 196:4286;129–136.
11 Sokol D. The Humane Lie: Acceptable deceptions in the doctor–patient relationship. *Consent and deceit in pain medicine* British Pain Society; Special interest group for philosophy and ethics. London: British Pain Society; 2009. pp5–15.
12 Polkinghorne J. *Theology in the Context of Science*. London: SPCK; 2008.
13 Porter R. *The greatest benefit to mankind*. London: Fontana; 1997.
14 Swayne J. *Homeopathic Method: Implications for Clinical Practice and Medical Science*. Edinburgh: Churchill Livingstone; 1998.
15 Orwell G. *The Collected Essays Journalism and Letters of George Orwell. Volume II*: My Country Right or Left 1940–1943. London: Harmondsworth-Penguin; 1970.
16 Lyng S. *Holistic Health and Biomedical Medicine*. New York: State University of New York Press; 1990.
17 Haslam D. Who cares? *Br J Gen Pract*. 2007; 57(545):987–993.
18 le Fanu J, Weatherall DJ. Is modern genetics a blind alley? *Br Med J*. 2010; 340 c1008:1008–9.
19 Bell IR, Caspi O, Schwartz G *et al*. Integrative medicine and systemic outcomes research. *Arch Intern Med*. 2002; 162:133–140.
20 Greenhalgh T. Not all those who wander are lost. *Br Med J*. 2010; 340 c4611:229.
21 Reeve J. Protecting generalism: moving on from evidence-based medicine? *Br J Gen Pract*. 2010; 60:576;521–523.

22 Firkins L. Setting research priorities: a layman's experience. *Br Med J.* 2008; 337 a212:114.
23 Walach H, Falkenberg T, Fønnebø V *et al.* Circular instead of hierarchical: methodological principles for the evaluation of complex interventions. *BMC Med Res Methodol.* 2006; 6:29.
24 Gabbay J, le May A. Evidence based guidelines or collectively constructed "mind-lines"? Ethnographic study of knowledge management in primary care. *Br Med J.* 2004; 329;1013–17.
25 Crump B, Landefeld S. Should we use large scale healthcare interventions without clear evidence that benefits outweigh costs and harms. *Br Med J.* 2008; 336:1267–1277.
26 Launsø L, Skovgaard L. The IMCO scheme as a tool in developing team-based treatment for people with Multiple sclerosis. *J Altern Complement Med.* 2008; 14(1):69–77.

19

LEARNING TO DO MEDICINE
The context and process of care

Summary

- A vocation to medicine is necessary, whatever the medical 'trade', (doctor, medical scientist, technician, administrator, etc.), if the individual is to have 'the passion necessary to practise it well'.
- This means that the medical system must allow, encourage and support that vocational instinct.
- Medical education must embrace the diversity of professions and disciplines that constitute the whole health care community, and acknowledge the actual landscape of contemporary health care.
- It is damaging to patients and to health care in general, for the medical establishment to restrict its vision of medicine and of medical education to what is provided by and for doctors and their mainstream professional colleagues.
- Increasing the scope and intimacy of interprofessional education (IPE) is essential to the evolution of health care. IPE improves patient care, and the working life and job satisfaction for practitioners.
- For improved collaboration to become a reality practitioners and educators must be *willing* to collaborate; changes in health care policy and organisation will be necessary; and medical education must become truly integrative and holistic.
- A prerequisite will be clarification and convergence of our understanding of the goals of medicine.
- Changes in the culture and curriculum of education for all healthcare professionals will be fundamental to any effective remodelling. These changes cannot be isolated from the wider context of culture and society that has already been discussed.

Vocation

The underlying premise of this book is that medicine is an activity whose goal is healing – through the prevention or relief of suffering, illness, sickness, disease and disability; an activity towards which people are drawn by the desire to serve that goal. That desire must accompany and justify, and perhaps transcend, whatever else there is in medicine that satisfies or gives expression to the interests, accomplishments or aspirations of the person who is drawn to it. It is what we call 'vocation', and why we call the practice of medicine in all its aspects 'a vocation'.

'Vocation' is not the prerogative of certain professions. Everyone has a vocational instinct towards some path in life that satisfies and gives expression to the interests and attributes that particularly motivate them, and that allows the fulfilment of their unique potential. We may have more than one vocation – as a mother, an athlete and a gardener, for example – one or other of which may come to the fore at different times in our lives. A vocation to medicine is necessary if the 'practitioner,' whatever the medical 'trade' (doctor, medical scientist, technician, administrator, etc.), is to have, in James le Fanu's words, "the passion necessary to practise it well".[1] It is necessary for the good of the patients, and for the good of the individual themselves.

This means that the medical system must allow, encourage and support that vocational instinct. Which for reasons that have been discussed in previous chapters at present it evidently does not. And it requires that medical schools and colleges, of whatever health care profession, take account of vocational motivation in their selection process; and that thereafter they nourish and develop it in the student and graduate, and guide it sensitively in the appropriate direction.

A medical *career* is about medical *care*; caring for and caring about patients. Any work in a medical environment is work in a care service. Hospital cleaners should be recruited with the capacity to care for, or at least to care about, the people under whose beds they clean, and that attitude should be encouraged by their management. This will not only be good for patients but will dignify the role of cleaner and encourage job satisfaction and 'the necessary passion to do the job well'. How much more vital must such motivation be to the role of someone with direct responsibility for patient care? It must surely be central to the education and training of any health care professional.

The question, 'Why do you want to be a doctor, nurse, physiotherapist, osteopath?' must never be a routine, tick-box question. The reason for asking it, the answer, the manner in which the answer is given and in which it is probed, must be based on insight into the vocational nature of health care and the foremost importance of a vocational instinct if a health care career is to be effective and fulfilling. I say 'effective' rather than 'successful' because success implies the possibility of secondary gains – opportunity to use particular skills or aptitudes for example, status or income perhaps – which may be legitimate, but which could be a distraction from patient care.

A high level of academic ability, demonstrated by school exam results has become an essential criterion for entry into medical school, and nursing is to be a degree entry profession in the UK now. (A development, it has been suggested, could fatally damage their traditional disposition as 'healers'; see Introduction).[2] In today's climate I doubt that my Advanced level examination marks would have been acceptable for a career as a doctor, and I believe I have been a good one. Such academic ability as I have developed came later. Medicine needs people of high intelligence and academic and technical expertise, but it doesn't only need them. It mostly needs people with *sufficient* intelligence, but with a variety of other attributes, including of course emotional intelligence. And underpinning all of these attributes must be vocation. Fortunately, courses to broaden the base of medical education to include students whose background or aptitudes have not provided the level of academic attainment usually required are being pioneered successfully, producing doctors of excellent and subtly different quality, and whose presence enhances the learning experience of fellow students along the way.[3]

Accepting that a vocation for healthcare will lead individuals in different directions as their education and training proceeds (see Figure 19.1), and that these different directions will require different skill sets and attributes, a common foundation is necessary. It will be necessary if the variety of professions that medicine needs is to be a *community* of care. This foundation will have two essential elements. One will be the early experience of working and learning with others, including tutors as well as fellow students, who represent an eclectic mix of attributes, aptitudes and aspirations. This 'interprofessional education' is necessary to develop the interprofessional awareness and respect and the collaborative care that will be discussed later in this chapter. The other, fundamental element of this 'foundation course' for health care and medicine will be shared vocational goals. These will be the glue that bonds students, and later practitioners, who bring different qualities and qualifications to this eclectic mix and subsequently proceed along different vocational and professional pathways. The common ingredient will be their vocation.

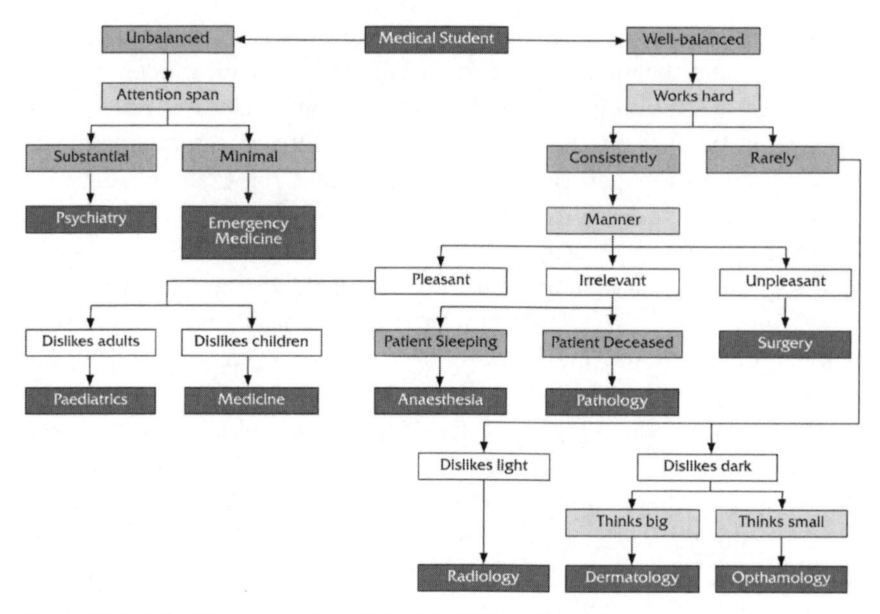

Figure 19.1 *A healthcare vocation will lead in different directions.*

A new perspective in medical education

This chapter is not just about medical education in the sense that it is usually applied to doctors. Medicine is the responsibility of the whole health care community; which is as extensive as the permutations of care that I discuss in Chapter 16 imply. 'Medicine' comprises a great diversity of professions and disciplines; whose professionalism and discipline, as well as their knowledge and skill, and their ability to care, constitute the 'musicianship' of good medicine. This medical, health care community of course includes the mainstream, non-doctor professions – nursing, physiotherapy, occupational therapy and so on, and medical education must be understood as encompassing their education and training. Indeed interprofessional education, discussed more fully later in this chapter, is now a required component of the education of all mainstream health care professionals – theoretically; as is familiarity with the main complementary medicine disciplines. And the modern health care community *de facto* includes complementary practitioners, who have schools and colleges, education and training. Many include modules teaching aspects of conventional medical knowledge and skill, often taught by conventional doctors. Several are established as departments in universities.

These university departments are decried by some mainstream medics and academics. But David Peters, Professor and Clinical Director of the

School of Integrated Health at the University of Westminster, makes the case for them eloquently, writing in the Times Higher Education:[4]

> Our range of courses is an authentic attempt to bring important areas of complementary therapies education, practice and research into the academic mainstream. Our aims are: to explore these therapies' role in augmenting conventional care and to produce the highest calibre of practitioners capable of critical thinking and safe practice and able to engage with the wider scientific and medical community. It is only through universities offering science-based complementary therapies degrees that the concerns of those who worry that practitioners are merely tricking their patients can be allayed.
>
> There is strong emphasis within the courses on reflective practice, which also forms the backbone of staff development programmes and clinical teachers' supervision groups.
>
> Complementary therapies underline philosophical problems – the mind-body relationship and the nature of experience – as well as hard scientific ones, such as how to research the therapeutic relationship and the organism's extraordinary capacity to self-regulate and occasionally heal itself against impossible odds. They raise sociological questions about complementary therapies' emergence and popularity, and about biomedicine's trajectory and sustainability. They also draw attention to the nature of complex interventions (and) how to teach and research (them).
>
> University departments where the practice of complementary therapies can be understood are ideal bases for the critical practice and research the field so badly needs.

BOX 19.1 *Learning to do medicine: the core curriculum*

- Learning to cure; learning about cure.
- Learning to care; learning about care.
- Learning to cope.
- Learning to heal.
  - holistic healthcare.
- Learning to collaborate.
  - interprofessional education;
  - integrative healthcare.

It is no longer good enough, in fact it is damaging to patients and to health care in general, for the medical establishment to restrict its vision of medicine and of medical education to what is provided by and for doctors and their mainstream professional colleagues. A model of medical education is required that acknowledges the actual landscape of contemporary health care, its actual 'cosmology'. (See Box 19.1.)

The pages that follow are written with that goal in mind, and several of the precepts they discuss are reflected in David Peters' article. Their argument has implications not only for practitioners, but for patients and the culture that shapes patients' attitudes to medicine, and for the political and administrative context and process of health care.

Learning to cure

There is immense satisfaction for a practitioner in ridding a patient of their complaint, or at the very least making it better than it was before. That is why we do what we do. And conversely there is disappointment when a patient does not respond to treatment, does not get better. We may feel we have failed. We may even feel let down by the patient. As a doctor and as a patient I have experienced this disappointment. And as a patient I have seen the disappointment in the face of the person treating me when I have not made the progress we were both hoping for.

This scenario will be familiar to all of us, and it reveals, or perhaps conceals, a number of truths:

- As practitioners we really do want people to get better. For some of us that may be only a technical challenge. But for many it is a vocation.
- As practitioners we have our professional pride. We have invested a lot in acquiring our knowledge and skill. We have high expectations of ourselves, and a strong desire for success in applying that knowledge and skill. Success is usually measured in terms of clinical outcome; our ability to control what is happening to the patient.
- These expectations are often too high. We know, or should know, that illness is a very complex phenomenon, and that the course of illness and treatment in any individual patient is fraught with uncertainty. And yet we may not make sufficient allowance for this when assessing the intended outcome.
- Consequently we may be excessively self-critical, and/or attribute the lack of success to some failing in the patient; or paradoxically to that complexity in the problem which we had not allowed for sufficiently when assessing the intended outcome.
- As practitioners we are creatures of the medical culture of cure and control. Even if our therapeutic method is unconventional, and seen as a stimulus to self-regulation, self-healing and health promotion, that is

the culture to which we still belong. A culture that pervades our own and our patients' thinking and expectations.

- Not surprisingly, when things go well, patient and practitioner are likely to feel duly grateful and gratified. But any honest practitioner will acknowledge that things have sometimes gone better than can be accounted for by the knowledge and skill they have brought to the task. There are many possible reasons for this, not least that the patient was going to get better anyway, and all the other contextual and 'meaning' effects that I discuss in Chapter 12 ('Natural medicine and natural healing'). But foremost of these reasons will have been our ability to care, rather than our ability to cure; the *caritas* that accompanied our *scientia*.

In other words, both practitioners and patients are caught up in a web of curing, caring and coping; a web of relationship and expectation that is difficult to manage, and that practitioners' training may not have equipped them to understand and manage well.

Learning about cure

Learning to cure means, of course, acquiring the knowledge and skill to achieve cure – remission or the relief of suffering and disability; to control the situation as far as possible. It also means learning the limits of those possibilities, learning to recognise those limits in particular clinical situations, and learning to cope with those limitations within the relationship with the particular patient. It means learning to come to an understanding with the patient, and helping the patient to cope with that understanding and to live with the implications. It means learning to understand and cope with the implications of what we can and cannot do.

For patients it is a matter of learning *about* cure and control. As patients we will learn from practitioners, and will come to expect what they teach us to expect. But we also learn from our culture – the culture of family, society, religion, and science. We learn from the plausibility structure, the paradigms, and the models we have grown up with, and which were mapped out in the Introduction. Our attitudes to death, disability and suffering, our aspirations and values, our view of human nature, will affect our attitude to medicine. And medicine will both reflect and shape those attitudes.

Learning to cure and learning about cure means learning about the limitations of medicine just as much as its achievements, and learning to be honest about them and to cope with them. And it means learning that whatever the limits of cure and control may be, there need be no limit to medicine's ability to *heal*. There *need* be no limit. But it does require a change of emphasis within the medical model, and within the system of medical education that sustains it.

Learning to care

It's not what you do; it's the way that you do it; that's what gets results.

The section, Natural Medicine and Natural Healing in Chapter 12 explains the importance of context and meaning in all therapeutic encounters, and we have seen how little we know about many of these effects and how to make best use of them. There is a great deal to be learned about the process of care and how to make it most effective. But we do know that one powerful element of this process is the doctor/practitioner–patient relationship, its 'meaningful' content, and the empathy and compassion it transmits. These qualities are no substitute for the knowledge and skill of the medical craft. But without them the power of that craft to cure, and above all to heal, is greatly diminished. And where that craft falls short or fails, they are essential to the healing that can still be achieved – the well-being that comes from the way "we relate *inwards* to ourselves and come to understand ourselves (and) *outwards* – to others, our community and our environment"[5] that can transcend the intractable problems of our physical health.

Those qualities are so fundamental to the value of health care that their development should be the foundation of the education and training of all health care professionals. They will be essential to the therapeutic repertoire of those who are involved in direct patient care, but also part of the *raison d'être* of those with an essential technical or supportive role who are not. There is no reason why pathologists examining tissue sections in the laboratory should not have compassionate insight into the feelings of the patient from whom it was taken and the clinician who is caring for her; insight that will enhance their commitment to the task and their vocational satisfaction.

And even more fundamental is something so obvious that it is shameful that we need even to consider it – the need for kindness. Do health care professionals need to *learn* to be kind? Or at least learn to remember to be kind; because we don't mean to be *unkind*, do we? But as Angela Jones reminds us in a catalogue of examples in a Personal View in the *British Medical Journal*, apparent unkindness is a too frequent experience in NHS medicine.[6] She contrasts the experiences related in anecdotes and official reports of poor treatment with the commitment in the 2009 NHS Constitution to:

> Respond with humanity and kindness to each person's pain, distress, anxiety or need. (To) search for the things we can do, however small, to give comfort and relieve suffering. (To) find time for those we serve and work alongside. We do not wait to be asked, because we care.

And she suggests that,

> What might seem to be a ridiculously touchy-feely notion becomes, on reflection, anything but. If we abolished unkind acts, trays of untouched food would no longer be taken away from debilitated patients on wards. Cries for help unheard and buzzers unheeded would become things of the past. Administrative delays leaving patients waiting for weeks or months in pain or fearing undiagnosed cancer would not occur. Concerned patients and relatives would no longer be brushed aside, ignored, or patronised. Furthermore, the universal application of kindness would mean that the needs of staff, in terms of training, support, and workload, would be acknowledged and met. This in turn would enable us to avoid the desensitisation that occurs when there are simply too many demands on our time and we feel forced to block out our patients' needs so as to function and survive.

This is indeed, sadly, a lesson that does need to be learned by everyone in involved in the education and training of practitioners and any aspect of the process of care, and those responsible for policies and management strategies that determine the context of care. Because as Dr Jones points out, it is training, support and workload that determine so much of our capacity to care; our sensitivity or contrasting desensitisation to the intimate needs of our patients.

Learning about care

Learning *to* care is the responsibility of health care professionals. But just as patients need to learn *about* cure, they need to learn *about* care. This is more likely to happen when the professionals demonstrate care, but it is also a matter of culture. The tendency to regard medicine and health care as a commodity and patients as customers or clients is seriously subversive to the goals and vocation of medicine. It undermines the *caritas*. This attitude is partly the product of a materialist culture, but it is also the product of healthcare and public health policy and 'surveillance medicine'. It is well exemplified by the increasing habit of referring to a check-up from one's doctor as an M.O.T., the abbreviation for the annual car safety check in the UK. The implication being that our health and well-being are mechanical functions to be routinely checked and legislated for and the faults repaired.

Patients as well as doctors need to know that the secret of caring for patients is to *care* for patients. The fact needs to be evident in the attitude and behaviour of health care professionals, certainly. But it also needs to be part of the understanding and expectation that patients have of them; an understanding that it is as important as their professional expertise. An understanding and an expectation that it will be there whether the expertise is curative, or palliative, and even, especially perhaps, when expertise is defeated by the complexity or intractable nature of the problem. And an understanding that care is costly. The milk of human kindness does not grow on trees – if you will pardon the mixed metaphor. It is the fruit of the human body, mind and soul.

And to repeat the vital point just made, this is a lesson that *must* be learned by health care policy makers and administrators too. The ability to care has to be sustained by the *process* of care, and the *context* of care. A system that is so focused on control and cure that it does not allow its practitioners the physical, mental and emotional space to care will destroy them, or at least their vocation, and fail its patients.

Learning to cope

Health care is costly, not just expensive. If it is truly health *care*, it is costly in human resources – of emotion, energy and commitment. For health care professionals this means learning to cope, and being helped to cope. This learning and help needs to start at the beginning of our education and training, modelled for us by our teachers, and to continue throughout our career by means of mentoring, supervision and peer support. And ideally it needs to be reflected in and sustained by the quality of our personal relationships outside work, which can be jeopardised by the stresses and costs incurred in our work.

Learning to cope begins with the acknowledgement of our own vulnerability and of the burdens of our shared humanity. It means being given permission to be vulnerable by teachers and colleagues who are aware of their own vulnerability, and do not pretend otherwise. Our vulnerability as carers is important. It makes us helpful to others. Understanding our vulnerability makes us stronger to bear their burdens.

This is not a matter of wearing our hearts on our sleeves, but of learning to be appropriately truthful, brave and loving in our relationships with ourselves and with one another. If we are to discover within ourselves the empathy and compassion that will make our therapeutic encounters most effective we need to learn to cope with ourselves, as well as with the feelings and experiences of the others whose burdens we share. As we come to achieve this personal well-being by the way we relate inwards to ourselves and come to understand ourselves, so we are better able to relate outwards to others, and so reap the dividends of greater well-being which that in turn yields.

Learning to cope is a process that many caring professions provide for in their training and in-service support. But it is not universal, and it is certainly not commonplace in the training and working lives of doctors. And it is not necessarily effective in all professional groups that do provide for it. A book that I was given to read at the beginning of a psychotherapy course warned that some professional care groups inhibit the insight they exist to foster, by replacing truthful awareness of themselves and each other with the interpretive language and professional 'games' of their school or method.[7] Professionals can avoid truthful self-awareness by recourse to what in another context has been called 'narrow speak';[8] jargon and the language of dogma.[i] The author of the psychotherapy book commends the family as the forum in which therapists are most likely to hear the truth about themselves!

To repeat: learning to cope involves self-discovery in a truthful, brave and loving environment. All health care professionals need and deserve this opportunity, in training and beyond, and it should be a basic ingredient of all strands of medical education.

And it is essential that professionals should learn to cope if they are to help their patients to be able to cope – with the challenge, distress or anxiety of their illness; which they have to be able to do. Practitioners have to help their patients to learn to cope; patients have to be willing to learn to cope. And here again is the dilemma at the interface of medicine with its society and its culture. Medicine and society collude in the illusion that medicine has, should have, or will have the answers; that the health service will provide. There is an unhealthy dependence on medicine, a debilitating intolerance of even mild inconvenience and distress associated with or attributed to illness. This is a social and cultural phenomenon that medicine has helped to create, by being able, or being assumed to be able to do so much, and by its collusion or acquiescence in that 'tyranny of health'.[9]

---

i The terms 'narrowspeak' and 'wholespeak' were coined by the Australian poet Les Murray. In an essay on religious poetry, *Embodiment and incarnation*: he writes of poetry as an agent of wholeness. *Wholespeak* is the language of poetry and dream, essential to our well-being. *Narrowspeak* embraces most of 'the administrative discourse by which the world is ruled from day to day', . . . 'based on the supposed primacy or indeed exclusive sovereignty of daylight reason; always in the service of some (ideology) at one or more removes'.

It is not always easy for people to judge when they need medical help (formal care) and when they do not; to know when and how to cope on their own or with the help and advice of family and friends (informal care). And people's ability to do so will vary according to their personal circumstances and attributes. But as with the earlier argument about health promotion, where the right relationship exists – a relationship of trust, proper authority, and empathy – practitioners can help them to learn. There is no 'top down' solution to this. Public health pronouncements won't change things. Medical education is not particularly effective in changing doctors' prescribing habits, and public health education is no more likely to change people's consulting habits or ability to cope. But enablement through a good practitioner–patient relationship evidently can do so, as we have seen.

Learning to heal

The relationship between medicine and healing is first discussed in Chapter 7, and explored further in Chapter 8. Chapter 12 sets out some general principles that distinguish healing from treatment and cure. There, healing was described as creative, a process that encompasses our natural capacity for self-regulation and repair, but that in its fullest sense has to do with the greater fulfilment of our potential as a unique human being, even in the face of intractable physical and mental health problems. Many skills and attributes equip us to assist this process in one another in ordinary relationships as well as in professional therapeutic relationships. But those of us with a professional therapeutic role have a particular responsibility to develop them.

We all have a healing instinct. It is represented in the healing of a wound – a natural process, but one that may need our assistance. It is also an instinct towards that greater fulfilment and wholeness. Whether we see it as a natural biological process or a more comprehensive aspect of human nature, it is innate, born in us. We can encourage it and assist it but we cannot of our own power heal. For that reason it is wrong for anyone to assume the title 'healer', as many do, including those who have subtle gifts of touch or presence that enable some aspect of the healing process.

Learning to heal means learning to assist the innate, instinctive healing process in others. It does not mean learning to be a 'healer'. It is learning to exercise a *responsibility* that we all have towards one another, especially in a professional role that involves direct patient care. This is the sense in which learning to give patients our full attention so that they know they have been 'heard', as well as the other attributes that equip a practitioner to be a better agent of healing, must be part of the curriculum of all medical education.

Learning to heal does, of course, involve learning the skills that assist the healing process. Learning first aid is learning to heal, as is learning neurosurgery. But the repertoire of technical skills is incomplete if it is not allied with the ability to employ the healing influence of context, meaning and relationship. It is incomplete unless it is accompanied by learning to care and learning to cope. It is incomplete unless we develop those attributes that equip us a *person* rather than just as a professional to enable and affirm the healing process in others.

Empathy and compassion, an understanding of natural healing and the ability to promote it – the healing qualities of our essential humanity – can be evoked and developed in the education, training and working lives of all involved in patient care. And they must infuse the whole culture of medicine, just as we need the humanities to do if medicine is to preserve its healing tradition.[2]

In that sense, learning to heal does not need to be a subject heading in the curriculum if it is recognised and represented as an aspect of *everything* that practitioners learn to do. An underlying question, explicit or implicit, should always be, 'How can I apply this knowledge or exercise this skill in a way that is most healing for this person?' For educators and trainers this is not primarily a matter of teaching technique but of attitude. And for clinical teachers it is a matter of demonstrating that attitude in their behaviour with patients. Unfortunately, the medical school experience seems to have the opposite effect. A study in *Academic Medicine* by Newton and colleagues adds to the evidence of this deleterious effects of medical education year on year on medical students capacity for empathy.[10] They conclude, "The significant decrease in vicarious empathy is of concern, because empathy is crucial for a successful physician–patient relationship".

The core 'virtues' of a healing profession may need to be proclaimed in the curriculum, but as the underlying ethos as well as a learning objective.

Learning to collaborate

I entered general practice at a time, the late 1960s, when the concept of the Primary Care Team, now well established, was quite new. The team was not just a vehicle for collaborative care, it was a learning experience as rich as any in the course of my medical training. Whether changing the bed of an incontinent stroke victim with the district nurse, helping a first time

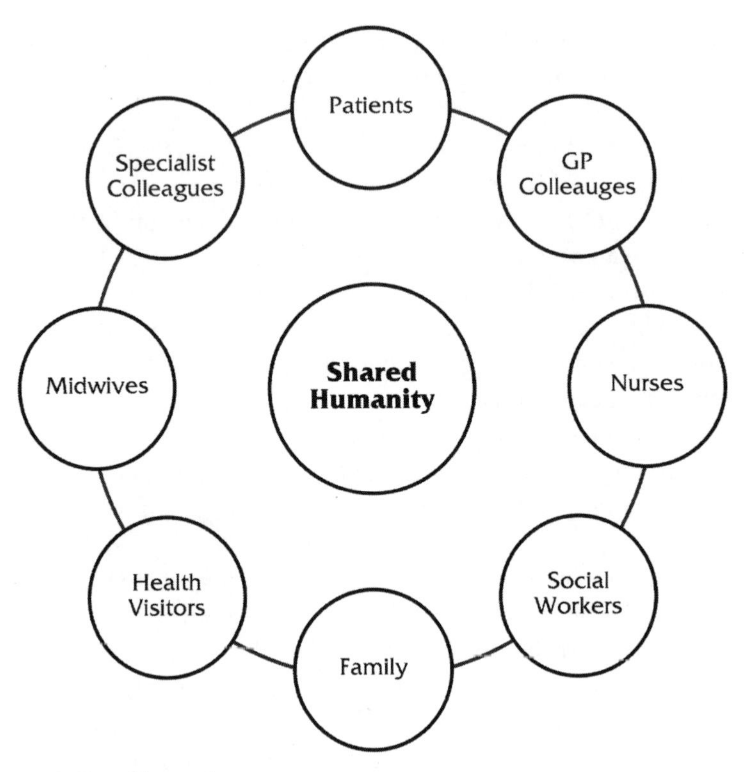

Figure 19.2 *Shared humanity.*

mother to cope with the fear and pain of childbirth with the midwife, or understanding the problems of a dysfunctional family with the health visitor, I was not just learning a new repertoire of skills and insights, I was gaining experience of our shared humanity (see Figure 19.2): the shared humanity of my colleagues and of our patients. At that time my sense of belonging to a health care community was enhanced by the ease and informality of access to consultant colleagues and the clinical departments in the local hospital, and to the social work and probation services. All this was facilitated by the convenient topography, but also by the health care culture. Over the years the experience of collaboration that I found so valuable was augmented by working in teams for the care of the elderly and for a community mental handicap service. This range of experience will be common for many doctors and their colleagues in other professions.

In the early days primary care teams were quite small. Now they are often much larger, incorporating a greater variety of professional skills; quite commonly counsellors, for example, and sometimes complementary therapists. One of the pioneering influences in this expansion of the primary care team was the Marylebone Centre Trust, set up by Patrick and

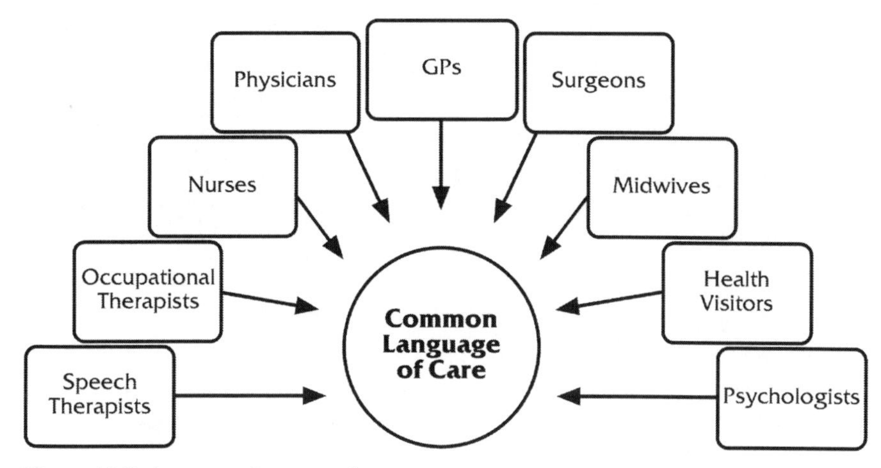

Figure 19.3 A common language of care.

Marilyn Pietroni in the early 1990's which established a primary care practice in St Marylebone Church in London committed to "a holistic understanding of interprofessional education and practice within which complementary therapies were assured of a place".[11] Such projects to explore and develop models of integrative care involving complementary therapies have been evolving for many years now, and are particularly well developed in the USA.

My own experience of interprofessional collaboration was further enhanced later in my career by two years working on the Read Codes. This was the original NHS project to develop a common terminology for use in electronic medical records. It was not just an academic exercise in medical terminology, but an opportunity to learn something of what it is like to be a surgeon, a gastroenterologist, a speech therapist, an occupational therapist. And to an extent to understand what it is like to be one of their patients; to have the sort of problem they strive to solve. Despite the technological nature of the product it was set up to develop, the project was a remarkable example of interprofessional collaboration; a challenging but rewarding exploration of the possibilities of 'a common language of care'.[12] Figure 19.3 illustrates this concept.

I may have been particularly favoured by the congenial interprofessional climate at the beginning of my career because the evolution of team work primary care and the interprofessional training to support it has been difficult and laboured; lead, or driven, by influential enthusiasts at a number of centres, but not gathering real momentum until the 1980s, and not entering the mainstream of professional education until the turn of the century.[10] I mention the influence of the Marylebone Centre Trust above.

In 1992 the Trust launched the *Journal of Interprofessional Care*, "destined to become the dedicated channel for national and later international exchange of scholarship in interprofessional education, practice and research", and delivered a Masters' programme incorporating the concept of interprofessional care validated at the University of Westminster, whose more recent work in this field was mentioned at the beginning of the chapter.

Effective interprofessional education and care is not yet a *fait accompli* in mainstream medicine, however. The paper from which I am quoting gives three excerpts from recent (2005–2009) statements from the Royal College of Physicians (RCP), the British Medical Association (BMA) and the General Medical Council (GMC) actively promoting the concept:

> Overall doctors have not spent sufficient time learning from other members of the health care team . . . we recommend that the GMC . . . and medical schools explore ways of strengthening common learning to enable better interprofessional education and training. (RCP)

> Emerging evidence suggests that interprofessional education can, in favourable circumstances and in different ways, contribute to improving collaborative practice, although further research is needed. Effective team working, collaboration and communication across professional boundaries are vital and interprofessional education a means to those ends. (BMA)

> 'Tomorrow's doctor' will, understand and respect the roles and experience of health and social care professionals in the context of working and learning as a multiprofessional team. (GMC)

It seems that these recommendations are still necessary despite the growing momentum of interprofessional education in the UK and internationally.

Interprofessional education

> Occasions when two or more (health and social care) professions learn with, from and about one another to improve collaboration and quality of care. (Centre for the Advancement of Interprofessional Education[13])

> Interdisciplinary training incorporates a collaborative and integrated program of care that celebrates and utilises the interdependent knowledge, skills, attitudes, values and methods each professional brings to the health care system. (Association of University Centers on Disabilities[14,15])

Interprofessional education (IPE) – variously labelled Interprofessional Learning (IPL) or Interdisciplinary Education (IDE), is now a core principle of undergraduate and continuing medical education for all health care professionals; for all mainstream health care professionals, that is. The

World Health Organisation (WHO) *Framework for Action on Interprofessional Education and Collaborative Practice* published in 2010 makes an emphatic case for this:[16,17]

> After about 50 years of inquiry, there is now sufficient evidence to indicate that interprofessional education enables effective collaborative practice which in turn optimises health services, strengthens health systems and improves health outcomes. In both acute and primary care settings, patients report higher levels of satisfaction, better acceptance pf care and improved health outcomes following treatment by a collaborative team. Research evidence has shown (that):
>
> Collaborative practice can improve:
> - Access to and coordination of health services.
> - Appropriate use of specialist clinical resources.
> - Health outcomes for people with chronic disease.
> - Patient care and safety.
>
> Collaborative practice can decrease:
> - Total patient complications.
> - Length of hospital stay.
> - Tension and conflict among care givers.
> - Staff turnover.
> - Hospital admissions.
> - Clinical error rates.
> - mortality rates

In response to national requirements for healthcare training programmes to be truly interprofessional, most universities in the UK are now planning or implementing IPE.[18,19]

The need for IPE

The goal of IPE is primarily to improve patient care, but also to improve the working life and job satisfaction for practitioners. The reasons for promoting IPE can be broadly described as 'strategic' or 'personal'.

'Strategic' reasons

The following excerpts from studies or reports on the development of IPE make the strategic need very clear:

> The need to train health professionals who can work across disciplines is essential for effective, competent, and culturally sensitive health care delivery. Health care students must be able to understand how colleagues are trained, what is covered in their curriculum, and what skills and competencies are associated with their clinical roles. Students should strive to understand and compare how other professional cultures define health, illness, the etiology of important health concerns, the role of biology, psychology, and social factors influencing these

> beliefs, the notion of cure or how change occurs, as well as the values and ethics that guide and direct their decision making and clinical practice.[14]
>
> Interprofessional education has been advocated by the government as a strategy to help overcome difficulties in communication and team working encountered within (different health care) settings. It is believed that IPE might help to change attitudes and dispel the stereotypes that exist between groups by increasing their knowledge and understanding of other professionals.[20]
>
> Students are immersed in both academic and practice settings during the course of their professional training and it is these environments that influence who they become as professionals. The environment in which we are trained and the people with whom we interact can profoundly influence our professional development. For example, if as nursing students they spend their days surrounded primarily by other nursing students and nurses they are likely to assume the professional values, attitudes and knowledge modelled for them. This is how they develop their professional identity. As they progress through their professional training they increasingly see the world through the eyes of their profession and as a result decrease the likelihood that they can see the world through the perspective of other professions. It is not that they lose the ability to see the perspective of the other. Rather, the lack of systematic exposure to other professions means that they often do not have the opportunity to learn that there is more than one valid way of seeing the world.
>
> We suggest that this narrowing of perspectives contributes to communication issues and misunderstandings that are seen regularly between the various health professions. How one interprets an interaction with a practitioner from another profession is dependent upon one's own profession's worldview. – An assumption may be made by them that if someone from another profession does not agree with them it is because the other person is wrong, misinformed or just not as well trained. This can lead at best to disagreement and at worst severe conflict. – the attitudes and beliefs we form during our early professional training become the basis for how we interact with our work environment and others in the future. (University of British Columbia – UBC[21])

Reasons personal to the patient

A particularly poignant account of the importance of a truly 'integrative' interprofessional approach to care comes from a study of the use of patient narratives to achieve a patient-centred approach to interprofessional learning in a stroke rehabilitation unit. Although it had a particular clinical focus, it revealed problems for patients that are likely to be common to any clinical situation where their care is divided amongst the members of a multi-disciplinary team lacking 'interprofessional awareness' centred on the needs of the individual patient. It noted the unease of patients and carers in occupying the position of being an object in the everyday milieu of an institution.

This seemed to be compounded by the size of the multiprofessional team. Interviews and conversations with patients revealed a sense of bewilderment resulting from the complex range of sometimes conflicting professional priorities that needed to be negotiated and satisfied in order to achieve discharge. One patient was puzzled, even annoyed, that he, as a patient had to bear part of the responsibility in conveying messages from one professional to another, while coping with the slow realisation that there were differing priorities and perspectives on caring and treatment amongst them. Many patients could not always gauge what would be an appropriate performance from them that would satisfy all the professionals.[22]

A critical feature of patient care confirmed by this study that is of particular relevance to rehabilitation after stroke but common to many health care situations, is the effect, for better or worse, of the manner in which care is given on the patient's sense of personal identity and meaning. It exemplifies the way in which good integrative medicine is literally integrative to the patient in the sense of encouraging or restoring a sense of personal wholeness. "Implicit in the interview data was the feeling that being subject to a range of professional perspectives was akin to a sort of 'dissection' of self. This could be a significant factor for patient rehabilitation since stroke often has a devastating effect on the individuals' sense of self." (But so can many other illnesses, not always necessarily so serious.) "It seems that being subject to the array of contrasting approaches in an interprofessional environment, could lengthen the process of reconstructing and asserting a fairly coherent new identity."

The authors conclude, "For us, these insights suggested that to attempt to provide education for better interprofessional care (needs) to be critically informed by patient experiences and perspectives". This view is echoed in an editorial in the *Journal of Interprofessional Care* by Professor JE Thistlethwaite from the University of Sydney: "Health care is complex. We now work within the philosophy that health care should be patient-centred. While this concept may be fairly well defined at the level of the individual patient-professional, what it means for an organisation is less clear, especially when the service is cash-restrained and patients' needs, let alone their wants, can never be fully met. Moreover how patient-centred is professional education? While patients are now involved in the assessment of students and health professionals, they are less likely to be involved in curriculum development and standard setting. We accept that modern health care is largely team delivered – but is the patient a member of the team, or rather only the recipient of its care? Teamwork will become more important as no-one practitioner is able to provide truly holistic care. Professionals will have to learn in teams to work in teams. How can we then hear 'the patient voice' in IPE?"[23]

Reasons personal to the practitioner

One theme that emerged from a study of interprofessional participation by Anna Forte and Patricia Fowler that I quote earlier that bears upon the personal needs of the practitioner is that of 'interprofessional awareness'.[18] This encompasses increased understanding of differences within role, learning and thinking styles, viewpoint, preconceived ideas, stereotyping and relevance to clinical practice. Another emerging theme is that of the 'impact on patient care'. In the study, students identified greater confidence in interactions with patients; improved communication between professional groups; greater awareness of care pathways; application of reflective practice; greater empathy developed from group work, role plays and discussion. The increase in empathy is especially worth noting.

There are helpful examples of both these benefits, first in a quotation from a GP member of a practice-based small group learning programme in Scotland:

> I think my learning needs are being met. I think the nurse balance helps because they are far better at sitting back and listening to people, initially. If (practice nurses) have said 'what does this do?', I haven't felt it has taken inordinate amount of time having to explain, and sometimes the things you are explaining, you are having to ask yourself why are we doing this, or why do we prescribe that? I think there is lots of different point of views, and it is amazing what patients are saying to nurses that we never hear.[24]

And in quotations from students in allied professions in the study by Forte and Fowler:[18]

> ... it is quite marked the differences in thought processes of the physios, OTs and the radiographers. It is interesting to see how we all approach things from those different angles. (Physiotherapy student)

> You're all there at the end of the day for the same person and that's the person you're caring for. There is a core set of things that we have to do, regardless of who we are or what profession. But I think there's more to be learnt from interprofessional learning than just that. (Occupational therapy student)

> It's more about the fact that you're building up a relationship with another team member who does a completely different job but you're both aiming for the same thing; about trying to build up a relationship with a professional and realising that you've got to work together as opposed to – Oh yes, you do your little bit and I'll do mine later. (Diagnostic radiography student)

Difficulties

Shared approaches to collective learning, understanding and achieving consensus, and developing the respect and trust necessary to effective and integrative interprofessional education and care are not easy to achieve.[25] The authors of the stroke rehabilitation study comment, "Usually, the problems caused by multiprofessional care as recorded in literature relate to the existence of different, sometimes irreconcilable disciplinary and theoretical perspectives within the clinical domain. (There is a need) to acknowledge and reconcile the tension arising from the fact that different professions may have different sets of criteria for patient care/rehabilitation that may not always match perfectly".[20]

The difficulty is illustrated by a contrasting quotation from another GP member of the practice-based learning group:

> I think the problem I have identified in the group is that we are coming from different backgrounds and different aspirations in terms of what we want to get out of it. I think we are discussing it at different levels . . . the nursing members in the group have different needs and knowledge base to the doctors in the group. And, therefore the level of intellectual or medicational content of the meetings can fall short of my aspirations.[22]

Reviewing the barriers of this kind to interprofessional training, a group in the US argue that the primary reason students are not trained across disciplines is related to the diverse cultural structures that guide and moderate health education environments. This profession specific "cultural frame" must be addressed if there is any hope of having interprofessional education accepted as a valued and fully integrated dimension of the curriculum. Each health discipline possesses its own professional culture that shapes the educational experience; determines curriculum content, core values, the meaning, attribution, and etiology of symptoms, even customs, dress, and the salience of symbols; and defines what constitutes health, wellness and treatment success. Most importantly, professional culture defines the means for distributing power; determines how training should proceed within the clinical setting; and the level and nature of inter-profession communication, resolution of conflicts and management of relationships between team members and constituents. It might be said that one factor limiting interdisciplinary training is *profession-centrism*. To achieve effective and fully integrated interdisciplinary education, we must decrease profession-centrism by crafting curriculum that promotes *inter-professional cultural competence*.[14]

Delivering IPE

The authors of this review go on to suggest that the essential first step in developing this competence is a willingness to enter into a dialogue with another professional. Within this conversation, students have the opportunity to explain their perceptions of assessment and treatment of a shared patient/client. Simultaneously, a culturally competent professional is able to be open to the views and approaches of their colleagues; altering their perceptions via the discussion when appropriate. Ultimately, the goal of interprofessional care is to do what is in the best interest of the patient/client.

Within the interdisciplinary setting, this often requires compromise, embracing the others perspective and rethinking your initial formulation. Students who are exposed to this type of interaction early in their training will be both skilled and more willing to carry this set of attitudes and behaviors into the practice environment post graduation. Attention involves the in-depth exploration of one's personal and professional, cultural background while simultaneously recognising one's biases, prejudices, and assumptions about individuals who are trained in different health care professions.

The University of British Columbia (UBC) had been exploring the need for IPE, and how to meet it for fifty years but without achieving an established place for it within the curriculum until the formation of the College of Health Disciplines in 2002. This comprised an eclectic collaboration of 15 health and human service programmes: Audiology and Speech Sciences, Counselling, Psychology, Dental Hygiene, Dentistry, Dietetics, Human Kinetics, Medical Laboratory Sciences, Medicine, Midwifery, Nursing, Occupational Therapy, Pharmaceutical Sciences, Physical Therapy and Social Work.

The recent report on the development of this curriculum, contends that in order to overcome or compensate for the inevitable narrowing of perspective inherent in uniprofessional training, students must be offered opportunities to interact meaningfully with members of other professions during the course of their training. And that the learning experience has to occur in such a way that it offers the student opportunities to be critically reflective in challenging their previously acquired attitudes and beliefs about other professions, and their own; to be challenged on an intrapersonal, interpersonal and community basis within the broader learning environment. In this sense, they say, community means within the 'community of professions' or the interprofessional context; which sounds close in concept to what I have called a healthcare community, or community of care.[21]

At UBC they achieve this by a process that begins at entry into training with exposure to the concept that there are multiple perspectives on a range of issues related to practice among various professions. At this stage, students are provided with opportunities to participate largely in parallel learning experiences with peers from other professions, with no expectation that they will fully understand or accept the positions of the other professions. This introductory stage takes into account the need to acquire a solid grounding in one's own profession before beginning to learn about other disciplines.

Thereafter the programme progresses gradually through increasing participation in the work of other professional groups – witnessing other professions in action; learning, in some detail, the perspectives and roles of other professions and the contributions they can make to patient care; learning more about the strengths and limitations of their own profession; reflecting on the experience so as to 'transform' their current perspectives on themselves, their own and other professions; acquiring an *interprofessional world view* that incorporates multiple perspectives and accepts and encourages the contributions of others; and eventually, at the graduate stage, mastering interprofessional concepts in such a way that they are incorporated in their daily professional practice.

Limitations

Broadly speaking, my admittedly limited exploration of the literature of IPE suggests that there are four ingredients of the interprofessional education necessary to a new medical 'cosmology', one or more of which is missing from all programmes of IPE. My apologies to any that do include all four, which are:

- An appreciation of the spiritual dimension of people's lives and its role in the dynamics of health and illness, and the representation of mainstream faiths (hospital chaplains, for example) amongst the professions included in IPE programmes.
- Explicit attention to the concepts of healing and holism, shared vocation, the goals of health care, the core principles of therapeutics, the development of empathy, and contextual healing, as 'foundation' themes to be introduced at the beginning of the programme.
- The essential inclusion of doctors, or students training to be doctors, alongside the other professions. One study involving 10 nurses, 2 physiotherapists, 2 occupational therapists, 2 therapy assistants, a nursing assistant and a speech and language therapist, regretted that

doctors were not available to participate, citing time pressures.[20] This epitomises a number of the problems that remodelling medicine needs to address.
- The essential inclusion of leading complementary medical disciplines implicated widely in the overall health care of patients within or parallel to mainstream health care.

The absolute importance of all these four 'ingredients' of any educational process promoting holistic and integrative practice is at least implicit and often explicit throughout this book.

One way or another, the *principle* of interprofessional education and collaboration and integrative care is widely established, and is being put into practice in many places and many clinical settings. In most cases the practice includes a mix of allied professions, such as Occupational Therapists, whose skill set and mind set are not primarily biomedical, and in many cases it involves practitioners whose skill set and mind set are not only not biomedical but also distinctly unorthodox. And yet, certainly in the UK, the medical landscape and the health care community remain predominately biomedical-doctor and bio-medical science orientated.

Policy and organisation

The principle, the practice and the value of collaboration, of shared inter-professional care, are well established – in theory. But is there any real sense of health care professionals belonging to a community of care? My impression is that this is actually less evident than it was in the early years of my career. The increasing specialisation and technical complexity of medicine has something to do with it. The closure of smaller clinical units such as Cottage Hospitals, and the concentration of resources in more geographically dispersed centres is another factor. It is suggested, "The relationship between primary and secondary care . . . is perhaps all the more fraught today, (because) with increasing demands on doctors in primary and secondary care, opportunities for contact across the divide are scarcer than ever".[26]

Commenting on the UK Coalition government's proposed NHS reforms, Professor Chris Ham draws attention to the need for greater collaboration. "Collaboration is especially important in areas such as urgent care and the provision of high quality cancer and cardiac services, where better outcomes depend on services being planned and provided in networks. General practitioners must also work more closely with hospital based specialists in clinically integrated groups to improve care for people with long term conditions. Recent NHS reforms have neglected the need for organisations to collaborate across local systems of care, and the capacity to do so in the proposed arrangements must be strengthened."[27]

The recent political emphasis on the 'market' in health care, on competition and league tables, and on an entrepreneurial spirit amongst health care providers is certainly not conducive to a sense of community. These various political and organisational influences are dis-integrative. They undermine the principles of collaboration and community in health care. But why do they have anything to do with learning to collaborate, and the general theme of this chapter – medical education? The reason is that it is health care professionals *themselves* who must shape the culture of health care that determines how they function and behave, and how they are allowed or encouraged to function and behave. And it is the way they are educated that will equip them, or fail to equip them to meet this challenge.

The way to learn to collaborate is to collaborate

This kind of rapprochement, whether between disciplines in mainstream medicine or between mainstream and unorthodox medicine, cannot be achieved simply by an exchange of doctrines, theories and methodological precepts. It has to be by shared experience, such as is achieved in the examples of collaboration and team work that I have given, when they are truly effective. Working alongside practitioners using an approach that may be different from our own, exploring the similarities and differences in order to understand them properly, and exploring them in dialogue with the patient as well, is the only reliable way of enlarging our perspective and gaining new knowledge and insight. It is essential if "the core knowledge and skills of each profession (are to) command the respect of each of the others (so that) liaison can be effective, and services become flexible and responsive"; which was the pre-requisite agreed by delegates to a seminar on interprofessional working in the early days of its evolution in primary care.[10] It is also the only reliable way of developing appropriate research strategies for investigating the clinical benefits of contrasting methods, of exploring the validity and value of the different precepts and insights that underpin them, and of understanding whether and how these may apply more generally in medicine.

This is particularly true of the need for collaboration in the field of complementary medicine. One of the aims of the work of David Peters' department at Westminster University, described in 'A new perspective in medical education' at the beginning of this chapter, is to equip complementary therapists for this kind of collaboration. But there are centres of excellence in the USA that are way ahead of us in this endeavour. One such is The Centre for Integrative Medicine in the Maryland School of Medicine in Baltimore, one of the centres of excellence supported by the National Institutes of Health to advance scientific investigation of the field of complementary and alternative medicine (CAM). The work of the centre comprises four main areas – research, patient care, informatics, and education – that mutually enhance each other and create a cohesive unit.[28]

The integration clinic at one of the university hospitals offers patients team care, coordinated by experienced integrative physicians; provides the research team with clinically relevant research ideas; expands the dialogue on health and healing through multi-cultural, multidisciplinary perspectives; builds bridges with colleagues through shared patient care; and offers opportunities for education and training.

The Centre does not just fund experts in research who have no CAM knowledge, nor those who are just experienced CAM practitioners but are not experienced in research. Its team approach brings together CAM experts, experienced clinicians (e.g. rheumatologists), methodologists, clinical trialists and statisticians to collaborate on study design, conduct and evaluation. One of its goals is to train a next generation of investigators who are dual qualified. Comparable initiatives in the UK are ad hoc and sporadic. There is no similar centre of excellence. Their nearest equivalents are the NHS homeopathic hospitals in London, Glasgow and Bristol, currently threatened by the prevailing hostility towards homeopathy within the medical establishment.

A different example of learning to collaborate by collaborating is the multidisciplinary integrative care project for patients with multiple sclerosis in Denmark described in Chapter 18. In the UK, the Marylebone Health Centre project that ran from 1990 to 2005 had a similar purpose of mutual learning between professionals of different disciplines, conventional and complementary, directed towards the choice of the most appropriate permutation of care for individual patients, and research based on the process and its outcomes.[10,29]

Holistic medical education

The proper understanding of the term 'holistic' is discussed in Chapter 12, and its application in practice in Chapter 14. Holism is a way of looking at people and the world, and at the way people inhabit and relate to the world. In medicine it applies to the understanding we seek of a patient's predicament – its depth and its breadth; depth in the sense of our understanding of the whole person as represented by the overlapping inner circles of Figure 1 in Chapter 12; breadth in the sense of the interplay of those 'inner' dynamics with the circumstances of the person's life represented on the perimeter, the 'outer' circle. General practice is pre-eminently a holistic medical discipline because the encounter between the doctor or primary care team and the reality of the patient's life, has the potential, not always fulfilled, to be comprehensive in those two senses. In other clinical situations, that encounter may be more circumscribed, but any clinician should at least have the 'bigger picture' in the back of their mind. Some complementary medical disciplines are explicitly orientated towards a holistic approach because of the comprehensive nature of the enquiry required to build up the 'case' or clinical picture that will determine the treatment strategy. But this could be simply an intellectual exercise without the empathy that is necessary to a truly holistic understanding of the other person.

So a holistic medical education must encourage:

- A vision of human nature in its fullness and in the wider context of a person's life.
- An understanding of the influence of those 'inner' dynamics and 'outer' relationships on the person's health and well-being.
- A willingness to engage with this personal reality.
- An empathetic ability to do so.

This is not such a tall order once these principles have become the living and breathing ethos of the curriculum. Indeed, you may be surprised that I am implying that this is not already and always the case. If it were, this book would hardly need to be written. When it is the case, we may expect that a key tutorial, seminar theme or even an examination question will be: 'Effective health care requires that all the above statements are true. Discuss.'

I have already made the point that a holistic perspective does not implicate any particular therapeutic technique, and that no particular technique guarantees a holistic perspective. Any student or practitioner, mainstream or complementary, needs to be able to discuss this theme perceptively to justify a claim to be holistic.

But the study and practise of complementary medicine does bring valuable assets to medical education. Brian Berman is Professor of Family Medicine and Director of the Centre for Integrative Medicine at Maryland University Medical School whose programme I have just described. Writing in the *British Medical Journal* in 2001, in the early years of that project, he recommended incorporating complementary medicine into the medical school curriculum to make teaching more holistic. Because, "We know from research that people are drawn to complementary and alternative therapy mostly our of a desire for a more humanistic, 'holistic' approach. Medical education should re-examine the emphasis it places on the importance of the integration of body, mind and spirit and acknowledge the role of social, cultural and environmental influences and the power of self care and healing. Healthcare professionals, patients, and our healthcare system can only benefit if medical education bridges the gap with complementary and alternative therapy".[30]

Complementary medicine in one or other of its manifestations, and regardless of the nature of the specific effects of the treatments, brings three essentials to a medical curriculum – an insistence on the narrative of illness, an awareness of the subtlety and complexity of the dynamics of health and illness, and an emphasis on our potential for self-regulation and self-healing. To take seriously in addition the implications of their therapeutic techniques as means of interpreting and acting upon the narrative, complex and self-regulatory elements of the process, and of stimulating the subtle and self-regulatory response, is to open up the possibility of new knowledge of human nature and biology to a most exciting degree; to a *scientifically* exciting degree. It is tempting to say, 'a scientifically as well as a humanistically exciting degree.' But that is to perpetuate the false dichotomy between scientific and humanistic; whereas they are, of course, co-inherent aspects of human reality and human aspiration.

To expand the medical curriculum in this way is not to do something new. These concepts have always been part of the spectrum of medical thought. But it is to give them new life; to rescue them from neglect. It is to shed new light on them from a different angle. It is to acknowledge and incorporate different ways of achieving the goals of which the biomedical and doctor orientated curriculum has lost sight.

Exposure to complementary therapies during training can be a welcome, even inspiring antidote to the narrowness of the conventional curriculum. I have quoted the comments of young doctors on their introduction to homeopathic medicine,[31] and described the process of transition of qualified doctors from a conventional repertoire to one incorporating homeopathy.[32] Medical schools in the UK now include some opportunity to experience complementary practice in their curriculum.

Those examples relating to homeopathy reflect my field of experience, but I would expect exposure to other complementary disciplines within the medical curriculum to be similarly illuminating. As essential nowadays, I

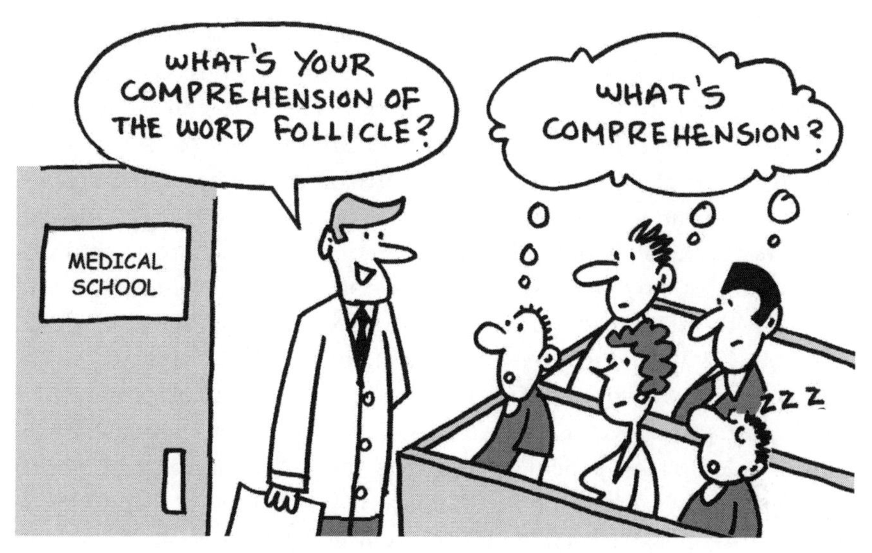

Figure 19.4 *Some elements of a core curriculum cannot be taken for granted.*

suggest, as the inclusion of basic medical knowledge in the education of complementary medical practitioners.

There is, however, an implication in all this that the lessons to be learned from complementary medicine are something to be injected into the conventional curriculum as a sort of dietary supplement. More to the point, to continue the metaphor, would be to regard them as contributing to a better general understanding of the basic principles of healthy eating. The real challenge is, in Brian Berman's words, "Some general consensus needs to be reached on the essentials of a core curriculum". It is a matter of incorporating insights from both mainstream and complementary medicine, which may be common to both or particular to one or the other, into a common core of knowledge as a foundation for all good medical practice. And as he says, this "highlights the need for Faculty development" – teaching the teachers; which can only proceed through collaboration.

From that common core an understanding of the possible permutations of treatment and care will underpin and infuse the later study of particular areas of medical knowledge and skill. Just as an understanding of anatomy and physiology was traditionally the starting point of conventional medical education, underpinning and infusing subsequent learning. That particular model is now old fashioned, and the move towards problem based learning, for example, provides a far more fruitful opportunity for developing the essential common core. It can pave the way for the eventual specialisation that individual vocation and service opportunities may recommend, while ensuring continuing interprofessional awareness, respect and collaboration; and hence effective integrative care and guided patient choice. (See also 'Practical implications' below.)

Cant and Sharma's book *A New Medical Pluralism* comprehensively surveys the relationship of alternative medicine, doctors, patients and the state.[33] They, too, emphasise the importance of mutual learning to achieve effective integration of knowledge, practice and roles. They, too, identify the areas of general theoretical knowledge – self-healing, empathy, individual characteristics of sickness and health, that lie in the common ground of all health care but that are neglected in conventional medical school, and about which complementary medicine has something to teach. Although they are writing about 'pluralism', their aim actually seems to be more integrative. Because they conclude, "We need a pluralism that will address the broadest patient needs, respectful of the diversity of patient experience and response, not one that has evolved entirely as a compromise answer to problems of public health care funding or as an ad hoc resolution of the occupational struggles of different groups of healers (biomedical or alternative)".

From her experience of integrating complementary therapies and approaches into clinical care, education and research, Kathi Kemper offers an interesting reflection on the way that a complementary medicine perspective can benefit the medical education and subsequent professional life of doctors.[34] She uses the traditional Chinese medicine model of Yin and Yang to illustrate the complementary qualities that are needed to make an effective clinician. For example, the Yang dominated biomedical culture restricts patients to one goal, treatment of the chief complaint. But if Yin-type goals are not met the patient feels dissatisfied and not heard. Poor bedside manner reflects lack of Yin sensitivity, not because the physician is hard-hearted, but because he has been trained to meet Yang-type goals. There is a Yang bias in selection for training as a doctor towards great intelligence and problem solving, at the expense of the Yin instinct to *be* with the patient, relieve suffering and extend compassion; an instinct that doctors need, not only to meet the needs of their patients and achieve better clinical outcomes, but also to meet their own needs and enhance their ability to cope.

Integrative medical education

If the whole spectrum of medical education is to recognise and reflect the diversity of the contemporary health care landscape, this cannot be achieved simply by bolting together modules with different labels. It will have to be truly integrative according to the highest ideals of interprofessional education that were discussed earlier in this chapter.

If the humanities in medicine are to humanise not only individual practitioners but the whole culture of medicine itself,[2] this will not be possible until a generation of teachers, trainers, supervisors and mentors has arisen who are themselves steeped in that humanising tradition, and able to model it for their students. It will not happen overnight. A similar process will be necessary if the insights and therapeutic potential of those areas of the medical landscape labelled 'unorthodox' and 'complementary' are to inform the evolution of health care and to play their part in it. Conventional medical educators will need to understand those methods, and their implications for our broader understanding of the dynamics of health and illness, in order that their students may do so and provide properly integrated care for their patients in the future.

But of course this has to be two-way traffic. The alienation of schools of unorthodox medicine must yield equally to the virtues and good influence of mainstream medicine. Not surprisingly in view of the legitimately cautious but sometimes and less excusably hostile attitude of the medical establishment, as well as their philosophical differences, there can be a defiantly separatist attitude amongst some complementary practitioners.

Patients, who make use of both of these medical 'worlds' in large numbers deserve the best of both. And that will only be possible when each of those worlds properly understands what is the best of the other. Then, eventually, the medical 'cosmos' will benefit from a repertoire of shared goals, values and insights that will underpin an effectively integrated and integrative repertoire of therapeutic methods.

Practical implications

The practical implications of all this are, of course, profound. For a start any move to change the curriculum of any pathway of medical education, conventional or complementary, let alone to bring about some convergence of different curricula, requires clarification and convergence of our understanding of the goals of medicine in the first place. It requires a significant shift in philosophical, cultural and moral attitudes for all concerned. It requires the realisation (the understanding *and* the making real) of medicine as a healing vocation whose goals are to be served by all who 'profess' it, whether in clinical care or in a technical, managerial or supportive role. It requires a similar realisation by all health care professionals of their 'co-inherent' membership of a community of care.

That agenda is challenging for all of us. For many it may seem barely feasible. For some it may seem actually undesirable. But I believe that for most of us, as health care practitioners or as patients, it is an inherently attractive agenda that represents what the goals of medicine actually should be and for most of us really are.

In a lecture to the Royal Society of Medicine, retired GP James Willis, whose books that I quote earlier,[35,36] makes a pertinent observation about this.[37] His misgivings about the way that modern medicine has gone astray, which are very similar to mine, are summarised in Chapter 9 ('A crisis of morale'). In the lecture he observes that many doctors feel as he does, but when push comes to shove, rather than resisting the unwholesome influences in medicine as he strove to do (eventually retiring when the compromises became untenable) they favour the prevailing 'wrong' paradigm. He says, "I found then, as I find now, that almost everyone agreed to some extent with my point of view. But this didn't stop them tipping, on balance for the diametrically opposite one. It was as if an invisible hand was pressing down on one side of the scales".

In this he is reflecting the paradox that I described in the Prologue to Part 2; the puzzling acquiescence of doctors in promoting and perpetrating a model of medicine that in their heart of hearts many deplore, and that some fervently, eloquently and publicly deplore. An acquiescence that is compounded by the institutional inertia, and all the other factors that contribute to the resistance to change are were discussed in Chapter 11.

All this being so, and being an incurable optimist, I can foresee that medicine is approaching a 'tipping point' at which the agenda or scenario I have just sketched out will become a motivating force for change. The desire for change will translate into a will for change and a willingness to change. I have quoted Schumacher's triad for promoting change – faith, awareness, and adequacy.[38] In this case the sequence is perhaps expressed better as awareness, faith and adequacy. The awareness of the need for change and the necessary direction of change, if not widespread is certainly in the hearts and minds of many involved in health care. There seems to be a lack of faith and courage in the possibility of effecting change. But I do not doubt the adequacy to achieve change once the faith and courage reach the critical level.

This critical level will be reached as more and more people involved in health care participate in collaborative care of various kinds, learning from one another in the process, and appreciating the benefit for patients to be gained by integrative interprofessional care. This clinical experience will be necessary to inform and develop the 'general consensus on the essentials of a core curriculum' that Brian Berman advocates, and that is obviously necessary. Those essentials will embrace the key concepts curing, caring, healing and coping, and the core principles of therapeutic relationships, informed by 'tributary' insights from a range of disciplines, orthodox and complementary. They will provide the basis for exploring and understanding the permutations that may best answer to the different health care needs of individual patients. They will provide the basis for exploring and understanding, and subsequently studying the essential core knowledge and skills for all clinical practice. In the process students will be encouraged and helped to discover the particular direction in which their vocational instinct, aptitude, character and abilities lead. And from that broad base they will diverge into the more specialised, but still partly integrated programmes of study and training required to follow that path.

The curricula of conventional medical schools are already developing flexibility and versatility that suggests that this more expansive scenario would not be beyond the wit, or the will of medical educationalists to achieve; even though the present outcome of the process is still a strongly biomedically oriented practitioner.

References

1 le Fanu J. *The rise and fall of modern medicine.* London: Abacus; 1999.
2 Greaves D. *The Healing Tradition.* Oxford: Radcliffe Publishing; 2004.
3 Garlick PB, Brown G. Widening participation in medicine. *Br Med J.* 2008; 336:1111–1113.
4 Peters D. Building bridges to health. *Times Higher Education* 2008 May 22nd.
5 Brown C. Alcoe J. The Heart of Well-being. *Journal of Holistic Healthcare* 2010; 7(1):24–28.
6 Jones A. Could kindness heal the NHS? *Br Med J.* 2010; 340:c3166;1363.
7 Guggenbuhl-Craig A. *Power in the helping professions.* Dallas: Spring bools; 1979.
8 Murray L. Embodiment and Incarnation. In: Murray L. *The Paperbark Tree.* Manchester: Carcanet Press; 1992.
9 Fitzpatrick M. *The tyranny of health.* Abingdon: Routledge; 2001.
10 Newton B, Barber L, Clardy J *et al.* Is there hardening of the heart during medical school? *Acad Med.* 2008; 83:244–249.
11 Barr H. Medicine and the making of interprofessional education. *Br J Med Pract.* 2010; 60:573;286–299.
12 Swayne J. A common language of care? *Journal of Interprof Care* 1993;7:29–35.
13 Centre for Advancement of Interprofessional Education. *Interprofessional education – A definition.* London: CAIPE; 1997.
14 Association of University Centers on Disabilities. *Interdisciplinary training guide.* Washington DC: Health Resources and Services Administration; 2001.

15 Pecukonis E, Doyle O, Bliss DL. Reducing barriers to interprofessional training: Promoting interprofessional cultural competence. *J Interprof Care* 2008; 22(4): 417–428.

16 World Health Organisation. *Framework for Action on Interprofessional Education and Collaborative Practice*. Geneva: WHO; 2010.

17 Barr H. The WHO Framework for Action. *J Interprof Care* 2010; 24(5):475–478.

18 Wright A, Lindqvist S. The development outline and evaluation of the second level of an interprofessional learning programme – listening to the students. *J Interprof Care* 2008; 22(5):475–487.

19 Department of Health. *Working together – Learning together*. London: The Stationery Office; 2001.

20 Forte A, Fowler P. Participation in interprofessional education: An evaluation of student and staff experiences. *J Interprof Care* 2009; 23(1):58–66.

21 Charles G, Bainbridge L, Gilbert J. The University of British Columbia model of interprofessional education. *J Interprof Care* 2010; 24(1):9–18.

22 Blickem C, Priyadharshini E. Patient narratives: The potential for "patient-centred" interprofessional learning. *J Interprof Care* 2007; 21(6):619–632.

23 Thistlethwaite J. The future of health professional education: Some reflections on possibilities and complexities. *J Interprof Care* 2008; 22(2):129–132.

24 Kanisin-Overton G, McCallister P, Kelly D, Macvicar R. The Practice-based Small Group Learning Programme: Experiences of learners in multiprofessional groups. *J Interprof Care* 2009; 23(3):262–272.

25 McMurty A. Complexity collective learning and the education of interprofessional health teams: insights from a university-level course. *J Interprof Care* 2010; 24(3):220–222.

26 Edgcumbe D. But there are no QOF points for Balint work. *B J Gen Pract*. 2010; 60(580);858–859.

27 Ham C. The coalition government's plans for the NHS in England. *Br Med J*. 2010; 341 c3790:111–112.

28 Berman B. Developing centers of excellence in complementary medicine research: The University of Maryland experience. *Complement Ther in Med*. 2004; 12(2–3):162–164.

29 Peters D, Chaitow L. Harris G. Morrison S. *Integrating Complementary Therapies in Primary Care*. Edinburgh: Churchill Livingstone; 2002.

30 Berman B. Complementary medicine and medical education. *Br Med J*. 2001; 322:121–122.

31 Reilly D. Taylor M. *Developing integrated medicine. Report of the RCCM Research Fellowship in Complementary Medicine: The University of Glasgow 1987–1990*. London: Research Council for Complementary Medicine; 1993.

32 Thompson T. *Homeopathy: exploring the popularity paradox. A multi-method study of the players process and outcome of homeopathic care by UK medical doctors*. Thesis (PhD). University of Bristol; 2005.

33 Cant S. Sharma U. *A New Medical Pluralism: Alternative medicine doctors patients and the state*. London: UCL Press; 1999.

34 Kemper KJ. The Yin and Yang of integrated clinical care. *Explore* 2007; 3:37–41.
35 Willis J. *The Paradox of Progress*. Abingdon: Radcliffe; 1998.
36 Willis J. *Friends in Low Places*. Abingdon: Radcliffe: 2001.
37 Willis J. James Willis' Website; 2010. Available online at http://www.friendsin-lowplaces.co.uk/
38 Schumacher E. *A Guide for the Perplexed*. London: Sphere; 1978.

20

LIVING TILL WE DIE
The context, process and practice of care

Summary

- What is the limit to what medicine can, or should, usefully, reasonably and compassionately do? What is the limit of what people should reasonably expect of medicine? What is the limit of what a society can, or should, reasonably and compassionately spend on medicine? What should or should not society allow, and medicine assist people to do with their bodies, their lives, and the lives of others? Where to draw the line?
- Medicine cannot divest itself of its responsibility for healing and wholeness because its task is to care for whole persons with spiritual aspirations as well as troubled bodies and minds.
- Medicine must understand that 'dying is a spiritual experience with medical implications', rather than the other way round, or even a medical experience with no spiritual implications at all.
- Decisions around prolonging life and assisting dying are a poignant challenge to health care. Whatever tools of medical science they may bring to it, this is one situation above all where science must not be allowed to become isolated from the rest of life.
- These matters are cultural and social problems with medical implications, and medical problems with cultural and social implications. This is true of medicine's role in commonplace events of medical care as well as more extreme dilemmas.

Where to draw the line?

This short chapter raises questions to which there are certainly no easy answers, and possibly no right answers; or no right answers that apply in all situations. But they are questions that confront medicine every day. They can be reduced to the single question, 'Where to draw the line?'

What is the limit to what medicine can, or should, usefully, reasonably and compassionately do? What is the limit of what people should reasonably expect of medicine? What is the limit of what a society can, or should, reasonably and compassionately spend on medicine? What should or should not society allow, and medicine assist people to do with their bodies, their lives, and the lives of others? Where to draw the line?

In one form or another these questions have recurred throughout the book, particularly in the discussion of medicine's cultural and social role and moral responsibility (Chapters 9 and 17). They revolve around another question that is a recurring theme, 'What are the goals of medicine? What is medicine *for*?'

Aspirations of the human spirit

The 'health care dilemma' that these questions represent is expressed clearly by Michael Fitzpatrick in the conclusion to his book *The tyranny of health*, that I quote earlier:[1]

> When health becomes the goal of human endeavour it acquires an oppressive influence over the life of the individual. If people's lives are ruled by the measures they believe may help to prolong their existence, the quality of their lives is diminished.

And he touches upon what I believe to be the crux of the matter when he goes on to say,

> The tyranny of health means the ascendancy of the imperatives of biology over the aspirations of the human spirit.

What we might all variously mean by 'the human spirit' is uncertain, although I represent my understanding of it in Chapter 12. But that we are all, in one sense or another and at various times in our lives moved by that spirit and by its aspirations is certain. And those aspirations are not always well served by the way we seek to manipulate our bodies and our minds, or expect medicine to do so for us. What is more, the disorders of body and mind that we look to medicine to remedy arise in part from threats or damage to those aspirations more often than we might suppose.

Medicine's responsibility

Medicine cannot divest itself of its responsibility for healing and wholeness because its task is to care for whole persons with spiritual aspirations as well as troubled bodies and minds. Its task is not to prolong the comfortable existence of a good looking body, or the uncomfortable existence of an aging and ailing body. Its task is not just to fend off premature death, and certainly not to delay timely death; but to help people to live as fully as possible till they die. That goal is particularly well exemplified by the hospice movement, a practical demonstration of the activity of the human spirit in the service of that spirit, promoting life in the midst of suffering and at the point of death; helping people to *live* until they die. It makes real the proposition that dying is a spiritual experience with medical implications[2] rather than the other way round, or even a medical experience with no spiritual implications at all.

Medicine's task is to manage pain and disability, certainly, but also to help people to live as fully as possible with pain and disability. To do so it has to recognise and acknowledge the spiritual aspirations and respond to *them* as well as to the biological imperatives. It must have the wisdom, courage and compassion sometimes to encourage and support the aspirations at the expense of the imperatives. Or rather to acknowledge that the biological, or biomedical, *possibilities* are not imperatives if they compromise the aspirations of the human spirit or diminish the fullness of life that depends upon them.

Doing too little; doing too much

This will involve coming to an understanding with patients and helping patients to come to an understanding with themselves in the manner I have discussed several times already. But principally it will require *practitioners* to come to an understanding with *themselves* about the proper limits of their clinical aspirations. They must recognise that in fulfilling their responsibility of trust towards their patient, while wishing, in Pellegrino and Thomasma's words, not to do too little, they must not intrude or presume too much (Chapter 8, 'Trust'). Practitioners need to be constantly aware that in their desire to do something for their patient, particularly when so much *can* be done, they will be tempted to do too much. This may be due to therapeutic zeal, professional pride, fear of negligence, or the desire not to fail; or to misjudgement of the patient's goals or expectations; or to an overestimate of medicine's power. Doing too much may result in unnecessary cost, inconvenience, discomfort or anxiety for the patient, increased risk of adverse effects, or additional expense and workload for the health service; or at worst, in the words of Paul Badham, "burdensome and futile medical interventions to prolong life, a situation in which some people are enabled to live on (when) they would actually prefer to die, rather than have any further extension of their earthly existence".[3] Or it may be directed to ends that the patient may not wish to pursue, which is when medicine becomes presumptuous. The practitioner's best intentions may not correspond to the patient's goals, which however misguided they may appear to him must be respected within the understanding that he and the patient arrive at together. He may be doing too much (see Box 20.1).

BOX 20.1 *Doctors doing too much*

Causes
- Therapeutic zeal, professional pride.
- Fear of negligence, fear of failure.
- Mistaken patient expectations.
- Family/carer expectations.
- Overestimate of medicine's power.

Effects
- Inconvenience, discomfort, anxiety for the patient.
- Risk of adverse effects
- Additional workload or cost.
- Burdensome and futile medical interventions.

As a zealous young GP, and rather forcefully perhaps, I encouraged a patient dying of breast cancer to be more generous in her use of the diamorphine mixture I had provided for pain relief. Her chastening response, albeit in a kindly tone, was "Don't you tell me what to do with my pain!" My good intentions and therapeutic zeal had disregarded her desire to manage her dying in her own way.

This example is in marked contrast to the more usual concern about the inadequacy of pain relief at the end of life. My patient almost certainly *suffered* less from her pain because she was at peace in herself, unafraid of dying. The most difficult deaths I have attended have been two patients whose suffering was hugely compounded by their fear of death.

Perhaps the most peaceful death I have attended was the most premature – a teenager dying at home of leukaemia. She had no fear and her symptoms were well controlled. Caring for her was actually quite a joyful experience. It was responding to her parents' anguish at the prospect of her death that presented the greater challenge.

Spiritual experience; medical implications

Death and dying are primarily adventures of the human spirit, whether or not you associate 'spirit' with God, the soul and an after-life. Birth and death are the two poles of our earthly existence. But the life that lies between those poles is more than mere existence, and "transcends our utility and function as biological human beings. Every human life is of unique and limitless value and should be cherished, treasured and defended, even (and especially) when that life is frail or vulnerable, oppressed or *in extremis*, or the object of contempt and marginalisation".[4] That is a statement with which, the author George Pitcher suggests, every secular humanist and human rights campaigner would concur without needing to invoke the 'added value' (my words) that comes with his Christian faith. It is in this sense, and from both a secular and religious perspective, that we can speak of death and dying as adventures of the human spirit. But they do have medical implications, sometimes very challenging ones, as does birth.

And it is doctors and nurses who have to bear the burden of those implications. This is not the same burden as that born by the patient, or that born by the patient's friends and family or other carers, whose burden is suffering or distress of a different order; although a compassionate and empathetic doctor or nurse will share in that. The medical implications, if they are at all challenging or complicated will compound whatever burden of suffering the patient has to bear, and whatever burden of distress and grief the loved ones and carers have to bear. But it is the doctors and nurses who will have to negotiate and implement decisions about the management of these medical implications. It is they who will have to come to an understanding first and foremost with the patient about what is happening and what is to be done, but also with others intimately concerned with the patient; and to help them to come to an understanding with themselves and one another. They may also have to negotiate with the requirements of medical ethics and the law. They are, of course, not alone in this. An understanding with the patient and with others is by definition arrived at in partnership; and it may be a partnership in which all concerned share. There will often be other professionals to listen, encourage, counsel and support. But when decisions are reached and the *medical* implications require action, it will be doctors or nurses who take it.

The decisions and the actions may be simple and straightforward. The 'negotiation' with my cancer patient required nothing more than that I should pay attention to her wishes rather than make myself feel more comfortable by attempting to do more (too much) for her pain. Her husband was entirely in tune with her wishes, so there was no need for any negotiation to reconcile him to her decisions about her care, which is often a considerable challenge when the family's sentiments do not coincide with the patient's. The negotiation required to reconcile the dying teenager's distressed parents to the fact that there was nothing more to be done medically for their daughter, other than tender loving care, was challenging for the district nurse and me.

Prolonging living; assisting dying

But that was a small burden compared with negotiations concerning actions that may prolong or shorten a patient's life. The dilemma arising from decisions of this kind is already acute and likely to get worse. It is most poignantly reflected in the debate about assisted dying, or assisted suicide, and euthanasia. Doctors and nurses are caught in the cross fire of this sometimes fierce debate, as well as having to wrestle with their own conscience when caring for individual patients whose predicament involves them directly in decisions that affect the end of life. For those who want to follow the debate I recommend two books I have quoted already, one by Paul Badham supporting assisted dying,[3] and one by George Pitcher opposing it.[4] Both authors are Anglican priests, the first a theologian and the second a writer and journalist who also has pastoral role. The fact that both argue their case from within the Christian faith reflects the complexity and degree of polarisation of the debate. But both explore the broader moral, ethical, social and political issues as well. This chapter is not concerned directly with this debate so much as medicine's responsibility within it and for some of the problems that give rise to it.

Everyone, medical and non-medical, involved in the care of the terminally ill and the dying will have some influence on the experience for the person who is dying and for those close to them, and consequently some responsibility for it. In fact everyone concerned is part of the experience, affecting it and affected by it. This is, of course, true of all human experiences, amongst which birth and death are of special importance. The point is that dying is a *communal* experience. It cannot be managed as a circumscribed and isolated event; or as in John Donne's poetic reminder that "no man is an island", as an 'insular' event. George Pitcher picks up a quotation from the poet Lucretius used by Catholic Archbishop Vincent Nichols writing about dying – "Life is given to no one as freehold, we all hold it on leasehold", and develops it like this: "You don't have to be religious to hold that view. You just have to be a human being – one who has lived and loved in community, one whose existence has changed the world for ever by touching others' lives. That's why our deaths don't belong to us any more than our lives do." Although those close to the dying person and their non-medical carers may have a great influence on the character and meaning of the experience, particularly as an experience of the human spirit, this is the context in which doctors and nurses have to manage the medical implications and play their part in negotiating whatever difficult terrain the experience may present.

Whatever tools of medical science they may bring to it, this is one situation above all where science must not be allowed to become isolated from the rest of life, in Mary Midgeley's words. But it is one situation in which doctors may attempt to do too much; partly because they feel it is their duty and that death is a failure, partly because it is what society or the patient's loved ones expect, partly because modern Western medicine is not good at coming to terms with death. The palliative care movement with its philosophy 'to accept the inevitability of death, to desist from burdensome and futile medical interventions and to help patients to live out their last days with as much comfort and dignity as possible',[3] is growing. At the same time medicine often does 'strive officiously to keep alive'.

Medicine's contribution to increasing life expectancy in the Western World (and it is only a contribution, not the whole story), and its success in keeping potentially fatal illness at bay have, in part, created the problems we now encounter at the end of life. Paul Badham quotes figures that show life expectancy in the UK between 1991 and 2001 increasing by 2.2 years, but by only 0.6 years of healthy life;[3,5] and that while expected years of ill health at the end of life are increasing by one year per decade in the UK, years of health have more or less stopped increasing. The consequence being that the average person in the West today can expect to die from a long drawn out degenerative disease and may often experience ten years of chronic disease and disability before death, and this figure is rising. Although I believe other data cast doubt on that rather alarming calculation, it does reflect many people's experience.

This is a distressing, profoundly challenging, and ironic dilemma for a profession whose goal is the relief of suffering and whose vocation is healing. The irony is compounded by the fact that elsewhere in the world very many children and young adults are dying prematurely of preventable diseases. The dilemma is made all the more poignant by controversy over the provision by the NHS of drugs that may increase the life expectancy of patients terminally ill with cancer, possibly by a few months or a year, but possibly by only a matter of weeks, and at great expense. And the irony of medicine's ambivalent role in life and death decisions is the coexistence, possibly within the same unit, of facilities for preserving the cherished life of extremely premature babies and for terminating the life of foetuses whose existence is, for one reason or another, unwelcome or unacceptable.

The culture of living and dying

These problems are cultural, social and medical. They are cultural and social problems with medical implications, and medical problems with cultural and social implications. They reflect a malaise of the developed Western world that like all illness is multi-factorial and multi-faceted. It has to do with the dilemmas that culture, society, science and medicine together have created; the dilemmas that Michael Fitzpatrick identifies of measures that people believe will prolong their existence but may threaten the quality of their lives, between the imperatives of biology and the aspirations of the human spirit. Medicine, medical science and medical technology are at the pivotal point of these dilemmas. Their resolution determines the fundamental 'therapeutic ratio' – the balance of good and ill in all health care interventions.

Medicine's role and influence are not only implicated in the more extreme dilemmas, such as end of life care, or abortion, or the rationing of expensive treatments, (not to mention a whole portfolio of other ethical problems). They have their effect in the more commonplace events of medical care such as those that affect our attitude to minor illness and the expectation that medicine can answer to all "the heartache and the thousand natural shocks that flesh is heir to".[7] Medicine's response to each problem presented to it, in every encounter, is not only a response to that individual predicament but also to expectations that are culturally conditioned, and that medicine has helped to shape. This point has been made before, but medicine's sometimes unhealthy collusive role in promoting measures that may compromise rather than enhance quality of living, and that elevate biological contingencies, let alone imperatives, above the consideration due to the human spirit, is thrown into high relief by problems of end of life care, and the management of increasingly prolonged and increasingly infirm old age. In its Promethean achievements medicine seems to have attracted to itself a Promethean fate.[i]

---

i A reminder that Prometheus was a demigod who stole fire from Olympus for the benefit of humankind and as punishment was chained to a rock to be preyed upon by vultures.

Of course medicine should not abandon its role in managing the biological contingencies of our existence even if it wanted to (which it wouldn't), and if the social and political structures that sustain it allowed it to (which they wouldn't). But if medicine rediscovers, or in some instances discovers for the first time its healing vocation, and applies itself to the understanding and profession of that vocation, it is capable of becoming the model and inspiration for others that Pellegrino and Thomasma suggest it could be. Health care practitioners are not to become priests, philosophers or gurus, but they can by their attitude to the body and the mind, and to the patient as a person, do much to nurture the human spirit as well as its unique biological home. In the process it may be able to reconcile itself and the people it serves to compassionate, respectful and courageous decisions not to do too much. Decisions which at their most difficult may require us to befriend death[ii], and for that matter disability, rather than seek to defeat them at all costs; because that may be at the cost of our true humanity.

At a conference of the Philosophy and Ethics Special Interest Group of the British Pain Society (doctors and other health care practitioners whose occupation is the management of chronic pain), there was unanimous agreement that the otherwise almost universal habit of speaking of the 'battle' against cancer is misguided. The war-like metaphor misrepresents the nature of the healing process that for all the increasingly effective tools that medical science can bring to bear, depends on the underlying resilience and self-healing ability of body, mind and spirit. Health care of any kind should never be a battle that makes our disordered body or mind an enemy to itself.

Whatever our personal philosophy life is a journey. It is always something of an adventure, always precarious, sometimes or from time to time tragic, sometimes or from time to time fraught with danger or suffering. Medicine's task is to help people accomplish that journey and to live it as fully as possible when it is threatened by the afflictions that medicine is equipped by its science and its humanity to treat or contain. It is a journey towards some kind of personal completion. Medicine has a responsibility to enable that process of completion so that it does not end prematurely, and is not wantonly constrained by disability. But at the same time medicine must understand and accept that death or disability do not necessarily render the journey incomplete or leave the person unfulfilled. Mabel Aghadiuno concludes her book *Soul Matters* with the intensely

ii *'Befriending Death'* is the title of a book by John Woodward, whose reference to dying as a spiritual experience with medical implications I quoted earlier.

poignant first person account, painful to read, of just such a journey, in 'Chiara M's story of illness'.[6] It is one of the features of the book that should make it compulsory reading for healthcare practitioners. One of the uplifting things about looking after my dying teenage patient was the conviction that her dying did not leave her life incomplete or unfulfilled.

A juggling act

Medicine has an almost, but not quite humanly impossible juggling act to perform. It is not humanly impossible because human life is not about the pursuit of perfect solutions. Human wholeness is possible despite error and imperfection, and healing is a process that embraces and reconciles error and imperfection. Medicine will be able to manage its near impossible juggling act when it is able to discriminate between its healing vocation and its desire to engineer our biological existence, and to put the second at the service of the first. For my part, I believe medicine will not be able to accomplish this task fully unless and until it comprehends that we are spiritual beings – bodies, minds *and* souls, as I have argued in Chapter 12. Acceptance of this proposition is not essential to our recognition of the biographical journey of the human spirit in a more general sense as the absolutely necessary concern of the *caritas and* the *scientia* of medicine and health care.

References

1 Fitzpatrick, M. *The tyranny of health.* Abingdon: Routledge: 2001.
2 Woodward, J. This new feeling never felt before: facing death with Christian hope. *The Church Times* 2010 August 27th; 20.
3 Badham, P. *Is there a Christian case for assisted dying?* London: SPCK; 2009.
4 Pitcher, G. *A time to live: the case against euthanasia and assisted suicide.* Oxford: Monarch; 2010.
5 Brown, G. *The Living End: The Future of Death, Aging and Immortality*. Basingstoke: Palgrave Macmillan; 2007.
6 Aghadiuno, M. *Soul matters: the spiritual dimension of healthcare.* Oxford: Radcliffe publishing; 2010.
7 Shakespeare, W. *Hamlet*, III, I, 56.

CONCLUSION

CONCLUSION

The model, the jigsaw puzzle and the bigger picture

It will probably be no surprise that this book does not conclude with a fully worked out and comprehensive specification for a new medical model. What I hope to have provided is a persuasive argument that change is necessary; that there has been a long-standing belief amongst many engaged in or concerned with medicine that this is so and that the momentum for change is growing. Against this background I have offered pointers to the direction that change should take. The permutations of care (Chapter 16) are so numerous that an evolving model of medicine will have something of the character of a three dimensional jigsaw puzzle; or even four dimensional if the changing pattern of those permutations over time is taken into account. It will have something of the character of a jigsaw puzzle because as in an ordinary puzzle each piece, each part of the model only has identity, value and meaning in relation to adjacent pieces and to the bigger picture as a whole. But the analogy breaks down because unlike an ordinary puzzle which holds its form and presents a constant picture once all the constituent pieces are correctly assembled the medical model must be dynamic, versatile and flexible. This is because it must accommodate two variables – the individual patients that are the model's raison d'être, and the personal and global circumstances of their lives. These variables introduce uncertainty and unpredictability that cannot be accommodated within any rigid model. And it is a limitation of biomedicine that it imposes a too rigid interpretive framework on health care.

In the various chapters of this book I have described pieces that do not comfortably fit the emerging model of the medicine of the future. Either because they simply do not belong in it, like some of the scientific or moral attitudes I have described. Or because they distort it by being misplaced, or by being given too much prominence within it. And I have suggested how these might be modified, and how other pieces might be rearranged or given greater prominence in order to achieve a model that is more harmonious, more wholemaking, more healing.

While dealing with these separate instances of principle and practice I hope a bigger picture has emerged of a truly holistic perspective of health care. A perspective that celebrates the biomedical approach and the benefits that its reductionist and mechanistic methods have brought us. But a perspective that accords it a more modest place amongst the permutations of care; a more modest place in our understanding and management of human suffering, illness, disease and healing. A perspective in which the biological events and imperatives are better understood in terms of their biographical significance and meaning; particularly in terms of 'the aspirations of the human spirit'. A perspective in which our proper concern with the disordered parts is a consequence of our 'worth-ship' of the whole.

If this is the bigger picture we are trying to build, and if we go back to the jigsaw puzzle as a metaphor for our model, what pieces can we put in place to give it some structure?

Uncertainty

It is easier to identify the separate pieces (sky, trees, houses, people, etc. in an ordinary puzzle), as in a sense I have done, than to see how they fit together to make a complete picture. A difficulty with this particular puzzle, as with most real life puzzles involving human affairs is that there is no picture on the box to guide us. We are creating the picture as we go along. Another difficulty is to identify the corners or edge pieces or other fixed points from which the picture can grow. The second of David Greaves' precepts for a new medical cosmology, "A better understanding of the boundaries of medicine and health care that acknowledges that these cannot be precisely defined", reflects this difficulty.[1] It is found in the uncertain demarcation between health, illness and disease, and between treatment, cure and healing. It is inherent in medicine's relationship with culture and society. It is an inevitable consequence of the complexity of human nature and of the freedom of the human spirit.

Medical science often disguises this uncomfortable fact with the illusion of certainty; the determined and confident pursuit of biomechanical remedies for the human condition. That is a generalisation, and like all generalisations it is not entirely true or fair because biomechanical solutions are not the only goal of medical science. And the search for those solutions is a worthy endeavour if it reduces suffering and disability. But we have too much faith in science's ability to produce 'magic bullets', breakthroughs that promise an end to some disease or disorder that blights our life. These breakthroughs are often real achievements. Some are of lasting benefit – aseptic surgical technique and anaesthetics to name but two. Some that promise so much, and at first at least may achieve much, prove of transient or limited benefit in the long run. Or they may bring new problems in their wake – antibiotics, steroids, non-steroidal anti-inflammatory drugs, statins, and successive generations of psychotropic drugs, for example, are powerful therapeutic weapons but two-edged swords. Stem cell therapy and gene therapy are the up and coming, if controversial solutions to some very serious diseases that may succeed. But we cannot be certain. All this is the inevitable consequence of the precarious and provisional nature of progress in medical science, detailed in an intriguing and exhaustive account by James le Fanu in his book *The rise and fall of modern medicine*.[2]

Though we are well aware of the social determinants of illness, in recent medical history biomedical science has seemed to provide the fixed points, the corner pieces and edges which we thought to use to compile the picture of health care. But the hoped for fixed points prove unreliable. They are important pieces within the puzzle, but by no means define its structure or pattern. They belong to the bigger picture but should not dominate it as they do. The boundaries of medicine and health care cannot be precisely defined because the biological imperatives that medicine confronts do not define the human condition. The certainties of science are frustrated by the rest of life. So the medical model of the future will have its biomedical parts and will continue to celebrate and use the insights of reductionist science. But it will not be a biomedical model. It will be a model that reflects the complexity and mystery of the human condition, and responds more imaginatively and effectively to it.

The fixed point

The need for a fixed point from which to begin the remodelling process brings us back to the question that is really at the heart of the matter – what is medicine, and indeed all health care, *for*? What are the goals and core values that give health care meaning and purpose and that should underpin the vocation of those who work in it, their 'passion to practise it well'[2]? This question is reflected in the first of David Greaves' precepts for a new medical cosmology, relating to the goals and values, visions and ideals that determine what medicine is for. Which he says must encompass more than a desire for biomedical and technological mastery of disease processes. But the core principle that provides the answer to this absolutely fundamental question is his fifth precept – the rehabilitation of healing as "central to any new system of medicine and health care, and seen as integral to all parts of it."[1]

I hope I have made my understanding of the concept of healing abundantly clear as the analysis of health care in this book has unfolded, and that many will share it at least in part. But if I had to choose one word to capture its essence it would be 'reconciliation'. Reconciliation places the emphasis firmly on relationship – the relationship with ourselves, with others, and with our world; personal, social, cultural and ecological. It describes the integrative, whole-making attributes of healing; and does so in its truly holistic sense, which embraces not only those personal, social, cultural and ecological dimensions, but also our biological constitution and its imperatives, and above all those aspirations of the human spirit. The concept of healing does not allow an exclusively materialist view of human nature, or even, for many, a secular view.

In short then, the rehabilitation of healing as the *raison d'être* of healthcare in general and medicine in particular has to be the fixed point from which to begin to compile the bigger picture. It has to be the foundation or cornerstone of the model. Goals, values, vision and ideals will be rooted in it. Medical education, clinical practice, and the fulfilment of medicine's social responsibility will depend upon it. The fact that the concept of healing is in large part philosophical and abstract is no excuse for not grappling with it as a fundamental theme of health care and all medical education. It is no more of an abstraction, in fact, than the use of pathology to define the illness in a sick person.

It is obvious that medicine has a limited role in achieving reconciliation in all aspects of life that affect our well-being. Though there are not many that lie outside its responsibility, at least for advocacy. You will find, for example, health professionals involved in addressing the problems of poverty, torture and climate change amongst other major challenges of our time. And I have discussed medicine's opportunity and responsibility to provide the kind of moral leadership so clearly defined by Edmund Pellegrino and David Thomasma.

Humble hubris, and willingness to change

Which brings us back to 'humble hubris': the hubris required if medicine is truly to fulfil – that is fully to realise (understand and make real) – its healing vocation in all these particulars; and the humility to accept its limitations in the face of the complexity and mystery of the lives of the people it serves. Medicine will continue to exercise a proper hubris in its desire to bring healing to humanity, and by its championing of 'the virtues in medical practice' to affirm essential cultural and social values. But it will be a humble hubris that seeks to enable rather than to control; that does what it can and should do; that does not presume to do too much; that does not expect and is not expected to have all the answers.

'Humble hubris' will be written into the mission statement of all programmes of education and training of all health care practitioners, into any future evolution of the Hippocratic Oath, and on the flysheet of every medical and scientific text book. And it will be stamped indelibly into the fabric of the medical model.

From this humble hubris, this dual realisation of responsibility and limitation, a better map of the boundaries of medicine and health care will emerge that acknowledges that they cannot be precisely defined but describes the landscape that does lie within them. This will be a different landscape from the one presently surveyed by the orthodox medical eye because it will feature more prominently, and as integral to it, approaches to healing that are still effectively 'fringe' medicine, even though some of them are actually integrated into some areas of conventional healthcare.

The rehabilitation of healing, and the remapping of the landscape of medicine will require and be reflected in the 'reconfiguration of medical knowledge' with regard to its many dimensions and different perspectives that is David Greaves' third precept. Medical education and research will be implicated in this reconfiguration, to achieve, in his words, "not a downgrading of factual knowledge and technical skills, but rather their appreciation within a different and wider context".

The remapping of the landscape of care, and the opportunities for integrative practice that it permits will not only yield insights that assist the progressive reconfiguration of medical knowledge, but also allow the reallocation of time and the provision of the more time with patients that all clinicians (and all patients) crave. Better integration will encourage better communication, and where there is shared care a better sense of continuity of care for the patient and an end to 'the collusion of anonymity'.

Better quality of care and improved clinical outcomes are implicit in all of this.

One corollary will be a change in the popular perception of the dynamics of health and illness and of the balance of medicine's role and the role of the individual in managing these; and by extension the role of society through its influence on the individual. The change has to be mediated by the quality of the relationship in the therapeutic encounter. This will often need to be more truthful, more courageous and more trusting on the part of both practitioner and patient. Which will be facilitated by the empathy of the practitioner – her or his ability to listen, understand and respond; to come to an understanding with the patient and to help the patient come to an understanding with him or herself.

The greater sense of responsibility in the practitioner for the healing aspect of their task must include the responsibility to encourage in patients their own sense of responsibility for their well-being; their 'health consciousness'. This is a demanding responsibility because it requires sensitivity to patients' existing perceptions of health and illness, which may be culture specific, and the willingness and ability to understand, acknowledge and respect these, and to support, moderate or challenge them as appropriate. It is demanding because it may involve sensitive life-style and behaviour issues, issues of coping and caring in disability and suffering, issues of death and dying. All of which practitioners will need to be able, or to be helped to cope with in themselves. The health care vocation is very privileged and very costly for all these reasons. And all education and training for it must be appropriate and adequate.

Realising the vision

The 'remodelling' that will promote the vision, goals, values and ideals exemplified in this book involves all three of the domains of health care that I have identified – clinical practice, the process of care, and the context of care. But it is practitioners – clinicians and health care professionals of every discipline, and those responsible for their selection, education, training and mentoring, who will have to initiate change.

They will have to draw upon the instinct for *caritas* that lead them to adopt the disciplines of *scientia* in order to serve others in order to recognise, acknowledge and amend what many, perhaps all in their heart of hearts, know to be wrong. They will have to draw upon their vocational 'passion to do the job well' to insist that things cannot go on as they are.

The momentum for change and the appetite for change are very strong. I could almost have composed this entire book out of quotations from committed and compassionate health care professionals, very many of them doctors, recommending change, sometimes pleading for change, and well aware of what needs to change. I profoundly hope that it will so reinforce that momentum and feed that appetite that all who think this way will be encouraged to make things happen. And I hope that those who may not yet have thought this way, or even thought about it at all, may be provoked to do so. Then the 'dissident voices' of past and present will become the orthodoxy of the future.

References

1 Greaves, D. Reflections on a new medical cosmology. *J Med Ethics* 2002; 28;81–85.
2 le Fanu, J. *The rise and fall of modern medicine.* London: Abacus; 1999.

INDEX